THE ECG IN ANESTHESIA AND CRITICAL CARE

THE ECG IN ANESTHESIA AND CRITICAL CARE

Edited by

Daniel M. Thys, M.D.
Associate Professor and Director
Division of Cardiothoracic Anesthesia
Department of Anesthesiology
Mount Sinai School of Medicine of the
City University of New York
New York, New York

Joel A. Kaplan, M.D.
Professor and Chairman
Department of Anesthesiology
Mount Sinai School of Medicine of the
City University of New York
New York, New York

CHURCHILL LIVINGSTONE
New York, Edinburgh, London, Melbourne 1987

Library of Congress Cataloging-in-Publication Data

The ECG in anesthesia and critical care.

Includes bibliographies and index.
1. Anesthesia—Complications and sequelae.
2. Heart—Diseases—Complications and sequelae.
3. Electrocardiography. 4. Critical care medicine.
I. Thys, Daniel M. II. Kaplan, Joel A. [DNLM:
1. Anesthesia—adverse effects. 2. Critical Care.
3. Electrocardiography. WG 140 E17]
RD87.3.H43E24 1987 617′.96 87–11698
ISBN 0–443–08426–2

Distributed in the United Kingdom by Churchill Livingstone, Robert Stevenson House, 1–3 Baxter's Place, Leith Walk, Edinburgh EH1 3AF, and by associated companies, branches, and representatives throughout the world.

Accurate indications, adverse reactions, and dosage schedules for drugs are provided in this book, but it is possible that they may change. The reader is urged to review the package information data of the manufacturers of the medications mentioned.

Copy Editor: Ann Ruzycka
Production Designer: Melanie Haber
Production Supervisor: Jocelyn Eckstein

Printed in the United States of America

First published in 1987

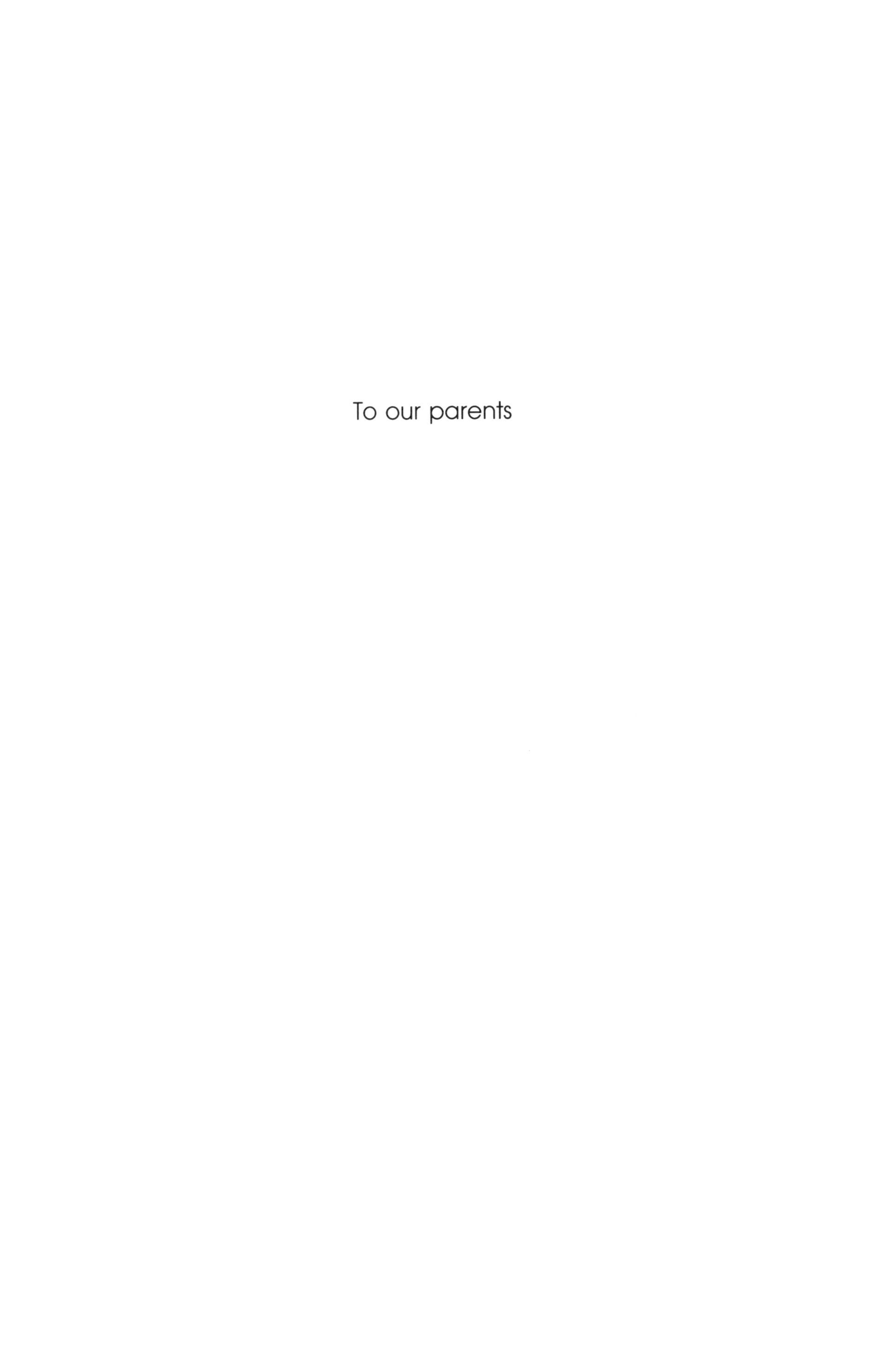

To our parents

CONTRIBUTORS

Jorge Camuñas, M.D.
Assistant Professor of Clinical Surgery, Division of Cardiothoracic Surgery, Department of Surgery, Mount Sinai School of Medicine of the City University of New York, New York, New York

John Dolman, M.D.
Fellow in Cardiothoracic Anesthesia, Department of Anesthesiology, Mount Sinai School of Medicine of the City University of New York, New York, New York

Ivan Dimich, M.D.
Associate Professor, Department of Anesthesiology, Mount Sinai School of Medicine of the City University of New York, New York, New York

James B. Eisenkraft, M.D.
Associate Professor, Department of Anesthesiology, Mount Sinai School of Medicine of the City University of New York, New York, New York

Barry Feinberg, M.D.
Assistant Professor, Department of Anesthesiology, Mount Sinai School of Medicine of the City University of New York, New York, New York

Richard M. Griffin, M.D.
Resident in Anesthesia, Department of Anesthesiology, Mount Sinai School of Medicine of the City University of New York, New York, New York

Jonathan L. Halperin, M.D.
Associate Professor of Clinical Medicine and Director of Clinical Services, Division of Cardiology, Department of Medicine, Mount Sinai School of Medicine of the City University of New York, New York, New York

Zaharia Hillel, M.D., Ph.D.
Assistant Professor, Department of Anesthesiology, Mount Sinai School of Medicine of the City University of New York, New York, New York

Joel A. Kaplan, M.D.
Professor and Chairman, Department of Anesthesiology, Mount Sinai School of Medicine of the City University of New York, New York, New York

Steven Konstadt, M.D.
Assistant Professor, Department of Anesthesiology, Mount Sinai School of Medicine of the City University of New York, New York, New York

John Manos, M.D.
Assistant Professor, Department of Anesthesiology, Mount Sinai School of Medicine of the City University of New York, New York, New York

Margaret Pratila, M.D.
Associate Professor of Clinical Anesthesiology, Department of Anesthesiology, Cornell University Medical College; Associate Attending Anesthesiologist, Memorial Sloan-Kettering Cancer Center, New York, New York

Vasilios Pratilas, M.D.
Associate Professor, Department of Anesthesiology, Mount Sinai School of Medicine of the City University of New York, New York, New York

George Silvay, M.D., Ph.D.
Professor, Department of Anesthesiology, Mount Sinai School of Medicine of the City University of New York, New York, New York

Daniel M. Thys, M.D.
Associate Professor and Director, Division of Cardiothoracic Anesthesia, Department of Anesthesiology, Mount Sinai School of Medicine of the City University of New York, New York, New York

Craig Weinstein, M.D.
Assistant Professor, Department of Anesthesiology, Mount Sinai School of Medicine of the City University of New York, New York, New York

Jacek A. Wojtczak, M.D., Ph.D.
Research Assistant Professor, Department of Anesthesiology, Mount Sinai School of Medicine of the City University of New York, New York, New York

PREFACE

One could wonder whether another book on electrocardiography is really needed. Every year numerous volumes are published on the subject, ranging from the most basic instruction manual to the very exhaustive and all-encompassing text. Yet, not a single work approaches electrocardiography from the viewpoint of the anesthesia care provider or addresses the specific problems concerning electrocardiography in the perioperative period. This book attempts to fill the void.

In most preoperative evaluations, the anesthesiologist will need to interpret standard 12-lead ECGs, and the decision to proceed with surgery will, in part, be influenced by the ECG findings. A thorough knowledge of the normal ECG patterns and some of the more common ECG abnormalities thus appears essential. We have not assumed any previous knowledge of electrocardiography, and the first chapter, therefore, describes very basic ECG concepts and simple methods to analyze the standard ECG. Subsequent chapters review some common pathologic ECG configurations.

Intraoperatively and postoperatively the major indications for the use of the ECG are the detection of myocardial ischemia and the recognition of dysrhythmias. Seldom is a complete 12-lead ECG available for this purpose, and pertinent information must often be derived from a single lead. Lead selection is thus crucial and has been extensively discussed in this text. Just as crucial is the rapid recognition and correct treatment of dysrhythmias. This topic has been discussed in more than one chapter, and a certain degree of repetition is intentional.

As the population ages, the implantation of pacemakers has become more frequent. These patients commonly require anesthesia, either for the actual implantation of the pacemaker or for unrelated disorders. Because numerous types of pacemakers are currently in use, a review of their various characteristics was in order. An expert in the field has provided an authoritative overview and has drawn our attention to some of the important anesthetic implications of pacemaker dependency.

One of our major concerns when agreeing to edit this book was our ability to gather original electrocardiograms. We were fortunate to enlist the cooperation of the electrocardiography department of Mount Sinai Hospital, and gratefully acknowledge their invaluable contribution. We are also particularly indebted to Ellen Felton, who provided most of the original illustrations, and to Rosalind Brathwaite, Teresa Villafana, and Francine Kurth, who remained good-humored through the numerous revisions of the manuscript. Without their gracious help this book would never have been completed.

Additional acknowledgments go to Norma Kaplan, who by now must be the world's leading proofreader in cardiac anesthesia, and to Toni Tracy and her staff at Churchill Livingstone. Without Toni's gentle but persistent admonitions we would most likely have abandoned this project a long time ago. She tolerated our numerous delays and postponements, and provided welcome encouragements whenever needed. She deserves a lot of credit for the completion of this book.

Finally, we would like to thank our families for giving us their continuous love and strength throughout the preparation of this text. Because of our busy professional schedules, time dedicated to them is often limited and additional commitments are only accepted with reluctance. They, however, gave us their wholehearted support and encouraged us whenever it was needed.

Daniel M. Thys, M.D.
Joel A. Kaplan, M.D.

CONTENTS

1

The Normal ECG

Daniel M. Thys, M.D.

Normal cardiac activity depends on the continuous transfer of sodium, potassium, and calcium ions across cell membranes. As these electrically charged particles move across the cell membranes, changes in electrical polarity in and around the cardiac cells are produced.

Not all cells are depolarized at the same time, however, and as a result electrical gradients are created. Along these gradients minute amounts of electrical current flow. The sum of all the currents flowing through the heart at a given moment represents the electrical potential of the heart, and electrocardiography is the science of recording and interpreting variations in cardiac electrical potentials.

A wide variety of electrical patterns have been observed in health and disease and the complexity of these variations tends to be somewhat overwhelming at first. With a systematic approach, however, the analysis of the ECG becomes much easier. The aim of this chapter is to review the normal patterns of cardiac electrical activity and to suggest a systematic method for analysis of the ECG.

THE LEAD SYSTEM

The presence of electrical activity in the heart was first demonstrated by Kolliker and Muller in 1855.[1] These workers placed a frog nerve–muscle preparation in contact with a beating heart and were able to show the presence of two distinct electrical changes at each beat of the ventricle. Numerous animal experiments followed these observations, but another 50 years had to go by before systematic electrical examination of cardiac patients became possible. Indeed, until 1903, when Einthoven introduced the string galvanometer, no instrument was available to record the human ECG.[2,3]

The string galvanometer, a predecessor of our current ECG recorders, is a device consisting of a string stretched between the two poles of a powerful magnet. Electrical current passing through the string will induce its deflection. The magnitude of the deflection will depend on the intensity and direction of the current. An image of this deflection can either be recorded on a paper strip or observed on an oscilloscope. The current is usually detected between two electrodes that form an electrical circuit with the galvanometer or electrocardiograph. One electrode acts as a negative pole, the other as a positive pole. Passage of the current in the direction of the positive pole will result in an upward deflection on the recording (a in Fig. 1–1), while flow in the opposite direction will produce a downward deflection (b in Fig. 1–1). The greatest deflection is obtained when the current flow is parallel to an imaginary line connecting the two electrodes. This line is called a lead.

As the angle between the current and the

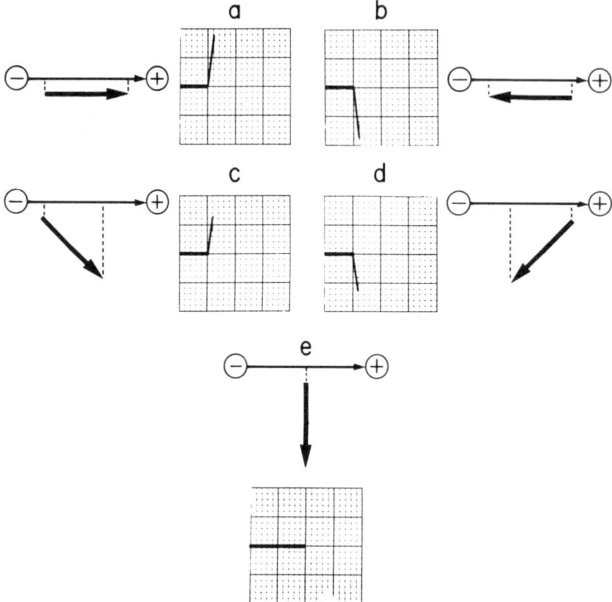

Fig. 1–1 In (a) and (b) the vectors are parallel to the ECG lead and produce the largest deflections. The deflection is upward in (a) because the current flows from the negative pole to the positive pole. Although the amplitudes of the vectors are unchanged, the deflections in (c) and (d) are smaller because the vectors are at an angle with the lead. In (e) no deflection is noted since the vector is perpendicular to the lead.

lead increases, the recorded deflection becomes smaller, although the amplitude of the current might remain unchanged (c and d in Fig. 1–1). If the current is perpendicular to the lead, no deflection will be obtained (e in Fig. 1–1).

In clinical electrocardiography this recording technique is applied in various leads, to permit accurate definition of the electrical activity of the heart. Analysis of the data, however, requires a number of assumptions. First, it is assumed that, at any moment, the sum of all electrical potentials can be represented by a single spatial vector. A vector is a symbol used to define both the magnitude and the direction of the electrical forces. Secondly, it is assumed that the vector, at all times, originates from an imaginary point at the center of the heart. Finally, it is postulated that projections of the vector on three perpendicular planes (defined by the X, Y, Z axes) can be adequately recorded with surface electrodes (Fig. 1–2). In clinical practice one usually limits the analysis to the frontal (X–Y axes) and the horizontal or transverse plane (X–Z axes).

THE FRONTAL PLANE

Bipolar Leads

Initially the study of the ECG was limited to the frontal plane. Einthoven postulated that the human body can be represented as a flat homogeneous plate in the form of an equilateral triangle.[4] Using his theory, the recording of electrical potentials is performed by electrodes placed at the angles of the triangle.

The surface electrodes are placed at the right arm, left arm, and left leg. The sides of the triangle are represented by three imaginary lines, the leads, connecting the three angles. By definition, lead I detects the current between the right arm and the left arm, lead II between the right arm and left leg, and lead III between the left arm and left leg (Fig. 1–3).

The midpoint of each lead forms the separation between the positive and negative zones of the lead.

At any given moment, the sum of the electrical activity of the heart can be represented as

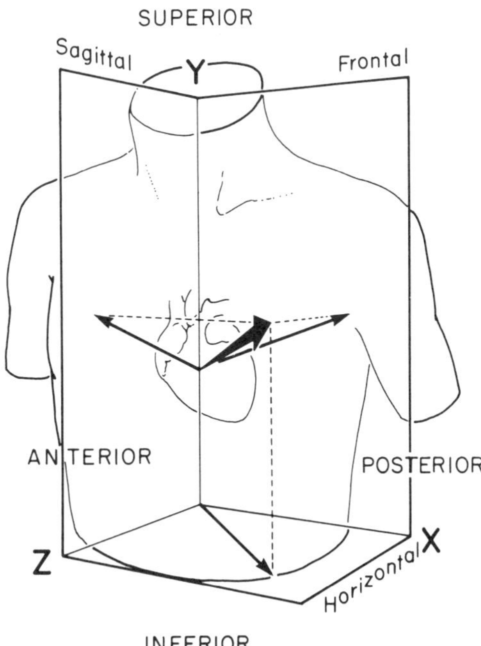

Fig. 1–2 Any cardiac vector can be projected on three perpendicular planes: frontal, horizontal, and sagittal.

a resultant or equivalent dipole vector located at the center of the triangle. Projection of the vector on each of the three leads yields a deflection in a particular direction and of a defined magnitude (Fig. 1–4). In clinical practice it is common to convert the equivalent triangle into a triaxial reference figure by superimposing the midpoints of the lead axes.[5]

Projection of the dipole vector on either the sides of the equivalent triangle or on the axes of the triaxial reference figure results in identical deflections (Fig. 1–5). Use of the triaxial reference figure is essential for determination of the electrical axes.

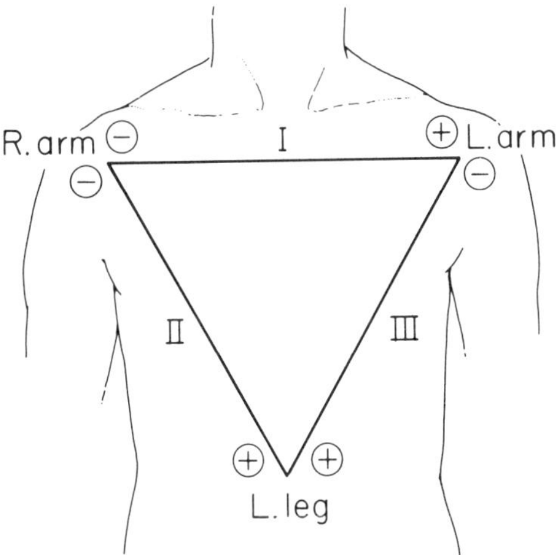

Fig. 1–3 The Einthoven triangle.

Unipolar Leads

Early investigators soon recognized that the recording of electrical activity in the three frontal leads was insufficient for the detailed diagnosis of cardiac abnormalities. To gain additional information on the electrical activity in the frontal plane, Wilson in 1934 introduced the unipolar limb leads.[6] The difference between a unipolar lead and a bipolar lead is that in the unipolar lead the negative or indifferent electrode is at zero potential. The positive or exploring electrode then records the absolute amplitude of

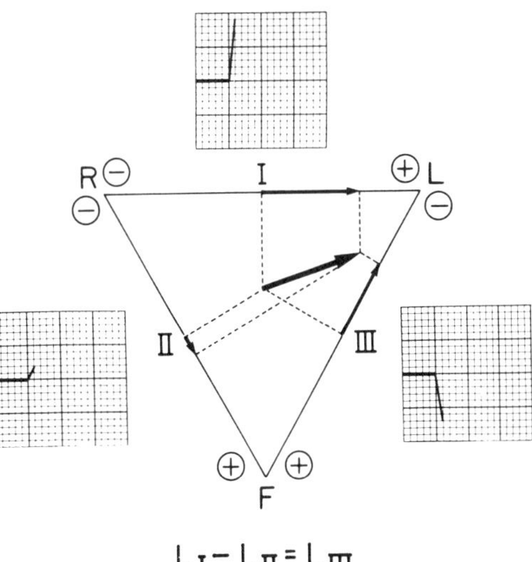

Fig. 1–4 Projection of a vector on the three limbs of the equilateral triangle. Note that the vector initiates at the center of the triangle, and therefore the projections begin in the middle of each limb.

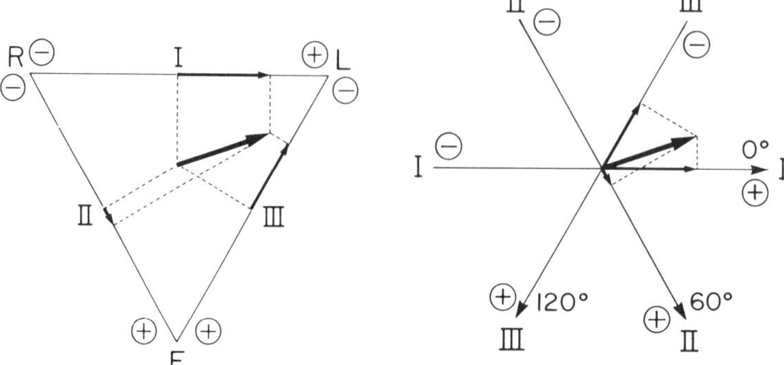

Fig. 1–5 Projection of an identical vector on the limbs of an equilateral triangle and on the triaxial reference figure.

the electrical potential rather than the difference in potentials recorded by bipolar leads. Wilson obtained the zero potential of the negative electrode by connecting the lead wires from the right arm, left arm, and left leg electrode at one central point. He called this point the central terminal. The central terminal has a zero potential because by definition the algebraic sum of the potentials at the three extremities must equal zero throughout the cardiac cycle.

Since the skin resistance under each of the surface electrodes varies, current could possibly flow between them and make interpretation of the recorded potentials impossible. To avoid this problem, Wilson inserted 5,000 Ω resistors in each of the electrode wires leading to the central terminal. The unipolar lead VR is obtained by measuring the potential difference between the central terminal and the right arm electrode (Fig. 1–6). VL and VF are recorded in a similar fashion.

A further modification was introduced in 1942 by Goldberger who removed the resistors from the lead wires and disconnected the exploring limb electrode from the central terminal.[7] The deflections thus obtained were much larger than those obtained with Wilson's model, these modified unipolar leads have since been called augmented leads, or aVR, aVL, and aVF (Fig. 1–7). In clinical practice it is common to record the three bipolar leads and the three augmented unipolar leads. These six leads then define the electrical vector of the heart in the frontal plane.

If the axes of the unipolar leads are added to the triaxial reference frame of the bipolar leads, a hexaxial reference frame is constructed (Fig. 1–8). The direction of a vector in the frontal plane can be described as inferior or superior and to the left or to the right. The direction of a vector is described as superior when it is aimed toward the half of the frontal plane above lead I. It is inferior when aimed toward the lower half. The direction of a vector is leftward when the vector is aimed toward the part of the frontal plane to the left of lead aVF. It is rightward when aiming to the right of aVF.

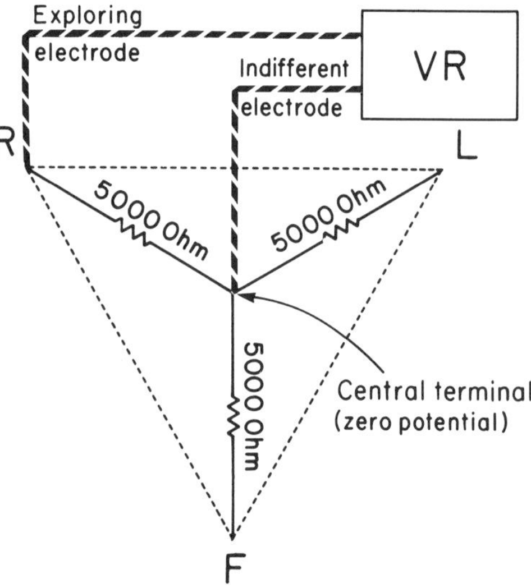

Fig. 1–6 Wilson's unipolar lead (VR).

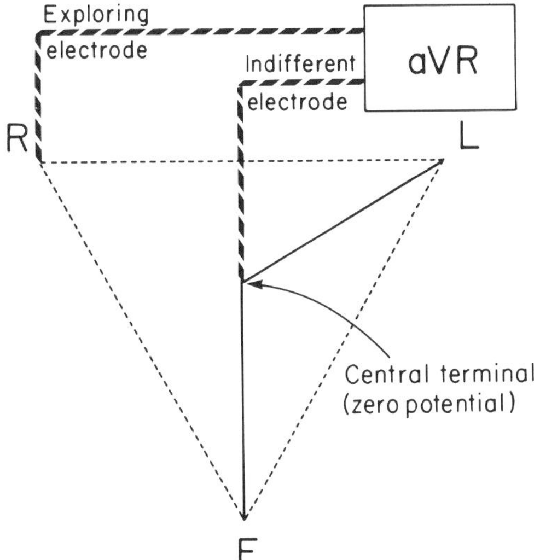

Fig. 1–7 Goldberger's unipolar lead (aVR).

THE HORIZONTAL PLANE

Having defined the limb leads of the ECG, we are now able to reconstruct the cardiac vector in the frontal plane (X, Y). The cardiac vector, however, is a spatial structure and thus requires a three-dimensional representation (Fig. 1–9). To achieve this, a third axis is required. In practice the information necessary to reconstruct the Z component of the vector is obtained by analysis of the unipolar precordial leads.[8]

Although one lead in the anteroposterior (AP) diameter would theoretically be sufficient to reconstruct the horizontal plane, it is common to record at least six precordial leads. These are unipolar leads with the negative or indifferent electrode at zero potential, while the exploring electrode is placed on the anterior surface of the chest (Fig. 1–10). V_1 is located at the level of the fourth intercostal space on the right sternal border, while V_2 is at the fourth intercostal space at the left sternal border. V_3 is midway on the line connecting V_2 and V_4. V_4 is placed on the midclavicular line at the fifth intercostal space. V_5 and V_6 are at the same level as V_4 but more laterally. V_5 is on the anterior axillary line, while V_6 is on the mid-axillary line.

In the horizontal plane the reference frame formed by the unipolar precordial leads is shown in Figure 1–11. The direction of a vector in the horizontal or transverse plane is described as anterior or posterior and to the left or the right. It is anterior when its direction is toward the half of the horizontal plane which is anterior to V_6. The direction of the vector is to the left when aimed toward the half of the horizontal plane that is on the left of V_2.

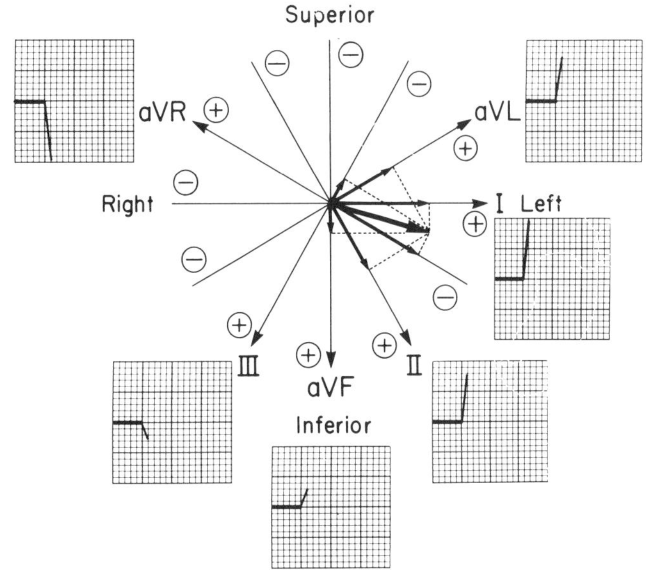

Fig. 1–8 Projection of a vector on the hexaxial reference frame. The axes of the unipolar leads are −150 degrees for aVR, −30 degrees for aVL, and +90 degrees for aVF. The direction of the vector in this figure is inferior and to the left.

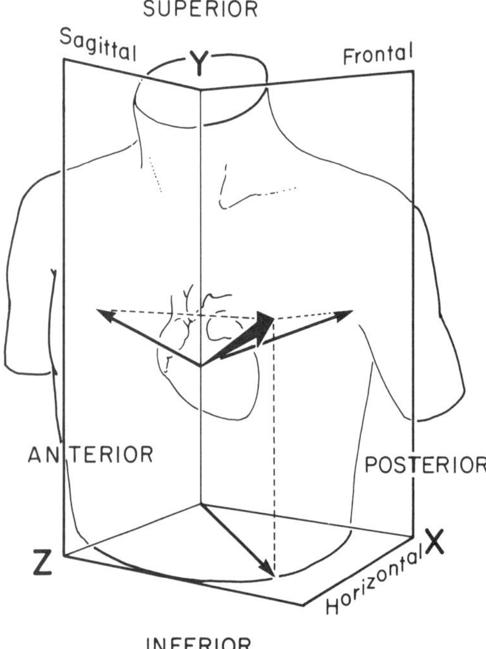

Fig. 1–9 The X, Y, and Z axes define the frontal and horizontal planes.

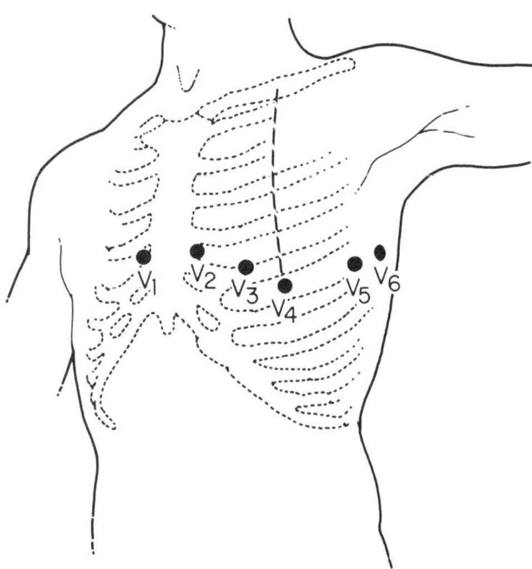

Fig. 1–10 Anatomic locations of the precordial unipolar leads. Occasionally right-sided precordial leads are recorded as well. They are labeled V_{3R}, V_{4R}, etc., and their location corresponds to the left-sided leads but on the right side of the chest.

Projection of any cardiac vector on the frontal plane will produce varying deflections in each of the six limb leads, while projection on the horizontal plane will do the same for the precordial leads. In a standard ECG recording the cardiac vector is represented on twelve individual tracings obtained from each of these 12 leads.

The ECG is normally recorded on special paper consisting of a grid of horizontal and vertical lines. By convention the recorder is set to run the paper at 25 mm/sec and the ECG is calibrated to show a 1-cm deflection for every 1 mV of electrical potential.[9] Provided the ECG has thus been standardized the distance between two heavy vertical lines represent the time-interval of 0.2 seconds and between the lighter vertical lines of 0.04 sec. The distance between two heavy horizontal lines equals 5 mm or 0.5 mV and the distance between two lighter lines is 1 mm or 0.1 mV (Fig. 1–12).

NORMAL PROGRESSION OF ELECTRICAL ACTIVITY

The P Wave

Numerous cells in the heart are capable of spontaneous depolarization. However, under normal circumstanccs thc sino atrial (SA) node, located at the junction of the superior vena cava and right atrium has the highest impulse frequency and is therefore the dominant cardiac pacemaker. From the SA node, the impulse spreads through the right and left atria. Specialized conducting tracts, the internodal tracts, can conduct the impulse to the AV node but they are not essential. On the ECG the depolarization of the atria is represented by the P wave. The initial atrial depolarization involves primarily the right atrium and occurs predominantly in an anterior, inferior and leftward direction. Subsequently, it proceeds to the left atrium located in a more posterior position.

In the frontal plane (limb leads) the mean electrical axis of the P wave is approximately

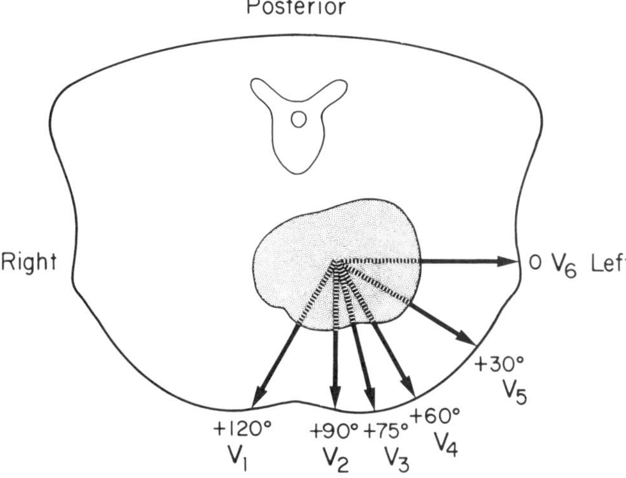

Fig. 1–11 Precordial leads in the horizontal or transverse plane.

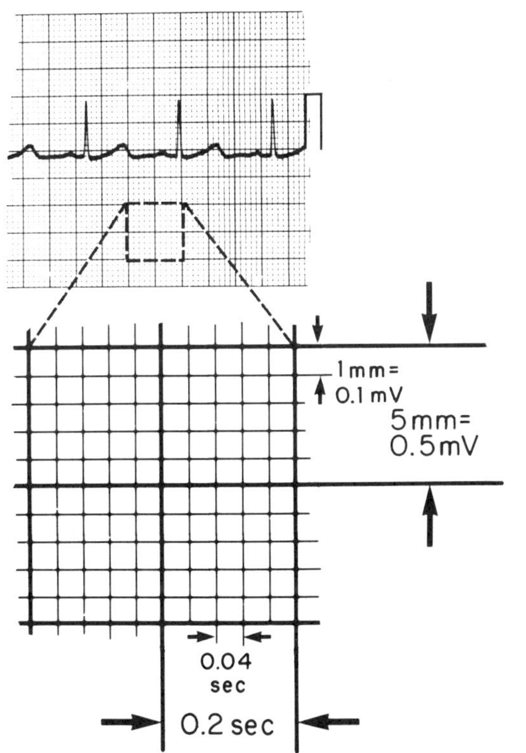

Fig. 1–12 Standard dimensions of ECG recordings. Note the 1 mV = 1 cm standardization mark on the right side of the ECG tracing.

60 degrees and is oriented along the axis of lead II. As a result the P wave is normally upward in I, II, and aVF and inverted in aVR. In III and aVL the P wave is variable and can be diphasic, inverted or isoelectric (Fig. 1–13). The electrical axis in the horizontal plane (precordial leads) is in general slightly anterior to +30 degrees. Therefore, the P wave is upright in V_4–V_6 and can be upright, diphasic or inverted in V_1. Once the depolarization reaches the AV node, a delay is observed. The delay permits contraction of the atria and ejection of blood into the ventricular chambers. The repolarization of the atria is represented by the T_p or T_a wave. This complex is usually buried, however, in the much larger ventricular depolarization wave: the QRS complex.

THE QRS COMPLEX

After passage through the AV node, the electrical impulse is conducted along the conduction pathways consisting of the common bundle of His, the left and the right bundle branches, the distal bundle branches, and the Purkinje fibers.

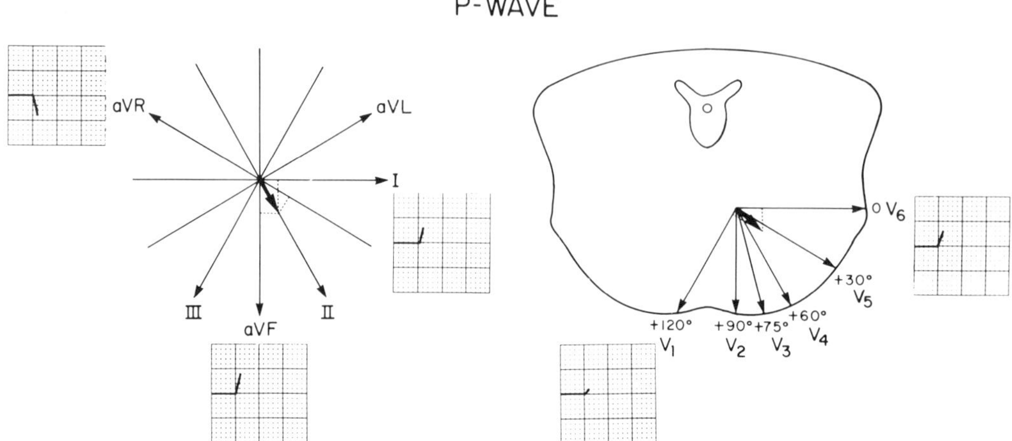

Fig. 1–13 The direction of the initial P-wave vector is inferior, leftward, and anterior.

For practical purposes, the spread of electrical activity from the AV node to the ventricles can be divided in four phases, each reflected by electrical vectors of differing magnitude and direction.[10]

The Septal Vector

Ventricular depolarization begins in the septum and spreads in a left to right direction. The depolarization of the septum is reflected by the septal vector, which is directed to the right in the frontal plane and anteriorly in the horizontal plane. The projection of this vector on the limb and precordial leads results in a small negative wave (Q wave) in I and V_6 and a small positive wave in aVR and V_1 (Fig. 1–14).

The Apicoanterior Vector

The impulse continues to spread in an apex to base direction along the distal part of the conduction system and penetrates the lateral wall of the right ventricle and apical portion of the left ventricle. The vector is oriented anteriorly, to the left, and inferiorly. The projection of this vector on the limb and precordial leads results in the initial upward portion of the R wave in I and V_6 and in a downward motion in aVR and V_1 (Fig. 1–15).

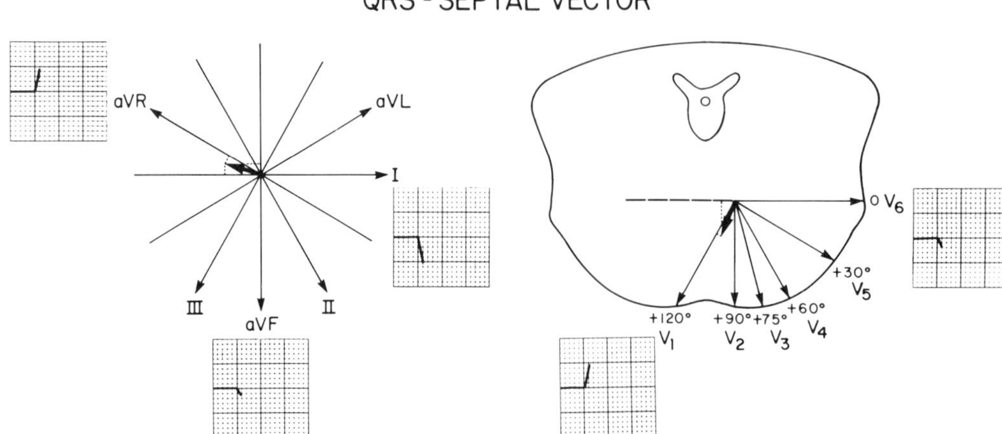

Fig. 1–14 The direction of the QRS septal vector is rightward and anterior.

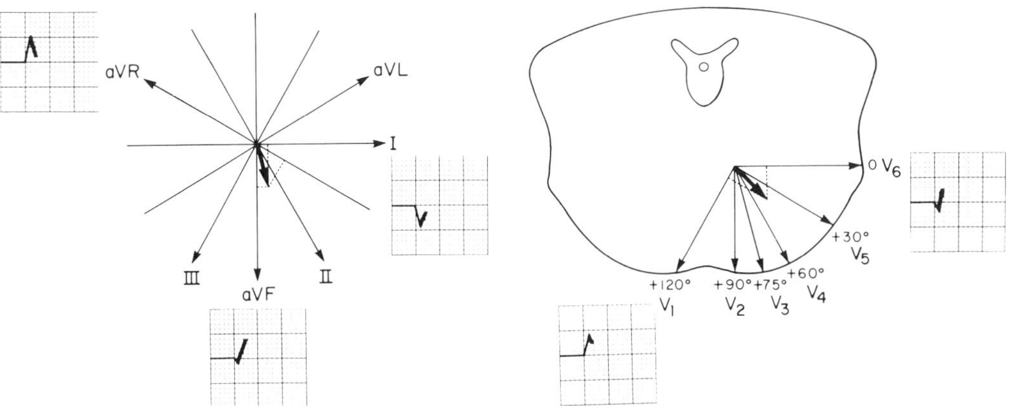

Fig. 1–15 The direction of the QRS apicoanterior vector is inferior, leftward, and anterior. The portion of the QRS corresponding to the apicoanterior vector is represented by the heavier line on the ECG tracing.

The Left Ventricular Vector

At about 0.04 seconds after onset of septal depolarization, the anterior wall of the right ventricle and septum have been completely depolarized. The electrical impulse now continues to spread through the thick anterior and lateral walls of the left ventricle. The direction of the vector is to the left, posteriorly, and slightly inferiorly.

In the limb and precordial leads, this vector produces the large upward part of the R wave in I and V_6 and the large downward portion of the S wave in aVR and V_1 (Fig. 1–16).

The Terminal or Basal Vector

The terminal vector is produced by the depolarization of the thick posterolateral and basal wall of the left ventricle. The direction of the vector is superior, to the left, and posterior. The projection of the vector on the limb and precordial leads produces the final upward por-

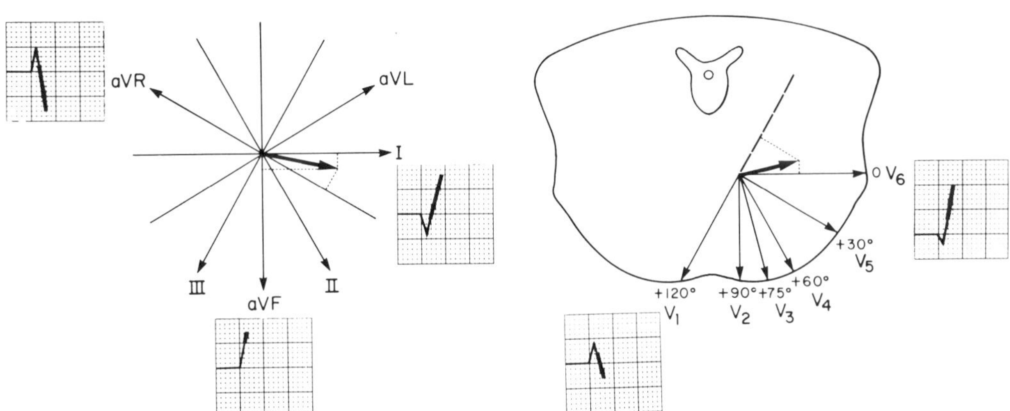

Fig. 1–16 The direction of the QRS left ventricular (LV) vector is leftward, slightly inferior, and posterior. The portion of the QRS corresponding to the LV vector is represented by the heavier line on the ECG tracing.

QRS - TERMINAL OR BASAL VECTOR

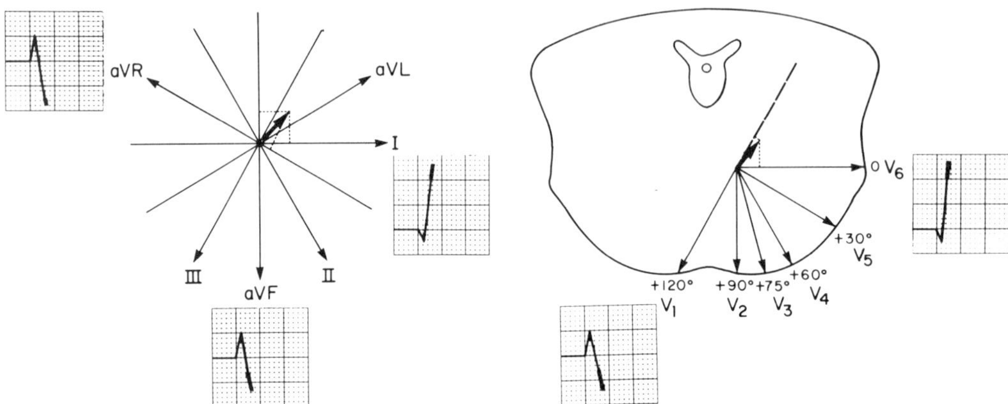

Fig. 1–17 The direction of the QRS terminal vector is superior, leftward, and posterior. The portion of the QRS corresponding to the terminal vector is represented by the heavier line on the ECG tracing.

tion of the R wave in I and V_6 and the final downward segment of the S wave in aVR and V_1 (Fig. 1–17).

After terminal depolarization, the ECG normally returns to baseline in all leads. Numerous variations in the pattern of the QRS complex are commonly observed and therefore it is essential to clearly define each of its components. By definition the first positive deflection represents the R wave. It can be preceded by a negative deflection called the Q wave or followed by a negative deflection called the S wave. If the S wave is followed by a sccond positive wave, it will be labeled R^1. To indicate the magnitude of a deflection, small and large letters can be used. Thus, qRs means that a large R wave is preceded by a small q wave and followed by a small s wave. Other variations are shown in Figure 1–18. In the precordial leads it is not uncommon to call the sharp deflection from the peak of the R wave to the baseline or to the nadir of the S wave, the intrinsicoid deflection. The time between the onset of the QRS and the beginning of the intrinsicoid deflection is important, since it reflects the time necessary for the ventricular depolarization to reach the epicardial surface under the site of the electrode. It is often prolonged in ventricular hypertrophy, ventricular dilatation, and bundle branch blocks. Repolarization of the ventricles begins at the end of the QRS complex and consists of the ST segment and the T wave.

The T Wave

Whereas depolarization occurs along established conduction pathways and is then propagated from cell to cell, the ventricular repolarization is a prolonged process occurring independently in each cell. Therefore, potential

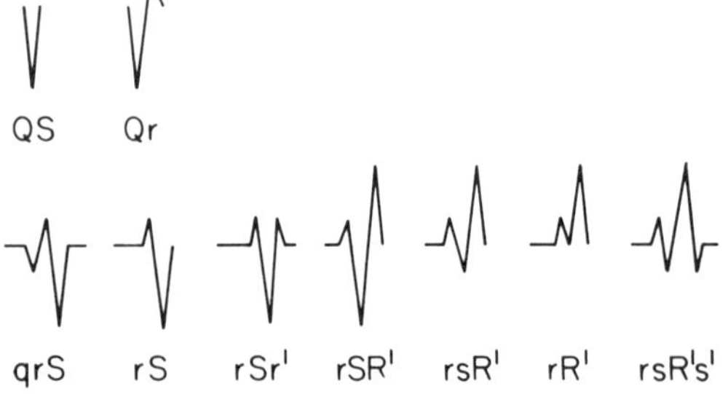

qRs qR Rs QRs RS RSr'

QS Qr

qrS rS rSr' rSR' rsR' rR' rsR's'

Fig. 1–18 QRS patterns.

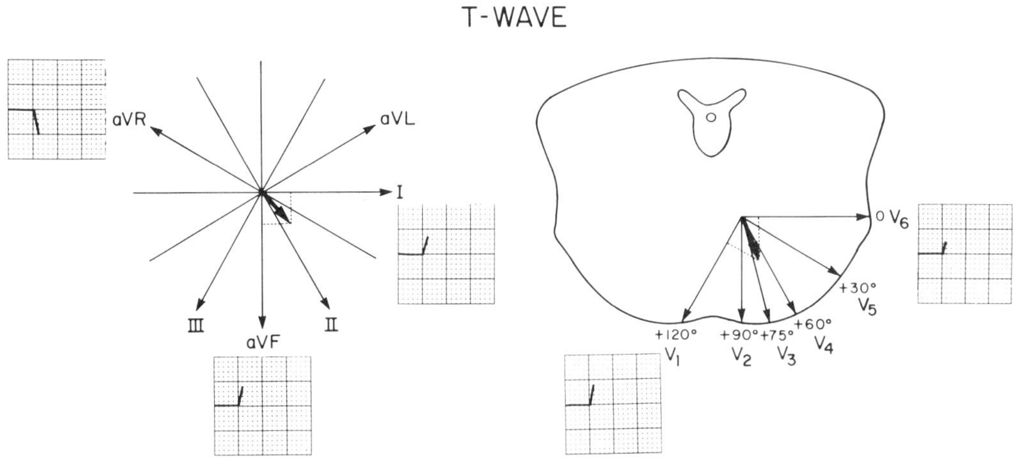

T-WAVE

Fig. 1–19 The direction of the T-wave vector is inferior, leftward, and anterior.

differences are oriented in many different directions and change frequently during recovery. Although a single vector can reflect the whole repolarization process it must be remembered that this represents a gross over-simplication of a complicated and diffuse process. On the ECG, the repolarization is represented by the ST segment, T wave, and U wave. The ST segment occurs during the plateau of the ventricular action potential (phase 2) (see Chapter 7), and is normally isoelectric.

The junction of the QRS and the ST segment is called the J junction. The T wave represents the uncancelled potential differences of ventricular repolarization. The vector of repolarization is oriented inferiorly, to the left and anteriorly (Fig. 1–19).

Projection of the T wave vector on the limb and precordial leads produces a positive deflection in I, V_1–V_6, and a negative deflection in aVR. The U wave is a small positive wave that follows the T wave. Its origin is not clear, but it is thought to reflect the potentials elicited by stretching of the ventricular cells during rapid filling of the ventricle.

PRACTICAL APPROACH TO ECG ANALYSIS

A systematic analysis of the ECG consists of the following steps:

1. Measurement of rate and rhythm
2. Determination of mean QRS axis in the frontal plane
3. Measurement of PR, QRS, and QT intervals
4. Morphologic description (P wave, PR segment, QRS complex, ST segment, T wave, and U wave)

Measurement of Rate and Rhythm

RATE

For regular rhythms, the rate can be determined by dividing 300 by the distance between two subsequent R waves (Fig. 1–20). This distance is expressed as the number of large squares and fractions thereof. Since by convention the paper speed is set at 25 mm/sec or five large squares per second, a 1-minute recording comprises 300 large squares. Therefore, if two subsequent QRS complexes are separated by one large square the rate must be 300 divided by one or 300 per minute. If five large squares separate each QRS complex, the rate is 60 per minute.[11]

If the rhythm is irregular, a longer ECG strip must be obtained and the number of QRS complexes on a strip of a determined duration must

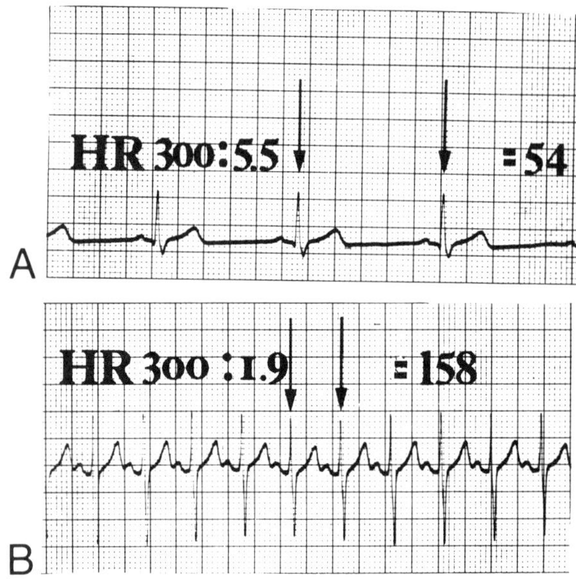

Fig. 1–20 **(A)** Two R waves are separated by five large squares and 2.5 small squares; the heart rate is therefore 300: 5.5 = 54 beats/min. **(B)** Two R waves are separated by one large square and 4.5 small squares; therefore the heart rate is 300: 1.9 = 158 beats/min.

be counted. If the number of QRS complexes on a strip of 60 large squares is multiplied by 5, the rate per minute is obtained (Fig. 1–21). If the rate is very rapid, a longer strip should be analyzed.

RHYTHM

When analyzing the rhythm, one must first establish whether a normal sinus rhythm is present. The conditions for a normal sinus rhythm are as follows:

1. Every QRS complex is preceded by a P wave that is upright in leads I and II and inverted in aVR.
2. Every P wave is followed by a QRS complex.
3. The heart rate is between 60 and 100 beats/min.
4. The PR interval is 0.12 seconds or more.
5. The sinus rhythm may be slightly irregular, but the longest and the shortest RR cycles differ by less than 0.12 seconds.

Determination of Mean Frontal Plane QRS Axis

The mean frontal plane QRS axis can be determined by reconstruction of the mean cardiac vector in the axial reference frame. If in any limb lead the algebraic sum of the QRS deflection equals zero or the QRS is very small, then the vector must be perpendicular to that lead. If the algebraic sum of the QRS is not equipotential in any of the leads, the vector must be

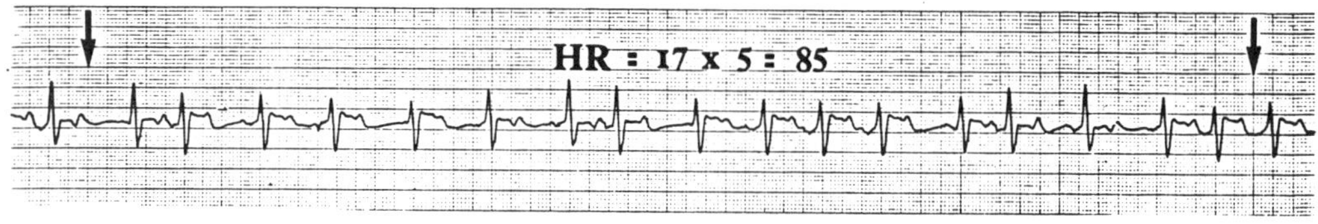

Fig. 1–21 Rate determination in irregular rhythms. The number of QRS complexes in a 12-second strip were counted. The paper speed is 25 mm/sec on five large squares/sec.

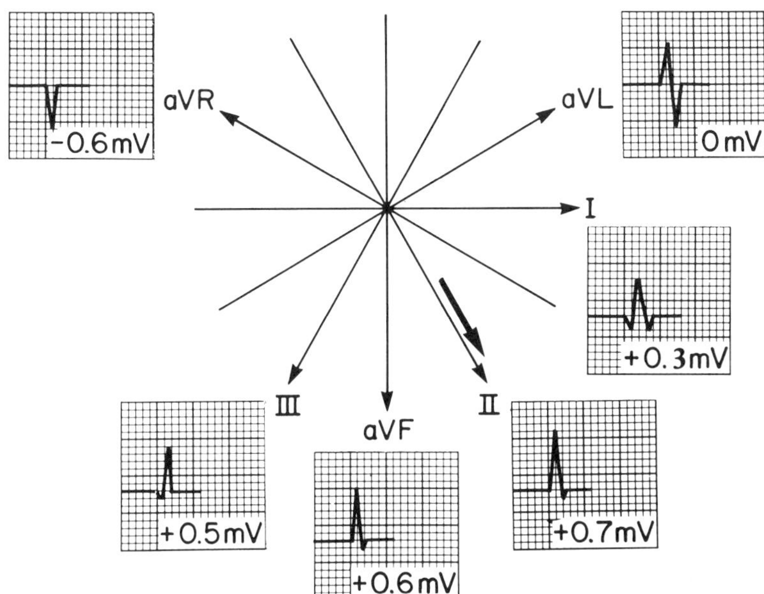

Fig. 1–22 Mean QRS frontal axis determination. The axis of +60 degrees can be confirmed by three methods. (1) The QRS potential equals zero in aVL, and therefore the axis is perpendicular to aVL. (2) The largest deflection is observed in lead II, and therefore the axis is parallel to lead II. (3) The mean QRS potential in I and aVF are positive and the deflection in aVF is twice as large as the deflection in I.

reconstructed from lead I and aVF (Fig. 1–22).

When the QRS deflections in I and aVF are roughly equal, the vector lies at a 45-degree angle of both leads. If the QRS in aVF is twice as large as the QRS in lead I the mean QRS axis lies at approximately 30 degrees from the aVF axis. When the QRS is twice as large in lead I as in aVF, the vector forms an angle of 30 degrees with lead I.

The mean frontal plane QRS axis is normally between −30 and +90 degrees in adults over the age of 30 and between 0 and +110 degrees in younger persons. An axis between −30 and −90 degrees (or 0 and −90 degrees in younger subjects) constitutes left axis deviation: an axis between +90 and −90 degrees is a right axis deviaton (Fig. 1–23).[12]

Measurement of Segments and Intervals

The PR interval is measured from the beginning of the P wave to the beginning of the QRS (see Fig. 1–24). It varies slightly according to age and heart rate but should normally range from 0.12 to 0.20 seconds. The PR segment lies between the end of the P wave and beginning of the QRS complex. It is seldom measured in clinical practice. The QRS interval is measured from the first deflection of the QRS from baseline (positive or negative) to the return to

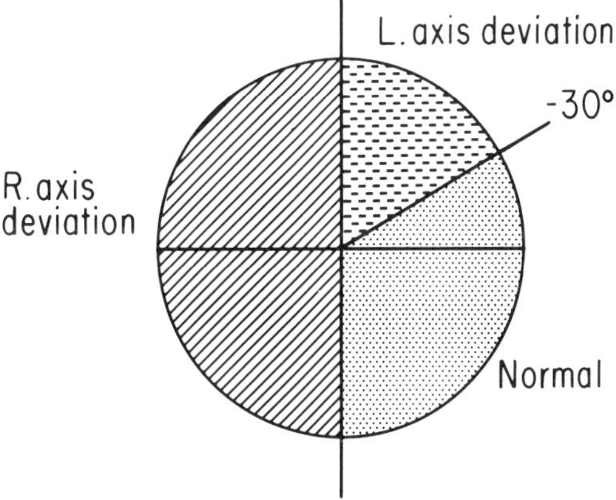

Fig. 1–23 Normal QRS frontal axis with limits for right and left-axis deviation.

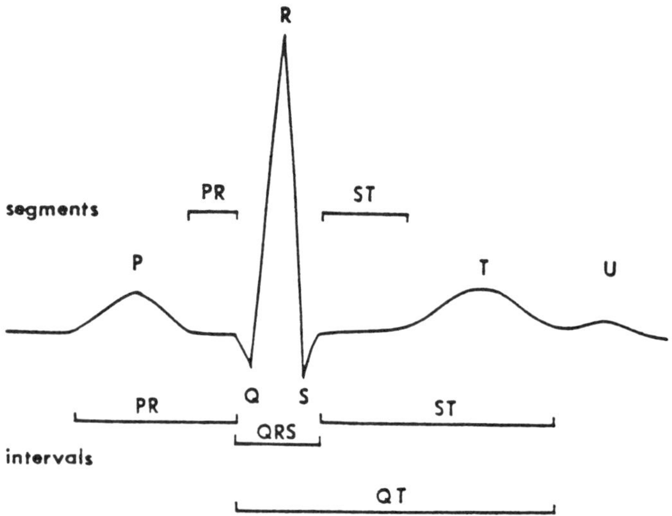

Fig. 1–24 ECG segments and intervals. (Horan E: Electrocardiography and vectocardiography in heart disease. In Braunwald E (ed): Heart Disease: A Textbook of Cardiovascular Medicine. WB Saunders, Philadelphia, 1980. Reproduced with permission.)

baseline. The QRS interval normally lasts 0.06 to 0.10 seconds. The ST segment is measured from the end of the QRS to the beginning of the T wave. While its duration is seldom measured its morphology is of the utmost importance in clinical diagnosis.

The QT interval is measured from the beginning of the QRS to the end of the T wave. Its length is markedly influenced by the heartrate and to determine whether it is within normal limits one should consult rate-correction tables or apply the formula

$$QTc = \frac{\text{QT interval}}{\sqrt{\text{RR interval}}}$$

The normal QTc interval should not exceed 0.44 seconds.

Morphologic Description

P WAVE

The normal mean frontal plane P wave axis is from 0 to +75 degrees. It is normally upright in leads I and II, aVF, and V_4–V_6. It is inverted in aVR and variable in the other leads. Abnormalities include inversions (upright where it should be negative and vice versa), increased amplitude, broader width, diphasicity, notching, peaking, or absence of P wave.

PR SEGMENT

The PR segment is normally isoelectric.

QRS COMPLEX

In additon to measuring the duration of the QRS complex, one should inspect its amplitude (total amplitude of 5 mm is too low and 25 to 30 mm is too high). One should also examine whether Q waves are present. A small narrow Q wave of 1 or 2 mm is a normal finding in leads I, aVL, and aVF and in V_5–V_6. Deep QS or Qr are normal in aVR, III, and V_1–V_2. The abnormality of Q waves depends on their depth and width and on the leads in which they appear.

ST SEGMENT

The ST segment is normally isoelectric.

T WAVE

The T wave is normally upright in leads I, II, and V_2–V_6. It can be flat, diphasic, or inverted in leads III, aVR, and aVF, whereas it is normally inverted in aVR and V_1. In younger individuals, inverted T waves are sometimes noted in V_1–V_3.

U WAVE

The U wave may be superimposed on the T wave. Its direction is the same as that of the T wave.

References

1. Kolliker A, Muller H: Nachweis der negativen Schwankung des Muskelstroms am natürlich sich contrahirenden Muskel. Verh Phys Med Ges. Wurzburg VI, 528:533, 1855
2. Einthoven W: Ein neues Galvanometer. Ann Phys IV XII: 1059, 1903
3. Lewis T: The Mechanism of the Heart Beat. Shaw and Sons, London, 1911
4. Einthoven W, Fahn G, DeWaart A: On the direction and manifest size of the variations of the potential in the human heart and on the influence of the position of the heart on the form of the electrocardiogram. Am Heart J 40:163, 1950; transl Pfluger's Arch 150:273, 315, 1913
5. Baily RH: On certain applications of modern electrocardiographic theory to the interpretation of electrocardiograms which indicate myocardial disease. Am Heart J 26:769, 1943
6. Wilson FN, Johnston FD, McLeod AG, et al: Electrocardiograms that represent the potential variations of a single electrode. Am Heart J 9:447, 1934
7. Goldberger E: Simple electrocardiographic electrode of zero potential and technique of obtaining augmented unipolar extremity leads. Am Heart J 23:483, 1942
8. Wilson FN, Johnston FD, Rosenbaum FF, et al: The precordial electrocardiogram. Am Heart J 27:19, 1944
9. Wilson FN, Kossman CE, Burch GE, et al: Recommendations for standardization of electrocardiographic leads: Report of committee on electrocardiography. Circulation 10:564, 1954
10. Cooksey J, Dunn M, Marsie E: Clinical Vectocardiography and Electrocardiography. 2nd Ed. Year Book, Chicago, 1977
11. Ritota M: Diagnostic Electrocardiography. 2nd Ed. JB Lippincott, Philadelphia, 1977
12. Lipman B, Dunn M, Marsie E: Clinical electrocardiography. 7th Ed. Year book, Chicago, 1984

2

ECG Lead Systems

Richard M. Griffin, M.D.
Joel A. Kaplan, M.D.

STANDARD AND PRECORDIAL LEAD SYSTEMS

The small electric currents produced by activity of the heart spread throughout the whole body, which behaves like a volume conductor, enabling the surface ECG to be recorded at any site on the body. Electrodes were first placed on the limbs in order to standardize the format of the ECG, and the potential differences between pairs of these electrodes became known as the standard leads. Knowledge of these basic leads and of their polarity is helpful in understanding the further modifications made in these leads for use in the operating room and intensive care unit (ICU).

Einthoven's triangle is a hypothetical equilateral triangle centered on the heart and formed by connecting the right arm, left arm, and leg electrodes, such that each lead is equal to the algebraic sum of the other two leads (Fig. 2–1).[1] The three standard limb leads are the most useful leads, with many dysrhythmias, heart blocks, and episodes of ischemia being easily identified. Lead I connects the right arm and left arm electrodes; lead II, the right arm and left leg; and lead III, the left arm and left leg. The right leg electrode usually serves only as a ground. The electrodes can be placed anywhere on the extremities. The polarity of the standard leads is also shown in Figure 2–1.

The standard leads are bipolar leads, since they record the potential difference between two electrodes. Additional information can be obtained by placing electrodes closer to the heart or around the thorax. If the three standard leads are connected through resistances of 5,000 Ω each, a common central terminal with zero potential is obtained. When this common electrode is used with another active electrode, the potential difference between them represents the actual potential. This is the basis of unipolar lead systems, with a neutral electrode formed by the standard leads and an additional electrode called the exploring electrode. The exploring electrode will theoretically give an accurate representation of electrical activity, since it is referred to a zero potential. Unipolar leads that have proved most useful are the precordial leads designated by a letter V and a numeral that corresponds to the location of the electrode on the chest wall:

V_1 just to the right of the sternum in the fourth intercostal space
V_2 just to the left of the sternum in the fourth intercostal space
V_3 midway between V_2 and V_4
V_4 in the mid-clavicular line in the fifth intercostal space
V_5 in the anterior axillary line lateral to V_4
V_6 in the mid-axillary line lateral to V_5

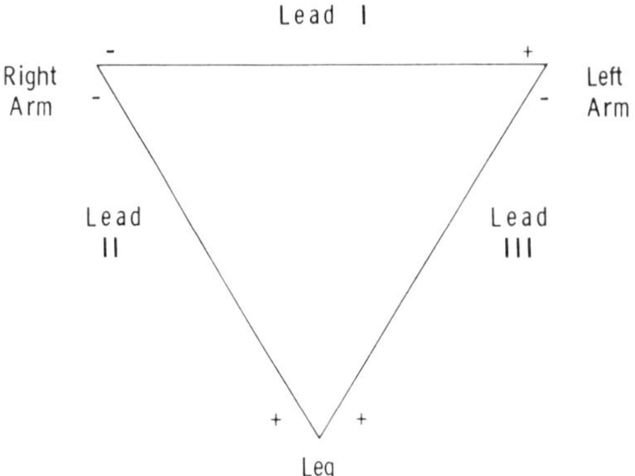

Fig. 2–1 Einthoven's triangle consisting of the three standard leads.

These leads are most useful in diagnosing rotational changes in the position of the heart, ventricular hypertrophy, bundle branch blocks, and ischemia of the anterior, anteroseptal, or lateral areas of the ventricles. Detailed analysis of myocardial ischemia has entailed the use of complex precordial lead systems with 35 leads, consisting of five vertical rows with seven leads on each row.

Precordial leads are more sensitive than the standard leads in detecting myocardial ischemia. Blackburn[2] clearly showed that the most sensitive exploring electrode is at the V_5 chest position, where 89 percent of the ST segment information contained in a standard 12-lead ECG is found. Mason et al.[3] showed that leads V_4, V_5, and V_6 were the most valuable and lead I the least informative for diagnosing ischemia. There is also good correlation between the site of coronary artery obstruction and the lead in which ischemia is detected.[4] ST-segment changes in leads II, III, and aVF correspond to disease of the right coronary artery, and changes in leads V_4–V_6 indicate ischemia from the left anterior descending or circumflex coronary arterial trees. In 1976, based on the above information, Kaplan and King[5] recommended that all patients with coronary artery disease should be monitored intraoperatively with a multiple-lead ECG system capable of recording at least leads V_5 and II.

The multiple-lead ECG system recommended by Kaplan and King[5] consisted of four electrodes on the extremities and a fifth electrode in the V_5 position (Fig. 2–2), which allows for selection of any of seven different ECG leads (I, II, III, aVR, aVL, aVF, or V_5). Leads II and V_5 are usually displayed simultaneously, allowing for observation of both inferior wall and anterolateral myocardial ischemia. This system

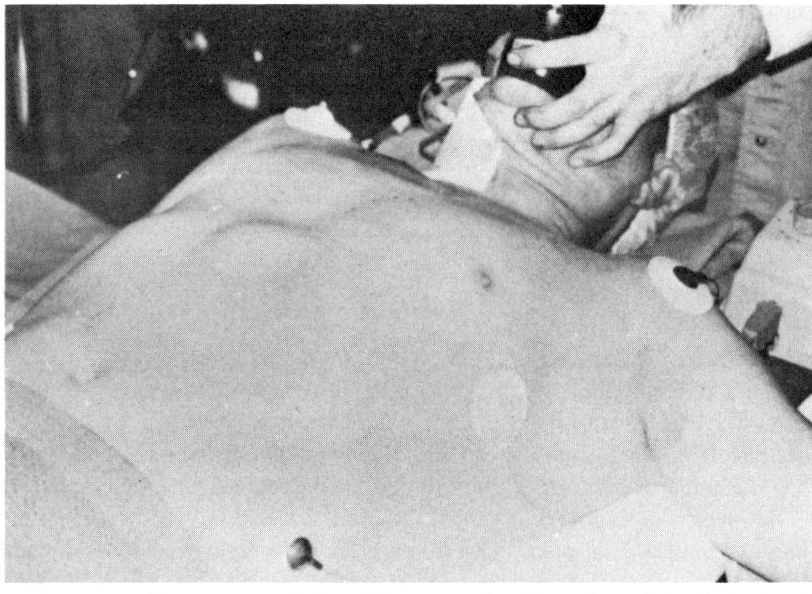

Fig. 2–2 Multiple lead ECG system consisting of four extremity electrodes and the V_5 lead. A lead selector switch is shown on the right side.

has become the standard way of monitoring patients with significant coronary artery disease over the past decade. The use of the unipolar precordial exploring lead (true V_5) requires a five-electrode system in order to produce the common central terminal. However, many operating room ECG monitors still have only a three-electrode system. These three-electrode systems can be adapted so that similar ECG information can be obtained using modified bipolar standard limb leads.

THE MODIFIED BIPOLAR STANDARD LIMB LEADS

In order to look at one particular area of the heart more closely, several modifications of the basic three-electrode bipolar chest leads have been devised (Fig. 2–3). The nomenclature and classification of these lead systems have evolved over time and can be confusing. Table 2–1 gives the principal bipolar leads useful in the operating room and intensive care setting. The nomenclature of these lead systems is based on that used for the precordial leads. In the precordial lead system, the indifferent electrode is placed on the central terminal and the chest electrode is the positive exploring electrode (e.g., V_5). In the modified bipolar lead system, the negative electrode is still designated as central (C), followed by its position (e.g., CL for left arm). A number (suffix) indicates the position of the exploring electrode on the chest (according to the usual precordial lead positions). The letter M before a given lead refers to modified (e.g., in lead MCL_1 the central lead has been modified by moving it down from the left arm to beneath the left clavicle).

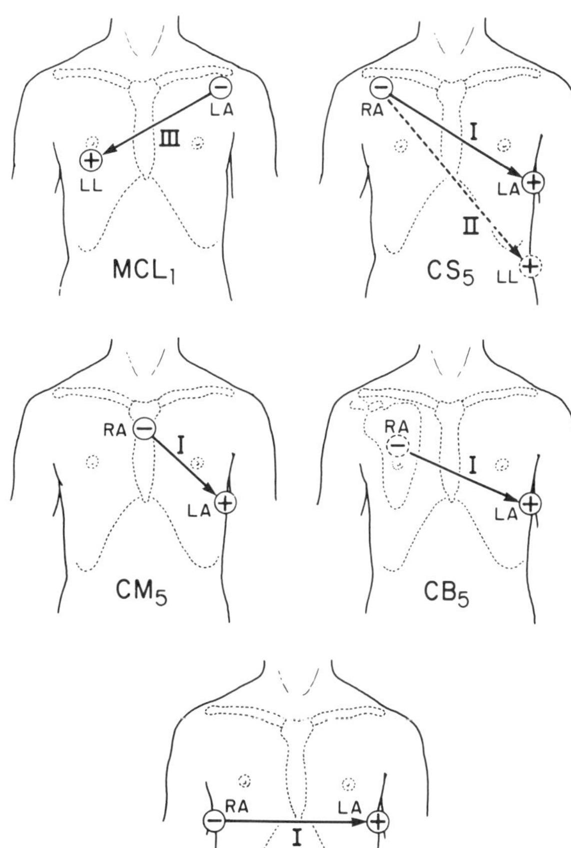

Fig. 2–3 Modified bipolar standard limb lead systems including MCL_1, CS_5, CM_5, CB_5, and CC_5. See text for details.

Table 2–1. Bipolar Leads for Use with Three Electrodes

Lead system	MCL_1	CS_5	CM_5	CB_5	CC_5
Right arm electrode	Ground	Under right clavicle (−) (subclavicular)	Manubrium sternum (−)	Center of right scapula (−)	Right anterior axillary line (V_5R) (−)
Left arm electrode	Under left clavicle (−)	V_5 (+)	V_5 (+)	V_5 (+)	V_5 (+)
Left leg electrode	V_1 (+)	Ground	Ground	Ground	Ground
Lead selected	III	I	I	I	I
Advantages and indications	Good P-wave and QRS complex; useful for diagnosis of dysrhythmias.	Monitoring for anterior ischemia	Monitoring for anterior ischemia	Monitoring for anterior ischemia; good P wave for diagnosis of dysrhythmias	Monitoring for ischemia

Note: +, positive electrode; −, negative electrode.

MCL_1 Lead (Modified Central Lead)

The modified central lead, MCL_1, is obtained by placing the left arm (negative) electrode under the outer third of the clavicle, the left leg (positive) electrode in the V_1 position (i.e., in the fourth intercostal space to the right of the sternum), and the right arm (ground) electrode in its usual position (Fig. 2–4). Lead III is selected so that the left leg lead becomes the exploring lead. This lead gives a good P-wave deflection and QRS complex which enables rapid and accurate diagnosis of atrial dysrhythmias, conduction defects, and bundle branch blocks. Consequently, it is the lead most commonly employed in coronary care units after acute myocardial infarctions. Since dysrhythmias and conduction abnormalities may occur during anesthesia, the MCL_1 lead would appear to be a useful lead to monitor in the operating room.

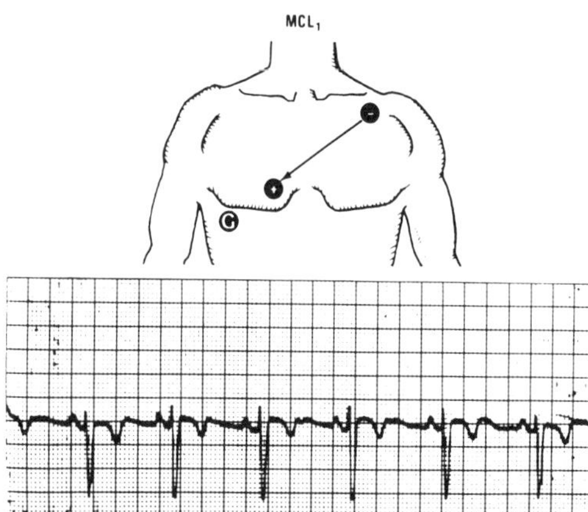

Fig. 2–4 MCL_1 lead system shown on top and a typical ECG tracing from this lead below. (McIntyre KM, Lewis AJ: Textbook of Advanced Cardiac Life Support. © American Heart Association, Dallas, 1981. By permission from the American Heart Association Inc.)

CS_5 Lead (Central Subclavicular)

The central subclavicular lead, CS_5, may be more correctly described as the MCR_5 lead according to the classification previously described. The right arm (negative) electrode is placed under the right clavicle, the left arm (positive) electrode in the V_5 position, and the left leg electrode remains in the usual position to serve as the ground (Fig. 2–5). Lead I is then selected. During stress test studies, this lead has been shown to be excellent for detection of anterior ischemia.[6] In the operating room, this CS_5 lead is the best and easiest alternative to the true V_5 lead for monitoring myocardial ischemia. One particular advantage of the CS_5 lead is that lead II can also be monitored using the same configuration of electrodes, since the left leg electrode is in its usual position. This enables periodic monitoring of the inferior wall of the heart for the development of ischemia, as well as using lead II for dysrhythmia detection.

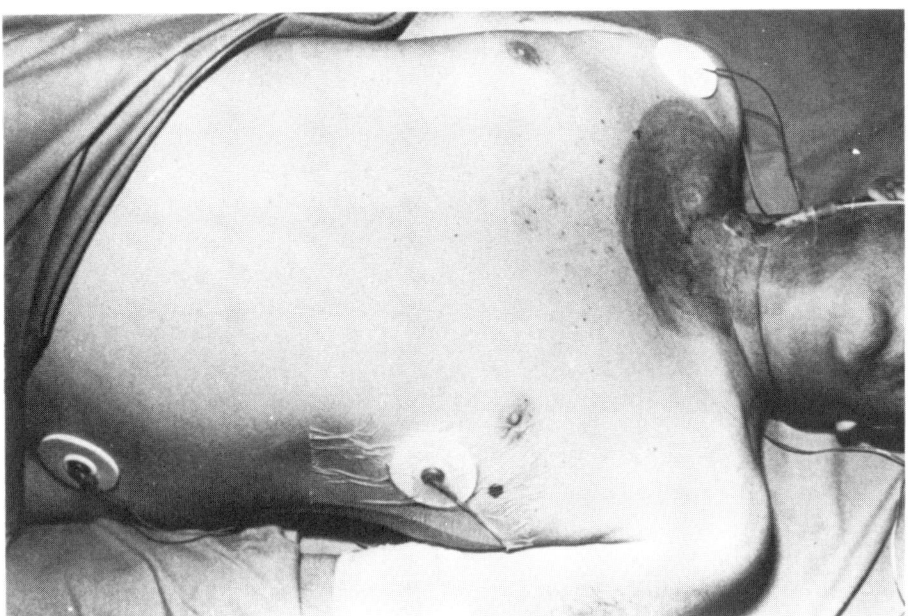

Fig. 2–5 The CS_5 lead arrangement is demonstrated. Standard lead I should be selected to monitor a modified V_5 lead.

CM_5 Lead (Central Manubrium Lead)

The central manubrium lead, CM_5, is obtained by placing the negative right arm electrode on the manubrium of the sternum, the positive left arm lead in the V_5 position, and the ground (left leg) electrode is usually placed in the left leg position. This lead essentially looks at the same vector as the CS_5 lead and provides similar information on ischemia.

CB_5 Lead (Central Back Lead)

The central back lead, CB_5, is obtained by placing the right arm (negative) electrode over the center of the right scapula and the left arm (positive) electrode in the V_5 position. The vector monitored by this lead is in the same direction as that monitored by a true V_5 lead (i.e., downward, leftward, and anterior). The P wave may not be seen on the true V_5 lead, since a certain proportion of the atria may lie to the right or posterior of the origin of the V_5 vector. However, the CB_5 lead, since it originates to the right of the atrium, produces a good P-wave deflection in addition to providing a similar QRS complex to the V_5 lead for detection of ischemia. A recent study comparing CB_5 and V_5 leads in patients with closed and open chests demonstrated a good correlation between ventricular deflections in both leads.[7] The ventricular deflection was 20 percent larger in the CB_5 lead, and, more significantly, the P wave was 90 percent larger (Fig. 2–6). Therefore, with this one lead, monitoring for supraventricular dysrhythmias and ischemia can be obtained. This may be useful in certain patients with ischemic heart disease who may be especially susceptible to the development of dysrhythmias during the perioperative period.

CC_5 Lead (Chest Chest Lead)

To obtain the CC_5 lead, the right arm (negative) electrode is placed on the right anterior axillary line over the fifth interspace and the

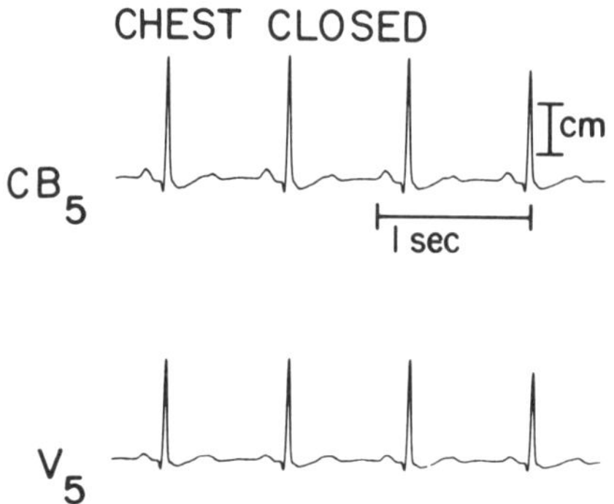

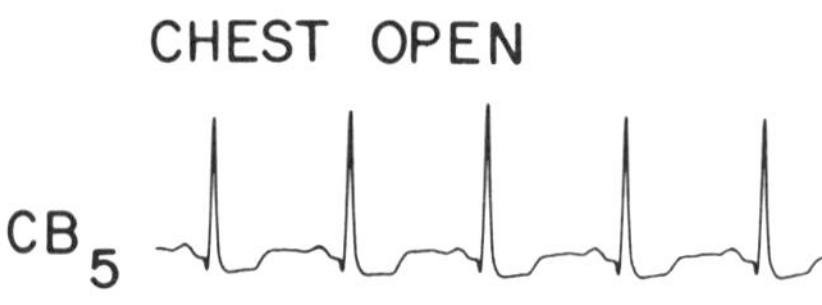

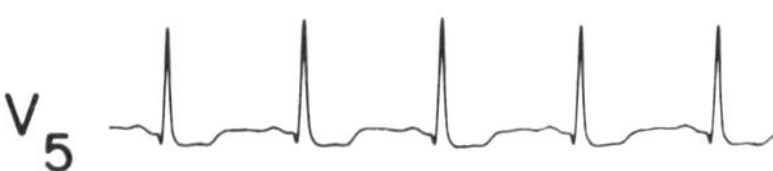

Fig. 2–6 CB_5 lead system is compared to V_5 in a patient with the chest closed and opened. (Reprinted with permission from the International Anesthesia Research Society from Bazaral MG, Norfleet EA: Comparison of CB_5 and V_5 leads for intraoperative electrocardiographic monitoring. Anesth Analg 60: 849, 1981.)

left arm (positive) electrode in the usual V_5 position. Lead I is selected. Using computerized techniques to monitor exercise-induced ischemia, Froelicher et al.[6] demonstrated that lead CC_5 was comparable to V_5.

INVASIVE ELECTROCARDIOGRAPHIC MONITORING

In addition to recording the electrical potentials of the heart from the surface of the body, they may also be obtained from body cavities adjacent to the heart (i.e., the esophagus and trachea) or from within the heart itself. This type of ECG monitoring is useful in the anesthetized patient, and each particular type of monitoring produces an ECG complex with certain advantages for the diagnosis of dysrhythmias or ischemia. Furthermore, these ECG leads are less susceptible to signal distortion by patient movement, baseline drift, and the electrocautery, but invasive monitoring is inevitably associated with some morbidity.

The Esophageal Electrocardiogram

The concept of placing an electrode in the esophagus, adjacent to the heart, in order to monitor the ECG is certainly not new. Cremer, in 1906, passed a 10 × 15-cm electrode into the esophagus of a professional sword swallower! Since then, numerous studies have confirmed the value of the esophageal lead in nonsurgical patients to facilitate the diagnosis of complex dysrhythmias.[8–10] The principal advantage of the esophageal ECG compared with the surface leads is the abilty to record a prominent P wave and thus identify the presence of atrial depolarization and its temporal relationship to ventricular activity. In addition, the esophageal ECG has been shown to be a useful monitor of posterior ischemia due to its close anatomic location to the posterior aspcct of the left ventricle.

The esophageal ECG may be monitored either as a unipolar or bipolar lead. The bipolar lead is more commonly employed since the P : QRS ratio is greater (i.e., there is greater augmentation of the P wave).[10] Interpretation of the esophageal ECG in isolation from other surface leads may be difficult, since the P wave may be larger, equal to, or smaller than the QRS complex and is sometimes difficult to distinguish from the QRS complex.[9]

A commercially available esophageal ECG electrode has recently become available that is suitable for use during anesthesia, in the recovery room, or in the intensive care unit. This esophageal ECG monitor consists of an 18-Fr. esophageal stethoscope with two external elec-

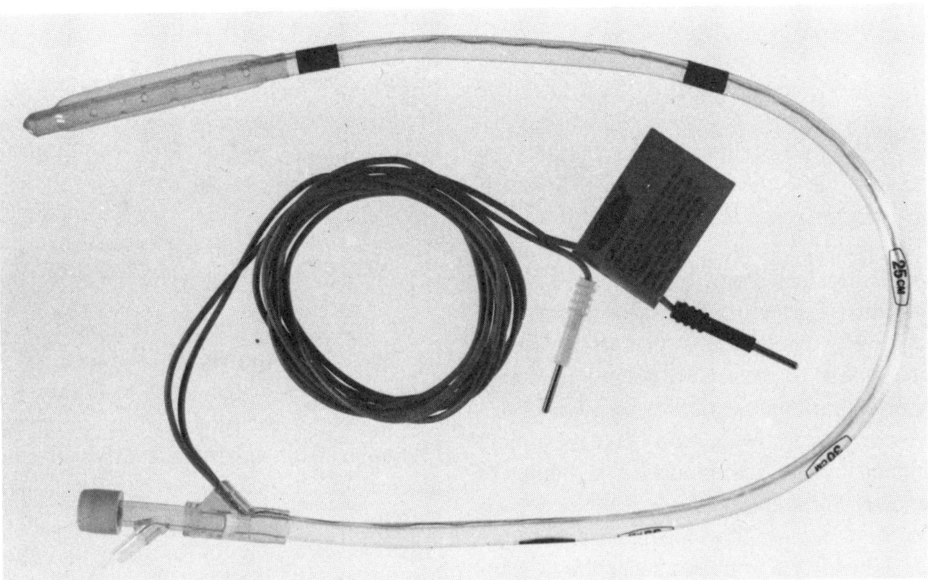

Fig 2–7 The Portex cardioesophagoscope. The esophageal leads are made of plastic. The ECG wires are attached to lead I of the ECG monitor.

trodes 7 and 20 cm from the distal end. The wires from the electrodes are extruded through the wall of the stethoscope and welded to conventional ECG lead wires at the proximal ends (Fig. 2–7). To observe a bipolar esophageal ECG, the leads are connected to the right and left arm terminals and lead I is selected on the monitor. A typical esophageal ECG tracing is shown in Figure 2–8, with lead V_5 for comparison. To minimize the risk of electrocution or esophageal burn injury, strict electrical safety precautions must be followed. All ECG monitoring equipment should be incapable of delivering more than 10 μA of leakage current to the patient. In addition, when electrocautery is used, a properly applied ground plate of sufficient surface area should be used and, as an extra precaution, an electrocautery protection filter capable of filtering radio frequencies greater than 20 kHz can be inserted between the ECG cable and the esophageal lead.

In a study of 20 patients undergoing coronary

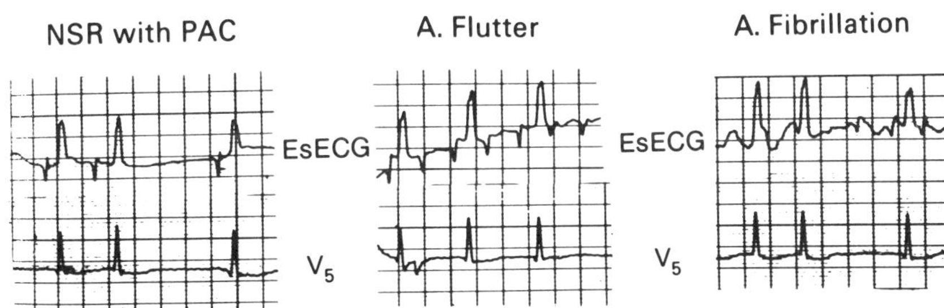

Fig 2–8 The esophageal ECG (EsECG) is shown on top and compared with a V_5 lead on the bottom. During cannulation of the heart, the patient progressed from a NSR to atrial fibrillation. (Reprinted with permission from the International Anesthesia Research Society from Kates RA, Zaidan JR, Kaplan JA: Esophageal lead for intraoperative electrocardiographic monitoring. Anesth Analg 61:781, 1982.)

artery bypass surgery, Kates et al.[11] compared the esophageal ECG with standard lead II, precordial lead V_5, and an intraatrial ECG obtained with a multipurpose Swan Ganz catheter that served as the gold standard for the definite diagnosis of dysrhythmias. The correct diagnosis was made from leads II and V_5 in 53.8 percent and 42.3 percent of cases, respectively, whereas the esophageal lead correctly diagnosed 100 percent of the dysrhythmias that occurred. The study clearly demonstrated that dysrhythmias may be missed or incorrectly diagnosed if only surface leads II or V_5 are employed (Fig. 2–9). However, leads MCL_1 and CB_5 give a more prominent P wave, and comparative studies of these leads with the esophageal lead are needed to confirm the value of esophageal ECG monitoring over all the conventional surface leads for diagnosing dysrhythmias. Kates et al.[11] also found one case of posterior myocardial ischemia with the esophageal ECG that was missed with leads V_5 and II (Fig. 2–10).

There have been only a relatively small number of patients monitored with an esophageal ECG, but so far there are no reports of postoperative symptoms related to the use of this monitor. In sum, the esophageal ECG appears to be a simple, safe method of monitoring the anesthetized patient that should be used in more cases, especially when there is a high risk of the development of dysrhythmias.

Intracardiac Electrograms

Recording of electrical potentials from within the heart itself produces prominent atrial (P wave) and ventricular (QRS complex) signals that allow for interpretation of complex dysrhythmias. Although more invasive than the esophageal ECG, there is less baseline wandering with the intracardiac electrogram. Several techniques are available for recording the intraatrial and intraventricular ECG.

SALINE-FILLED CARDIAC CATHETER

In 1949, Hellerstein et al.[12] described a method of obtaining intracavitary potentials with a single-lumen catheter. The catheter was

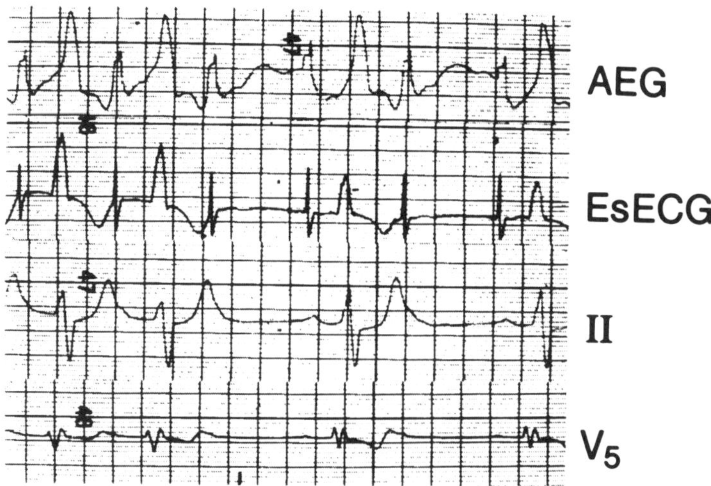

Fig 2–9 Four ECG leads are demonstrated in a patient after cardiopulmonary bypass. AEG, atrial ECG; EsECG, esophageal ECG. The patient progressed from a normal sinus rhythm with first-degree heart block to a Mobitz type II block. The type of bradycardia was misdiagnosed from leads II and V_5 as sinus bradycardia, while the AEG and EsECG show the heart block. (Reprinted with permission from the International Anesthesia Research Society from Kates RA, Zaidan JR, Kaplan JA: Esophageal lead for intraoperative electrocardiographic monitoring. Anesth Analg 61:781, 1982.)

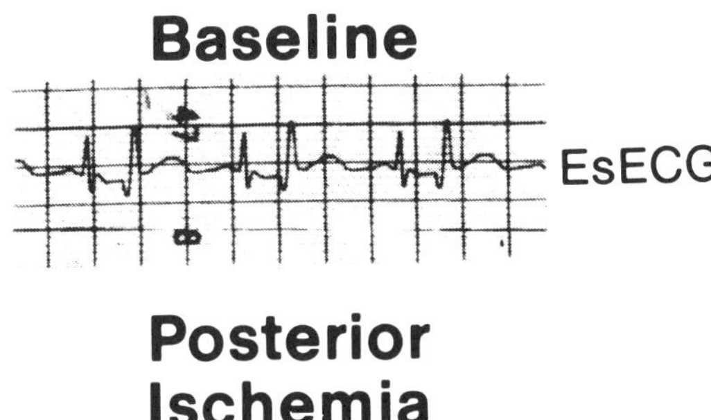

Fig 2–10 Posterior myocardial ischemia during cardiopulmonary bypass diagnosed on the esophageal ECG lead but not seen on leads II and V_5. The baseline EsECG is shown at the top. (Reprinted with permission from the International Anesthesia Research Society from Kates RA, Zaidan JR, Kaplan JA: Esophageal lead for intraoperative electrocardiographic monitoring. Anesth Analg 61:781, 1982.)

passed into the heart while connected to a heparinized saline drip and a simple electrode was then passed 2 to 4 cm into the proximal end of the catheter and connected to the exploring lead of the ECG. The saline acted as a conductor to transmit the electrical potentials to the ECG electrode. The potentials obtained from the saline electrode were identical in form to those obtained simultaneously from a wire electrode inserted into the right ventricle. However, the amplitude of the complexes obtained with the wire electrode was greater than those with saline due to the greater resistance of saline or blood, and alternating current interference was a frequent problem that could not be completely overcome. Use of hypertonic saline has been shown to provide a better electrode and may be used to locate the distal end of a ventricular–atrial shunt for hydrocephalus.[13] The saline-filled electrode has also been used to locate a catheter in the right atrium or superior vena cava to facilitate aspiration of air during procedures in which there is a high risk of air embolism.[14] Thus, the principal uses of the saline-filled electrode have been to locate probes in the heart on a short-term or long-term basis for diagnostic or therapeutic purposes. The use of the electrode as an ECG monitor is limited by susceptibility to artifact and electrical interference.

INTRAVASCULAR WIRE ELECTRODE

The indications for use of an intravascular wire electrode are essentially similar to those for the saline-filled catheter electrode. The wire electrode may be inserted percutaneously via any of the usual venipuncture sites. Richards and Freeman[15] first described the use of a metal stylette inserted into the intracardiac tubing of a Holter valve shunt to form a rigid probe and locate the tip in the atrium. A bipolar lead I was recorded from the intracardiac electrode by connecting the proximal end of the metal stylette to the right arm terminal via an alligator clip and a length of sterile wire. More recently, a J-tipped wire guide has been used as the intravascular ECG lead to position a catheter tip in the right atrium.[16] The increased rigidity of the wire/catheter combination, compared with the saline-filled electrode, results in less artifact caused by catheter whipping during insertion. Moreover, the wire guide has a lower electrical resistance and is therefore less sensitive to AC interference.

MULTIPURPOSE PULMONARY ARTERY CATHETER

Chatterjee et al.[17] first described the use of a modified balloon-tipped flotation catheter for recording intracavitary ECGs. They used a standard 7 Fr. Swan-Ganz catheter with two pairs of electrodes situated 17 to 18 cm and 28 to 29 cm from the catheter tip for the ventricular and atrial electrodes, respectively. The wires from the electrodes were insulated and conveyed via the third lumen of the catheter to its proximal end. The atrial and ventricular electrograms were recorded as bipolar leads by attaching the electrode wires to the arm leads and selecting lead I. With the catheter tip properly located in the pulmonary artery, the proximal and distal pairs of electrodes should come to lie in the upper atrium and right ventricle, respectively. In a series of 43 patients with various cardiac diagnoses, stable tracings were obtained which greatly facilitated the diagnosis of complex dysrhythmias. When necessary, atrial, ventricular, or atrioventricular (AV) sequential pacing was promptly initiated.[17] Mantle et al.[18] modified the thermistor-tipped pulmonary artery catheter to incorporate two electrodes at 25 and 26 cm from the tip of the catheter to record the intraatrial electrogram. The catheter was found to be useful for the diagnosis and treatment of dysrhythmias in 30 patients with serious cardiac disease. On average, the catheter was left in place for 3 days without the development of serious complications.

The multipurpose pulmonary artery catheter that is currently available has five electrodes: two intraventricular electrodes situated 18.5 and 19.5 cm from the distal end, and three intraatrial electrodes situated 28.5, 31.0, and 33.5 cm from the distal end (Fig. 2–11). Incorporation of a third intraatrial electrode has enabled the electrodes to be properly positioned in heart chambers and great vessels of varying sizes. The multipurpose pulmonary artery catheter provides for comprehensive hemodynamic monitoring (pulmonary artery pressure, wedge pressure, central venous pressure, and cardiac output), stable intraatrial and intraventricular ECG monitoring, and the capability of atrial, AV sequential, or ventricular pacing, if necessary. The ease of insertion and pacing capabilities of the catheter were evaluated in a series of 30 patients undergoing cardiac surgery.[19] The catheter was easily inserted on each occasion, and AV sequential pacing was successful in approximately 70 percent of patients. The high-fidelity tracings

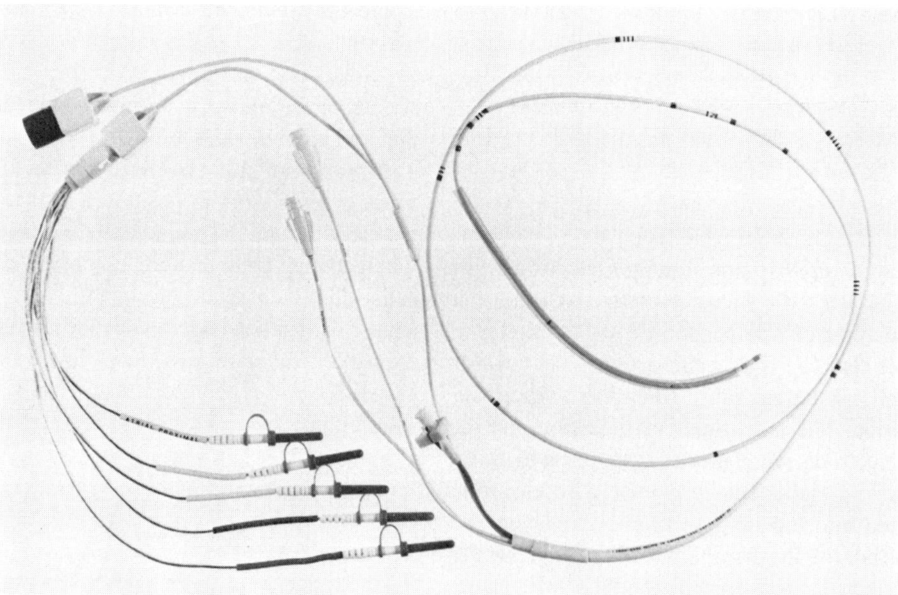

Fig. 2–11 The multipurpose pacing Swan Ganz catheter. Three atrial and two ventricular electrodes can be seen.

obtained from intracardiac electrodes are particularly suitable for computer analysis and reliable, consistent operation of any device requiring QRS triggering mechanisms (e.g., the intraventricular electrogram provides a large voltage spike that can be used for triggering an intraaortic balloon pump).[20] The application of the multipurpose pacing catheter, however, should not be limited to cardiac surgical patients and should be considered whenever critically ill patients with serious cardiac disease present for noncardiac surgery.

THE ENDOTRACHEAL ELECTROCARDIOGRAM

The endotracheal ECG provides a route for monitoring the ECG in situations in which it is difficult or impossible to use surface ECG leads. The esophageal ECG can play a similar role, but may not be acceptable in small infants. The endotracheal ECG comprises a standard endotracheal tube with distal (1.2 cm long) and proximal (6 cm long) electrodes shrunk onto the exterior of the tube (Fig. 2–12).[21] The electrodes were connected in a Teflon-coated wire, through a 47,000 Ω resistance, to a battery-powered ECG with an isolated preamplifier that was shown to conform to the current recommended electrical safety standards. Endotracheal ECG tracings were obtained from three pediatric patients and compared with lead II tracings (Fig. 2–13). An inverted QRS complex was obtained with a low amplitude P wave compared with lead II. Alternating current interference was a major problem which could be improved by use of a reference electrode (a two-electrode system was used for simplicity), improved common mode rejection in the amplifier, and better matching of input impedances. Position and movement of the tube also were critical factors in the quality of the signal.

The endotracheal ECG offers advantages for monitoring small infants where surface electrodes cannot be used (e.g., with certain surgical sites, following extensive trauma or burns, and in long-term critical care, where surface electrodes may cause skin irritation or hamper temperature maintenance).

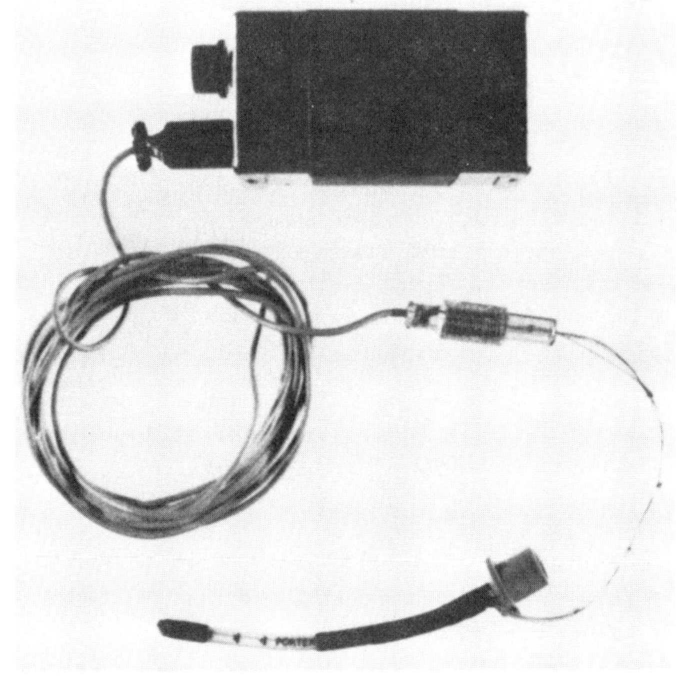

Fig. 2–12 Endotracheal ECG system using a 3.5-mm endotracheal tube. (Mylrea KC, Calkins JM, Carlson J, Saunders RJ: ECG lead with the endotracheal tube. Crit Care Med 11:199, 1983. © 1983 The Williams & Wilkins Co., Baltimore.)

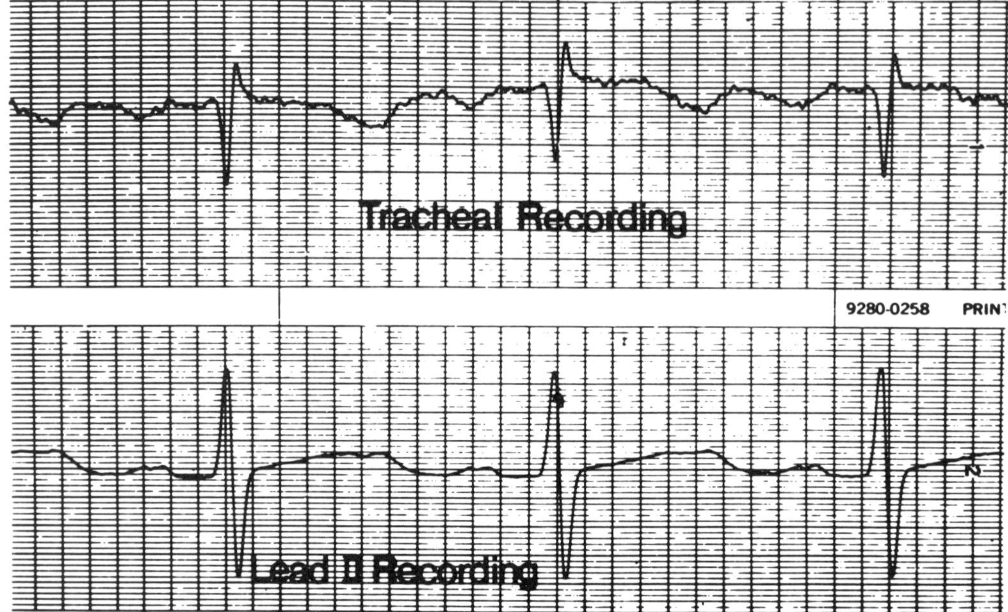

Fig. 2–13 Comparison of an endotracheal ECG (top) with a standard lead II in an 11-month-old child. (Mylrea KC, Calkins JM, Carlson J, Saunders RJ: ECG lead with the endotracheal tube. Crit Care Med 11:199, 1983. © 1983 The Williams & Wilkins Co., Baltimore.)

ARTIFACTS AFFECTING THE ELECTROCARDIOGRAM IN THE OPERATING ROOM

Electrocardiographic monitoring in the operating room is subject to many types of interference that may prevent reliable interpretation. Artifacts simulating dysrhythmias may occur and even lead to inappropriate therapeutic intervention. Some of the artifacts produced are common to ECG monitoring outside of the operating room, while others are problems unique to the operating room environment.

Artifacts Related to the Patient

1. Muscle tremor produces a characteristic fine fibrillatory pattern on the ECG. It may be evident in anxious patients prior to induction of anesthesia and also in the awake, shivering patient on emergence from anesthesia.
2. Movement of the patient may cause sudden changes in potential differences between the electrodes or may disturb the electrode contacts.
3. Hiccoughing and movements of the diaphragm produce a motion artifact on the ECG.
4. Respiratory-induced variations in the electrical axis may be produced during spontaneous or controlled ventilation.
5. Assumption of the lateral or Trendelenburg position may cause axis deviations.

Artifacts Related to the Lead Systems and ECG Monitoring Equipment

1. Loose electrodes and broken leads may produce a variety of artifacts which may simulate dysrhythmias, Q waves, or inverted T waves.[22] Pregelled disposable Ag/Ag chloride electrodes are usually used in the operating room. It is important that all the electrodes be moist, uniform, and not out of date. To ensure

good contact between the electrode and the skin, the electrical resistance of the skin should be minimized (i.e., rub with alcohol) and excess body hair removed. Some ECG monitors have built-in cable testers, enabling a lead to be tested by plugging in the distal end. A high resistance causes a large voltage drop, indicating that the lead is at fault.

2. Abnormal waveforms may be produced due to incorrect placement of the leads. If the right and left arm leads are reversed, a minor image of the normal lead I will be produced and leads II and III will be reversed.

3. A simple fault in the ECG monitor, such as weak batteries, may simulate a dysrhythmia.[23]

Artifacts Produced by External Sources of Interference

1. During cardiopulmonary bypass the roller pumps can produce an artifactual trace resembling atrial flutter (Fig. 2–14). Automatic infusion pumps may cause similar problems.

2. Direct contact with the patient by other operating room personnel.

Electrical Interference

1. Electrocautery is the most important source of interference on the ECG in the operating room, since usually the electrocautery completely obliterates the ECG tracing. Analysis of the electrocautery has identified three component frequencies.[24] The radiofrequency between 800 and 2,000 kHz comprises most of the interference, coupled with 60 Hz AC frequency and 0.1 to 10 Hz low-frequency noise from intermittent contact of the electrosurgical unit with the patient's tissues. Preamplifiers may be modified to suppress radiofrequency interference, but these filter circuits are still not widely available in the operating room.

2. All equipment in the operating room should be properly grounded, otherwise 60 Hz alternating current can produce gross interference.

MONITORING AND RECORDING THE ELECTROCARDIOGRAM

The function of the ECG monitor is to detect, amplify, display and record the ECG signal. The changes of potential produced by the heart between two electrodes is of the order of 1 mV and has a rapid time course (normal QRS complex is less than 0.12 seconds). Moreover, the skin has a potential of 20 mV with a slow time base and must be separated from the ECG signal, thereby enabling an output signal to drive a recording or display system. The ECG is usually displayed on an oscilloscope, and several monitors now offer nonfade storage oscilloscopes. These offer no advantages over the use of direct writing recorders which enable accurate interpretation of difficult ECGs and provide a written record for the patient's chart. The capability of recording the ECG on paper should be available in every operating room.

The advent of computer technology has led to the development of various types of trend

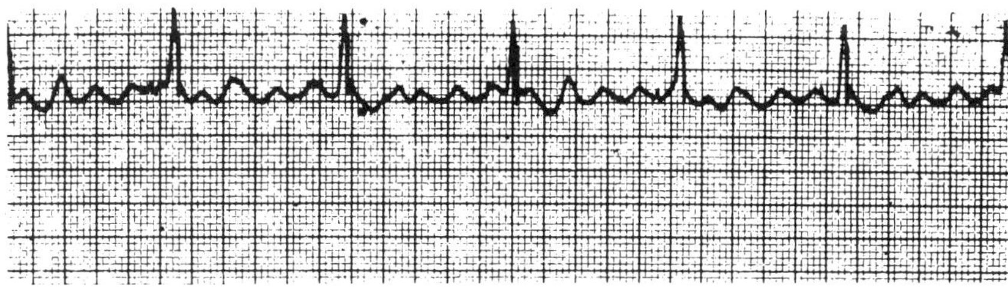

Fig. 2–14 Electrocardiogram showing artifact due to the roller heads on cardiopulmonary bypass that could be mistaken for atrial flutter.

monitoring. The ECG can be displayed as a trend for the previous 2-, 8-, or 24-hour period, identifying heart rate and abnormal beats. Some monitors have an edit/recall facility that enables the user to scan the dysrhythmias for the preceding 24 hours. Trend monitoring has a wider application in the intensive care unit than in the operating room.

The ECG may also be monitored by radiotelemetry. Essentially, the ECG signal is used to frequency modulate an appropriate carrier signal for emission by a miniature transmitter. The carrier signal is a radiowave which is detected by a receiver and converted back to an ECG signal. The advantage of the system is the lack of any lead connection to the patient. This is especially useful in neurodiagnostic procedures (e.g., pneumoencephalography) in which the patient may be turned through 360 degrees or other procedures in which access is difficult (e.g., radiation therapy).

REFERENCES

1. Kaplan JA: Electrocardiographic monitoring. p. 117. In Kaplan JA (ed): Cardiac Anesthesia. Grune & Stratton, Orlando, Florida, 1979
2. Blackburn H: The exercise electrocardiogram: technological, procedural, and conceptual development. p. 220. In Blackburn H (ed): Measurements in Exercise Electrocardiography. Charles C Thomas, Springfield, Illinois, 1969
3. Mason RE, Likar I, Biern RO, et al: Multiple lead exercise electrocardiography. Circulation 36:517, 1967
4. Robertson D, Kostok WJ, Ahuja SP: The localization of coronary artery stenosis by 12-lead ECG response to graded exercise test. Am Heart J 91:437,1976
5. Kaplan JA, King SB: The precordial electrocardiographic lead (V_5) in patients who have coronary artery disease. Anesthesiology 45:570, 1976
6. Froelicher VF, Wolthius R, Keiser N, et al: A comparison of two bipolar exercise ECG leads to lead V_5. Chest 70:611, 1976
7. Bazaral MG, Norfleet EA: Comparison of CB_5 and V_5 leads for intraoperative electrocardiographic monitoring. Anesth Analg 60:849, 1981
8. Brown WH: A study of the esophageal lead in clinical electrocardiography. Part I. Am Heart J 121:306, 1936
9. Kistin AD, Bruce JC: Simultaneous esophageal and standard electrocardiographic leads for the study of cardiac arrhythmias. Am Heart J 53:65, 1957
10. Copeland GD, Tullis IF, Brody DA: Clinical evaluation of a new esophageal electrode, with particular reference to the bipolar esophageal electrocardiogram. Am Heart J 53:862, 1959
11. Kates RA, Zaidan JR, Kaplan JA: Esophageal lead for intraoperative electrocardiographic monitoring. Anesth Analg 61:781, 1982
12. Hellerstein HK, Pritchard WH, Lewis RL: Recording of intracavitary potentials through a single lumen, saline filled cardiac catheter. Proc Soc Exp Biol Med 71:58, 1949
13. Robertson JT, Shick RW, Morgan F, Matson DD: Accurate placement of ventriculo-atrial shunt for hydrocephalus under electrocardiographic control. J Neurosurg 18:255, 1961
14. Michenfelder JD, Terry HR Jr, Daw EF, Miller RH: Air embolism during neurosurgery: A new method of treatment. Anesth Analg 45:390, 1966
15. Richards CC, Freeman A: Intra-atrial catheter placement under electrocardiographic guidance. Anesthesiology 25:388, 1964
16. Westheimer DN: Right atrial catheter placement: Use of a wire guide as the intravascular ECG lead. Anesthesiology 56:478, 1982
17. Chatterjee K, Swan HJC, Ganz W, et al: Use of a balloon-tipped flotation electrode catheter for cardiac monitoring. Am J Cardiol 36:56, 1975
18. Mantle JA, Massing GK, James TN, et al: A multipurpose catheter for electrophysiologic and hemodynamic monitoring plus atrial pacing. Chest 72:285, 1977
19. Zaidan JR: Experience with the pacing pulmonary artery catheter. Anesthesiology 53:S118, 1980
20. Lichtenthal PR: Multipurpose pulmonary artery catheter. Ann Thorac Surg 36:493, 1983
21. Mylrea KC, Calkins JM, Carlson J, Saunders RJ: ECG lead with the endotracheal tube. Crit Care Med 11:199, 1983
22. Borello G: ECG artifacts simulating atrial flutter. JAMA 223:439, 1973
23. Shapiro LA, Jejeikin R, Hoffman S: Misdiagnosis due to ECG failure. Anesthesiology 60:166, 1984
24. Doss JD, McCabe CW, Weiss GK: Noise-free data during electrosurgical procedures. Anesth Analg 52:156, 1973

3

The Preoperative ECG: Changes in Chamber Size

Zaharia Hillel, M.D., Ph.D.
Daniel M. Thys, M.D.

This chapter describes basic ECG representations of abnormalities in the size of the heart. Vectorcardiographic analysis of ECG abnormalities has been limited to the frontal plane (e.g., right- or left-axis deviation, vertical or horizontal orientations), since most anesthesia personnel are familiar with this type of analysis. Vector loop analysis has been omitted.

ATRIAL ENLARGEMENT

Electrical depolarization of the right and left atria (RA, LA) produces the P wave on the ECG. It therefore seems reasonable that abnormalities in atrial chamber morphology or atrial function will primarily be reflected in the P wave. However, changes in atrial repolarization and even changes in QRS pattern have been shown to reflect atrial abnormalities.

The diagnosis of atrial chamber enlargement by ECG is complicated because P-wave changes can reflect additional atrial abnormalities such as increased intraatrial pressure, increased atrial volume, abnormal intraatrial conduction, and changes in the state of the autonomic nervous system.[1] It has been observed that, in the same person, the configuration of the P wave may change in response to different physiologic stimuli. Furthermore, unequivocal ECG evidence of atrial enlargement has been found in patients in whom other diagnostic criteria failed to show the same. Conversely, normal P waves have been found in the presence of atrial disease. Finally, enlargement of the right atrial chamber can be simulated by enlargement of the left atrial chamber. Thus it becomes clear that diagnosis of atrial enlargement or hypertrophy using the ECG alone is not simple because false-positive as well as false-negative diagnoses can be made. Since the ECG representation of normal atrial activity may not be well known to most readers, a detailed description follows.

During a normal cardiac cycle, the sinus node initiates electrical activity for the entire heart in the RA. The RA is the first chamber to depolarize and therefore contributes to the initial and mid-portions of the P wave (Fig. 3–1A). Left atrial depolarization follows and contributes to the mid- and terminal portions of the P wave. Normal P-wave characteristics are as follows (Fig. 3–1A):

1. The normal P wave is upright in leads I, II, aVF, and V_4–V_6 and inverted in aVR; it has variable polarity in leads III, aVL, and V_1–

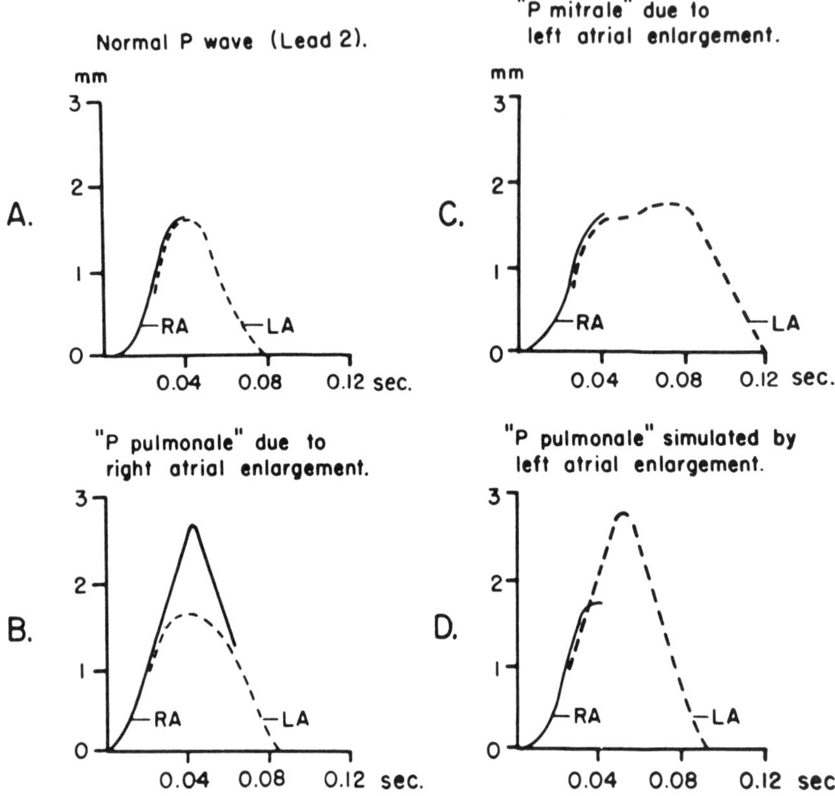

Fig. 3–1 Normal P-wave morphology, P pulmonale, P mitrale, and the mechanisms proposed by Chou and Helm for the appearance of a P-pulmonale pattern in left atrial hypertrophy. (Chou TC, Helm RA: The pseudo-P pulmonale. Circulation 32:96, 1965. By permission of the American Heart Association, Inc.)

V_3. Thus the P vector points down and to the left and may either be in or point away from the frontal plane.

2. The amplitude of the P wave does not exceed 2.5 mm in any lead.

3. The maximum duration of the normal P wave is 0.07 second until age 1 year, 0.08 second between 1 and 12 years of age, 0.09 second between 12 and 16 years, and 0.10 second in older children or adults.

4. The P wave is rounded at the top without being unduly pointed. Notching of the P wave (Fig. 3–2A) is not abnormal unless the distance between peaks exceeds 0.03 second and the P wave is abnormally wide.

5. For P waves that are biphasic in lead V_1 (i.e., they exhibit positive and negative deflections), the terminal force is normally between −0.01 and −0.03 mm-sec (Fig. 3–3), while the duration of the intrinsicoid deflection is 0.03 seconds or less (Fig. 3–4).

6. Normal ratio of the P-wave duration to the PR segment is 1.0 to 1.6.[1]

Atrial repolarization produces the atrial ST segment (ST_A) and the atrial T wave (T_A). The ST_A occurs during the PR segment, while the T_A wave is usually masked by the QRS complex with which it overlaps. In cases of prolonged AV block or AV dissociation, the T_A may be identifiable and has the opposite direction of the preceding P wave.

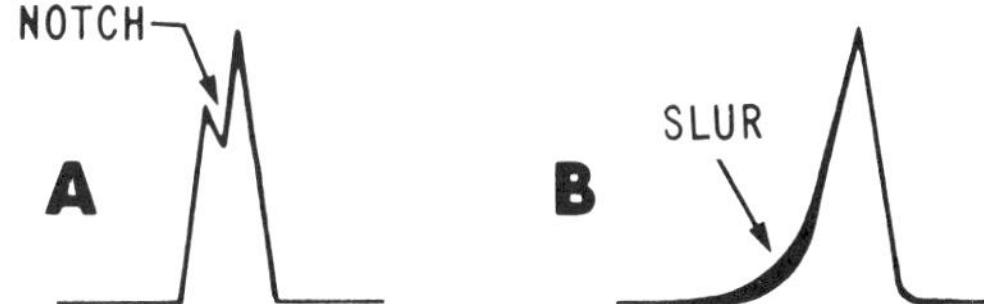

Fig. 3–2 Schematic representation of notching and slurring. (Friedman HH: Diagnostic Electrocardiography and Vectorcardiography. © 1977 McGraw–Hill, New York. Reproduced with permission.)

RIGHT ATRIAL HYPERTROPHY

Right atrial enlargement, or hypertrophy (RAH), is seen usually in association with the conditions listed in Table 3–1. RAH produces a P vector heading anteriorly and inferiorly. This is a right and anterior shift from the normal P-wave orientation. The criteria for RAH are as follows[1,2]:

1. A P wave in leads II, III, and aVF that has a height of more than 2.5 mm (Fig. 3–5).
2. A P-wave duration of less than 0.11 second.
3. A rightward shift of more than +70 degrees in the mean electrical axis of the P wave.
4. Biphasic P waves, with initial voltage components often exceeding 2.5 mm in the right precordial leads (Fig. 3–6). (This does not apply in emphysema, in which the entire P wave or its terminal component may be inverted.)
5. The presence of a qR complex in lead V_1 or a small QRS voltage in lead V_1 that increases abruptly in lead V_2 (to > 3×) in a patient without myocardial infarction. Both abnormalities are seen in Figure 3–7.

The diagnosis of RAH based on the presence of a qR complex in lead V_1 correlates best with echo-determined RAH. The abrupt increase in QRS voltage from lead V_1 to V_2 is most useful

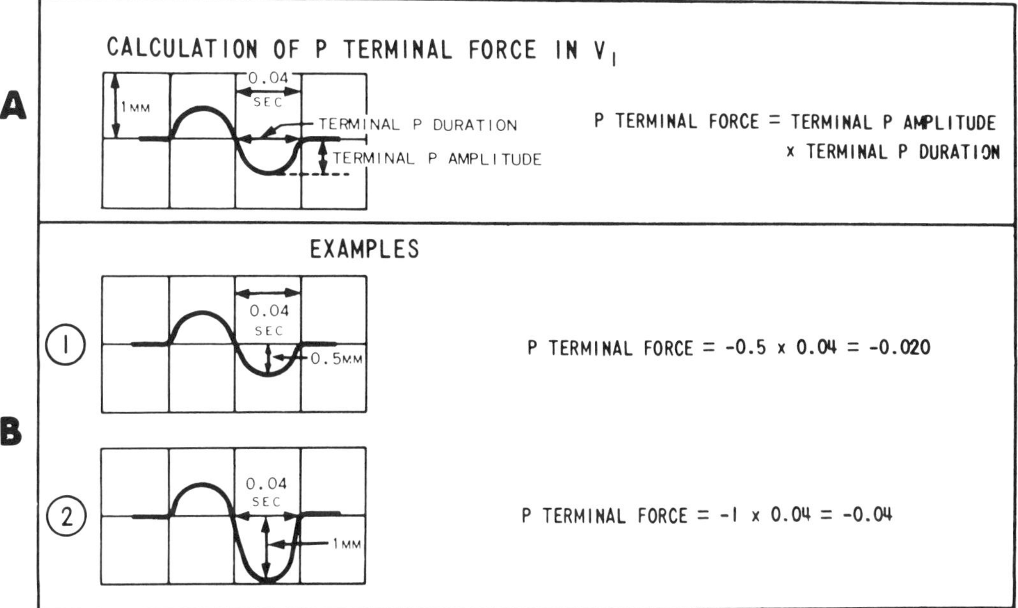

Fig. 3–3 Measurement of the P-terminal force in lead V_1. (**A**) The P wave is divided into initial and terminal portions. The biphasic duration (in seconds) and the amplitude (in millimeters) of the terminal component are measured. The P-terminal force is the algebraic product of these two values and is expressed in millimeter-seconds. (**B**) Examples: (1) normal P-terminal force; (2) abnormal P terminal force. (Friedman HH: Diagnostic Electrocardiography and Vectorcardiography. © 1977 McGraw-Hill, New York. Reproduced with permission.)

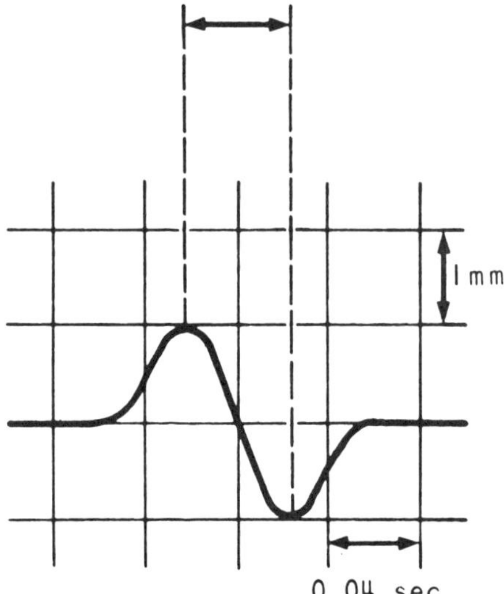

Fig. 3–4 Measurement of the duration of the intrinsicoid deflection of a biphasic P wave in lead V_1. The duration is measured from the peak of the initial component to the nadir of the terminal component. (Friedman HH: Diagnostic Electrocardiography and Vectorcardiography. © 1977 McGraw-Hill, New York. Reproduced with permission.)

in the presence of atrial fibrillation or flutter, wherein P waves cannot be identified. In the patient with atrial fibrillation, the presence of coarse, relatively large fibrillatory waves, especially in lead V_1, suggest RAH. This pattern contrasts with that seen in atrial fibrillation complicating arteriosclerotic or hypertensive heart disease, in which the fibrillatory waves are fine and often not identifiable.[2]

In the adult, the most common cause of RA abnormalities is chronic obstructive pulmonary disease (COPD). Increased pulmonary vascular resistance may lead to right ventricular hypertrophy, reduced right ventricular compliance, and RAH. The accompanying P-wave abnormalities are classically described as P pulmonale (Figs. 3–1B and 3–8B). By definition, the axis of a P pulmonale is > +70 degrees. However, patients with COPD can show this right shift of the P axis without RAH. This is due to the changes in pulmonary anatomy resulting from a vertical heart position. For this and other reasons, the P-pulmonale tracing is nonspecific for RAH, and the term pseudo-P pulmonale has been introduced to describe the presence of an RAH-like P pulmonale in the absence of atrial enlargement. Pseudo-P pulmonale can be found in association with coronary artery disease, with angina pectoris, with acute LV failure, and occasionally in the absence of heart disease, but in association with hypoxemia.[1] It has also been suggested that in some cases the presence of a pseudo-P pulmonale in predominantly left heart disease reflects an increase in the left atrial component of the P wave (Fig. 3–1D).[4] The presence of left ventricular hypertrophy (LVH) and an abnormal P-terminal force in lead V_1 suggest pseudo-P pulmonale rather than true P pulmonale and a situation in which left atrial hypertrophy (LAH) simulates RAH. RVH or pulmonary disease and a P pulmonale suggest RAH.[1] ECG tracings for which the differential diagnosis includes LAH with a pseudo-P pulmonale pattern are shown in Fig. 3–8A,C. In another unusual situation, the right atrial appendage may be so enlarged that it extends leftward across the front of the heart. On the ECG, this may result in an inverted P wave in V_1, creating the illusion of LAH[2] (Fig. 3–9).

In RAH secondary to tricuspid valve disease, the P waves may be tall and notched with the first peak of the P wave taller than the second (P tricuspidale). This is demonstrated in leads II, V_3, and V_4 of the ECG shown in Figure 3–10.

Table 3–1. Conditions Associated with Right Atrial Hypertrophy

Chronic obstructive pulmonary disease (COPD)
Rheumatic valvular heart disease
Isolated tricuspid valve disease
Mitral valve disease
Congenital heart disease
Atrial septal defect
Transposition of the great vessels
Tricuspid atresia
Tetralogy of Fallot
AV canal lesion
Pulmonary hypertension

LEFT ATRIAL HYPERTROPHY

Changes indicative of LAH are frequently seen in the presence of mitral stenosis, mitral regurgitation, and aortic valve disease. They

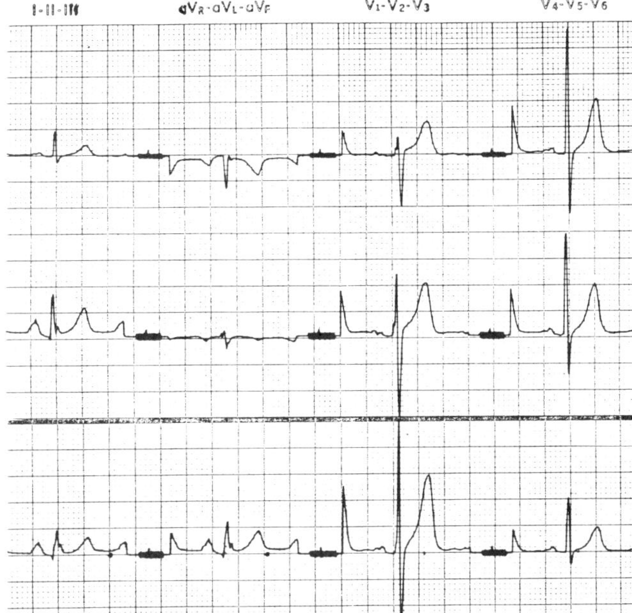

Fig. 3–5 Right atrial hypertrophy. Note prominent P waves in leads II, III, and aVF. The P-wave axis is 75 degrees.

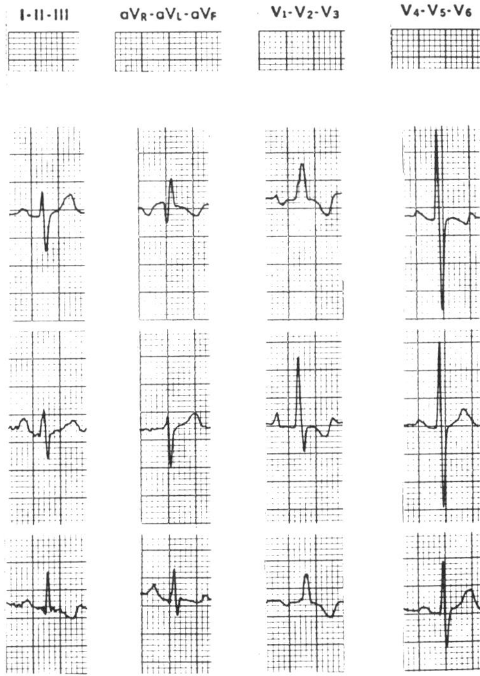

Fig. 3–6 Secundum ASD in a 4-year-old. The tracing demonstrates right axis deviation (RAD), right atrial hypertrophy (RAH), and right ventricular hypertrophy (RVH). Note the biphasic P wave in lead V_1 and the large P waves in leads II, aVF, and V_2. RV strain is seen in leads III and V_1–V_4.

may also occur in association with the conditions listed in Table 3–2. Criteria for LAH are as follows:

1. The duration of the P wave exceeds the normal values noted above (often greater than 0.12 second), causing shortening or absence of the PR interval. The P wave is notched and slurred in leads I and II.
2. The mean axis of the terminal component of the P wave in the frontal plane is shifted leftward to $<+30$ degrees, producing positive terminal P-wave deflections in leads I and aVL and negative deflections in leads III and aVF. The initial P-wave forces are usually unchanged, but occasionally the mean axis of the entire P wave shows a leftward shift to between $+45$ degrees and -30 degrees.
3. The right precordial leads show biphasic P waves with wide and/or deep terminal components, the terminal force of which is more negative than -0.04 mm-sec. This is a reliable sign of LAH or strain except in emphysema.
4. The duration of the intrinsicoid deflection of the biphasic P wave in lead V_1 is >0.03 second.

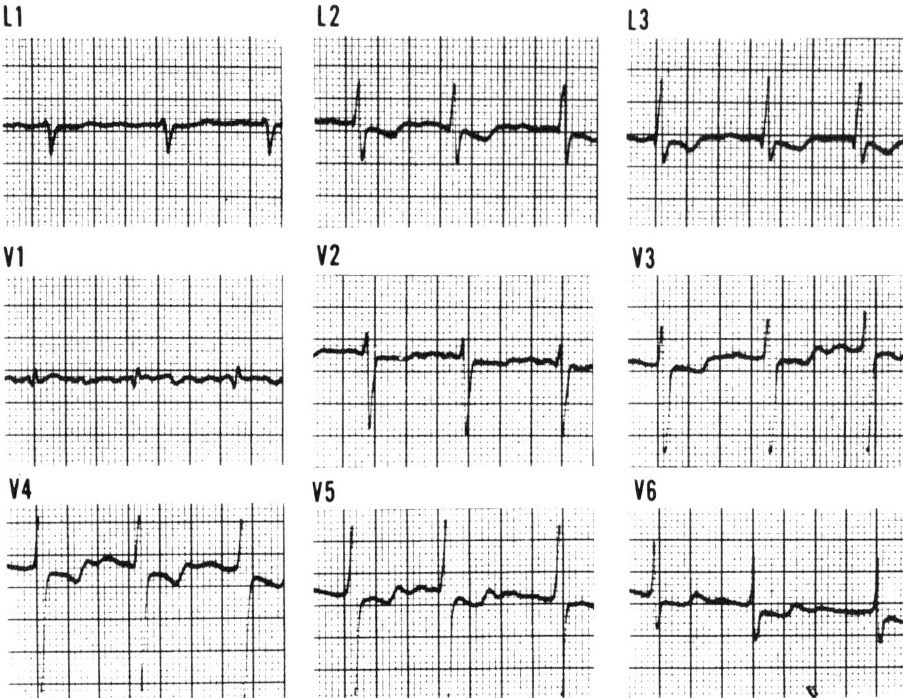

Fig. 3–7 Right atrial hypertrophy in a patient with rheumatic valvular heart disease and tricuspid regurgitation. The basic rhythm is atrial fibrillation. The right axis deviation, squatty QRS in lead V_1 and clockwise rotation are consistent with mitral valve disease. The QR pattern in V_1 reflects the right atrial intracavitary potential and indicates a regurgitant tricuspid valve. (Reprinted with permission from Braunwald E: Heart Disease. WB Saunders, Philadelphia, 1984.)

The ECG pattern of LAH may be due to intraatrial conduction disturbances rather than to chamber enlargement. However, it sometimes reflects both left atrial conduction disturbances and enlargement. Three examples of LAH and RVH are demonstrated in patients with mitral disease. In Figure 3–11A, notching, slurring, and a long P-wave duration with loss of the PR interval are well demonstrated in leads I, aVL, V_5, V_6. Figure 3–11B shows slurring and a clearly biphasic P wave with an abnormal P-terminal force and an abnormal intrinsicoid deflection in lead V_1. A different example of LAH secondary to LV diastolic overloading in a patient with rheumatic mitral regurgitation is shown in Figure 3–12, where the P-mitrale pattern is evident with broad notched P waves (Fig. 3–1C) and a remarkable left axis shift of the entire P wave, not just its terminal component, to −15 degrees (note the nearly isoelectric P wave in lead II).

COMBINED ATRIAL HYPERTROPHY

Hypertrophy of both right and left atria can be seen in patients with the conditions listed in Table 3–3. In combined atrial enlargement, both the amplitude and the duration of the P wave are increased using the criteria for enlargement of the individual chambers. Left axis deviation of the terminal P-wave component is also seen.

An example of biatrial enlargement associated

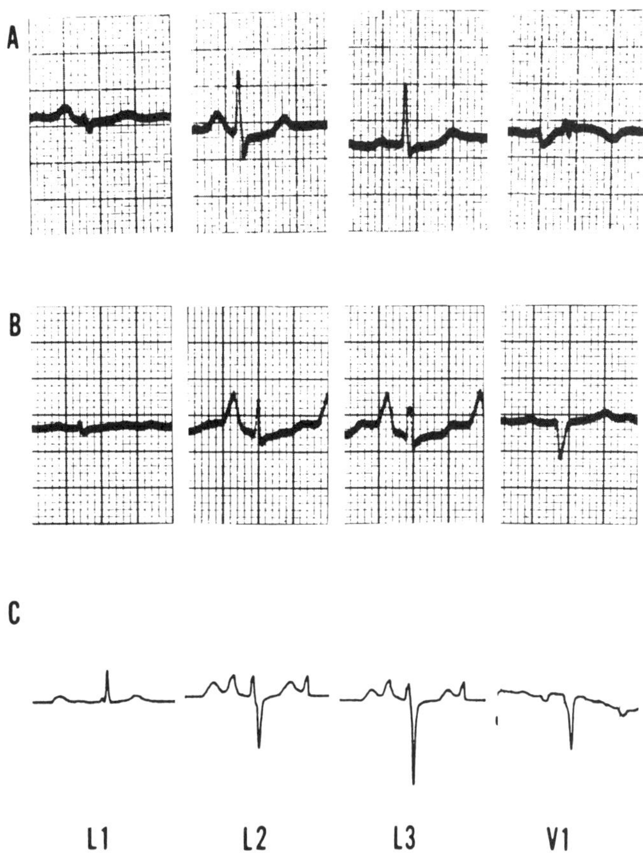

Fig. 3–8 (**A**) Recording from a patient with mitral stenosis showing biatrial hypertrophy manifest by a tall P wave in lead II, a notched P wave with left axis deviation of the terminal component in lead III and a pronounced large biphasic P wave in lead V_1. (**B**) Recording from a patient with chronic obstructive pulmonary disease (COPD) showing right atrial hypertrophy manifest by right axis deviation of the P wave and a tall, peaked P wave in leads II and III. (**C**) Recording from a patient with hypertension showing left ventricular hypertrophy (LVH) and possible left atrial hypertrophy (LAH) with a pseudo-P-pulmonale pattern. The P-terminal force is −0.04 mm-sec. (A and B reprinted with permission from Braunwald E: Heart Disease. WB Saunders, Philadelphia, 1984.)

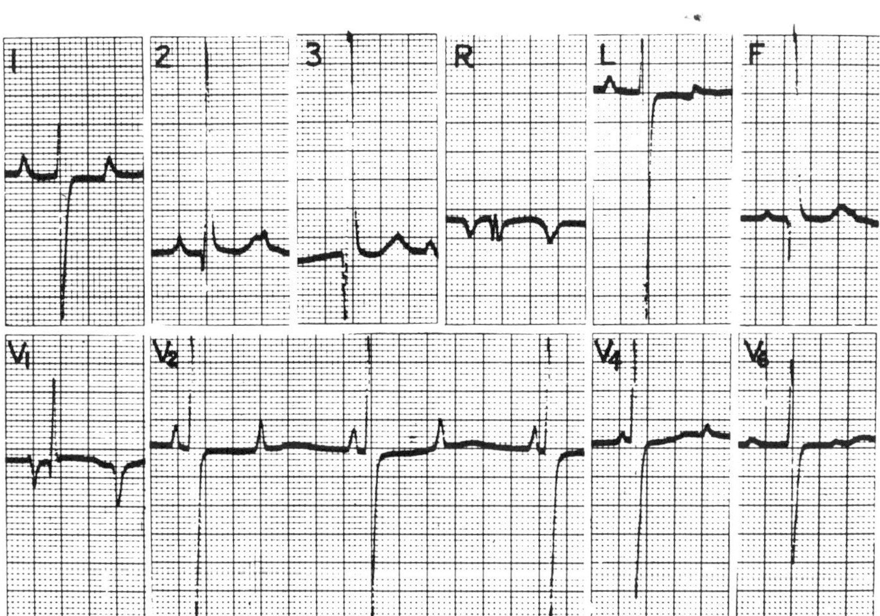

Fig. 3–9 RAH simulating LAH in a patient with corrected transposition of the great vessels. (Marriott HJL: Practical Electrocardiography. © 1983 The Williams & Wilkins Co., Baltimore.)

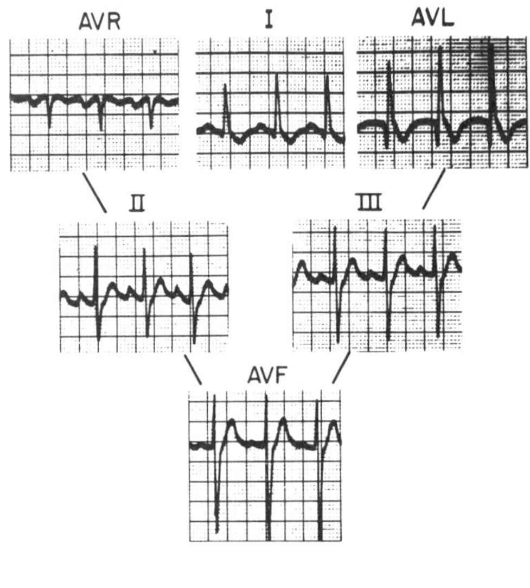

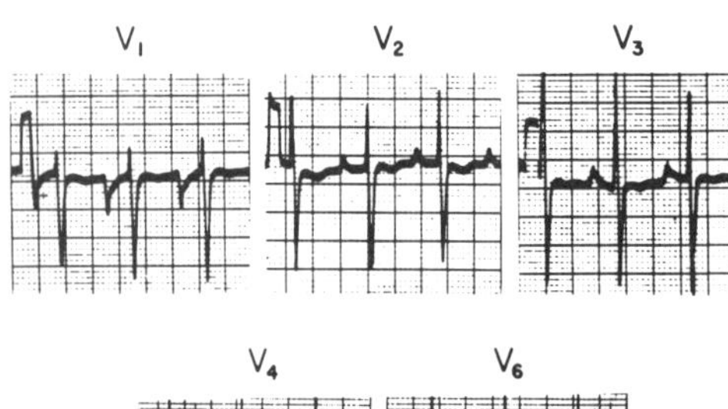

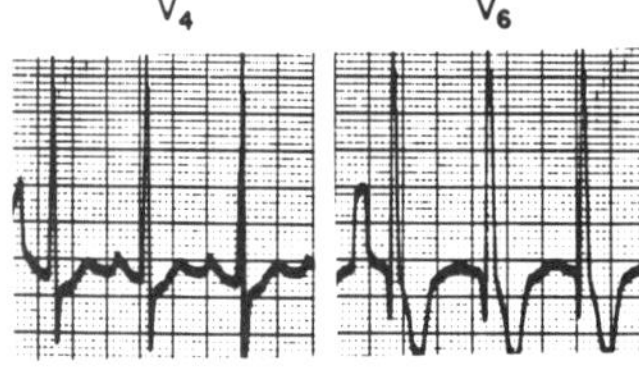

Fig. 3–10 Atrial enlargement secondary to tricuspid atresia. The ECG also shows left axial deviation (LAD) and left ventricular hypertrophy (LVH). (Reprinted with permission from Braunwald E: Heart Disease. WB Saunders, Philadelphia, 1984.)

Table 3–2. Conditions in Which the ECG May Show Left Atrial Hypertrophy

Mitral valve stenosis
Mitral valve regurgitation
Aortic valve disease
Coronary artery disease
Acute myocardial infarction
Acute coronary artery disease
Constrictive pericarditis
Idiopathic hypertrophic subaortic stenosis
Coarctation of the aorta
Endocardial cushion defect
Systemic hypertension
Congestive heart failure

with mitral stenosis is shown in Figure 1–8A, where the P wave shows a large amplitude and duration, notching, profound biphasic contour, and an abnormal terminal force as well as abnormal duration of the intrinsicoid deflection. Figure 3–13 shows ECG evidence of biatrial enlargement in combined mitral and tricuspid stenosis. The biatrial enlargement ECG pattern in idiopathic hypertrophic subaortic stenosis (IHSS) is shown in Figure 3–14. In this case, however, an isolated LAH abnormality producing a pseudo-P pulmonale pattern cannot be ruled out.

LEFT VENTRICULAR HYPERTROPHY

The left ventricle enlarges when it has to perform increased work secondary to valvular disease, hypertension, or cardiomyopathy (Table 3–4). Hypertrophy occurs by an increase in the size of the individual myocardial fibers and not by an increase in the number of fibers. LVH is seen in congenital heart disease such as aortic stenosis, coarctation of the aorta, ventricular septal defect (VSD), patent ductus arteriosus (PDA), hypertrophic cardiomyopathy, and tricuspid atresia. An enlarged left ventricle has a thickened wall and larger surface area. As a result, it generates greater electrical forces. In addition, an enlarged left ventricle is closer to the chest wall because of its increased size; it therefore inscribes larger potentials in the precordial leads. Because the muscle mass is larger, electrical depolarization and repolarization of the left ventricle are slower, thus making the duration of the QRS complex slightly longer. For the same reason, travel time of the depolarization wave from the endocardium to the epicardium is lengthened, making for a longer intrinsicoid deflection. More importantly, since the oxygen demand of an enlarged heart facing a larger work requirement is greater than that of a normal heart under normal workload, relative coronary insufficiency may develop because of an inadequate myocardial oxygen supply–demand ratio. This relative ischemia is said to produce the LV strain pattern on the ECG, char-

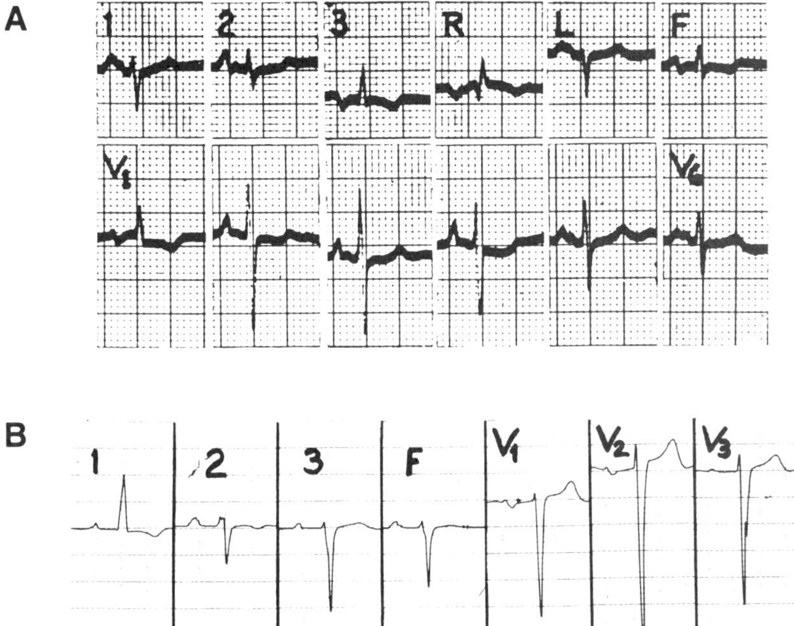

Fig. 3–11 (**A**) Evidence of left atrial hypertrophy (LAH) and right ventricular hypertrophy (LVH) in a patient with severe mitral disease. Note P mitrale with wide notched P waves, marked right axis deviation (RAD) (+150 degrees) with prominent R in V_1. (Marriott HJL: Practical Electrocardiography. © 1983 The Williams & Wilkins Co., Baltimore.) (**B**) Left atrial and left ventricular enlargement in a patient with hypertension. The P waves are slurred or biphasic, and there is first-degree AV block.

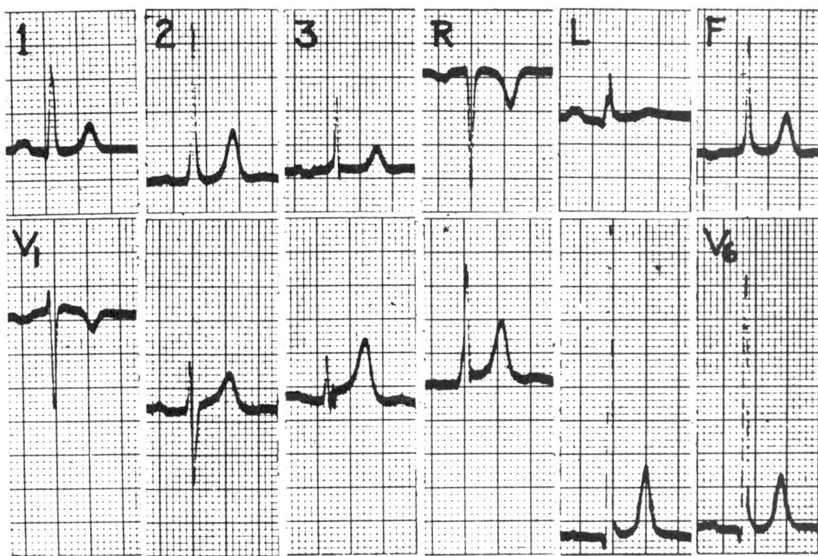

Fig. 3–12 Left ventricular diastolic overloading, in a patient with rheumatic mitral regurgitation. R waves in V_5 and V_6 are unusually tall and are accompanied by tall and pointed T waves. The P waves show a P-mitrale pattern, being rather broad and notched with a leftward axis shift to about −15 degrees. (Marriott HJL: Practical Electrocardiography. © 1983 The Williams & Wilkins Co., Baltimore.)

Table 3–3. Conditions That Can Lead to Combined Left and Right Atrial Hypertrophy

Isolated mitral stenosis
Combined mitral and tricuspid stenosis
Idiopathic hypertrophic subaortic stenosis
Congenital heart disease
Tricuspid atresia
Endocardial cushion defect
Ventricular septal defect
Patent ductus arteriosus with pulmonary hypertension
Transposition of the great vessels
Truncus arteriosus

acterized by abnormal repolarization of the LV. In the presence of LV strain—a misnomer, since the ECG does not record hemodynamics—the ST segments are depressed and convex upward, while the T waves are asymmetrically inverted in the left precordial leads, V_4, V_5, and V_6, and several limb leads (Fig. 3–15A). The anatomic and ECG consequences of LVH differ from person to person and depend on the patient's age, the original orientation of the heart, and either coexisting cardiac or noncardiac disease, or both. Since the surface of the ventricle is symmetrically enlarged, there may be little change in the orientation of the QRS vector. For this reason, the presence of LVH in young people, who have relatively vertically oriented hearts, will mainly produce large increases in the mean spatial QRS vector in the vertical limb leads (leads II, III, aVF). By contrast, in older people, who usually have more horizontal hearts, LVH will produce a larger increase in the horizontal component of the mean spatial vector (limb leads I, aVL, and lateral chest leads). Similarly, in a person with a vertical mean QRS vector, the ST-segment depression and the T-wave inversion produced by LV strain will be seen in limb leads II, III, and aVF (Fig. 3–15B), while in a person with a horizontal mean QRS vector they will be seen in leads I and aVL (Fig. 3–16).

The LV strain pattern is not specific for LVH. It can be seen with digitalis, coronary artery disease, electrolyte disturbances, and myocarditis. Neither is increased voltage specific for LVH, as it can be found in thin or normal elderly persons or young adults or in the absence of LVH. Conversely, in certain patients who have LVH, the ECG may fail to record abnormally large voltages. This can occur because of body habitus, emphysema, pericardial effusion, or even coronary artery disease. Because of such false-positive and false-negative diagnoses, multiple and complex criteria have been established for LVH. Although quite specific, these criteria lack sensitivity. The ECG criteria are estimated to have a limit of 60 percent sensitivity

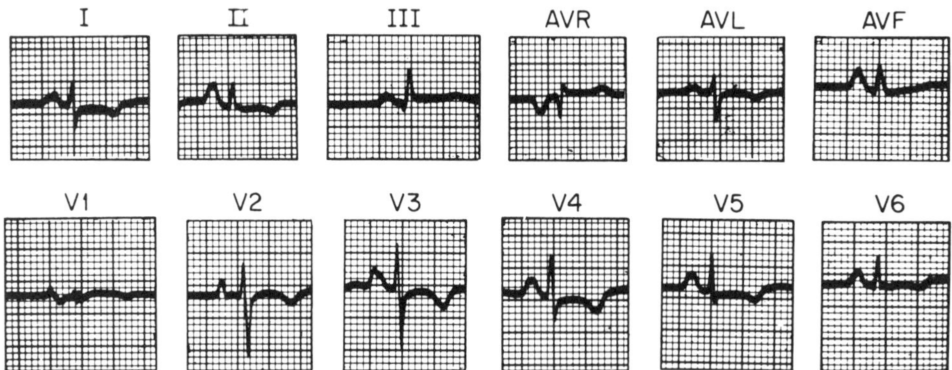

Fig. 3–13 Biatrial enlargement and right ventricular strain in a patient with mitral and tricuspid stenosis. The P waves are both abnormally broad and tall. Right ventricular strain is manifested by the inverted T waves in the precordial leads and can be considered evidence of right ventricular enlargement. (Friedman HH: Diagnostic Electrocardiography and Vectorcardiography. © 1977 McGraw-Hill, New York. Reproduced with permission.)

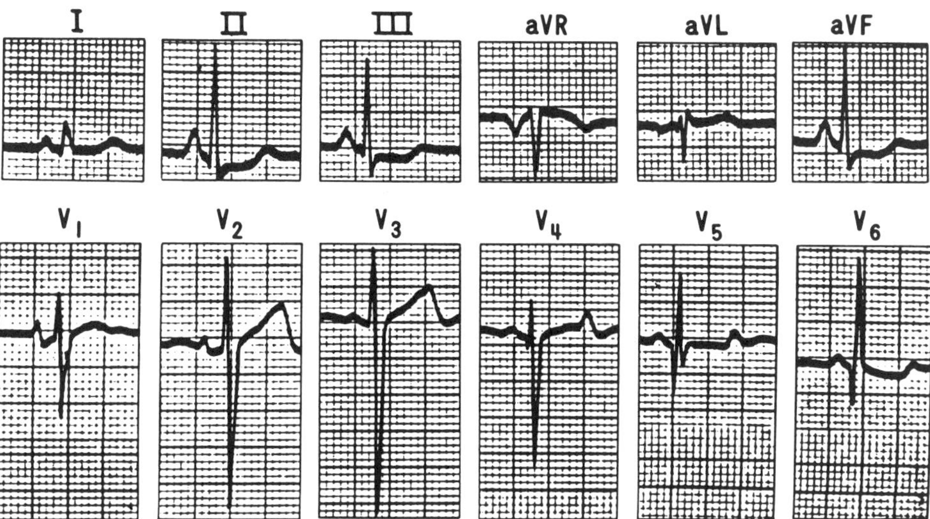

Fig. 3–14 Hypertrophic obstructive cardiomyopathy simulating myocardial infarction by the presence of prominent Q waves in leads V_5 and V_6. The diagnosis of left ventricular hypertrophy is suggested by voltage changes and by the criterion $R_{v5} < R_{v6}$. Tall and broad P waves are seen in leads II, III, and aVF, and the P terminal force in lead V_1 is increased. These findings indicate either biatrial enlargement or a pseudo-P pulmonale pattern caused by left atrial hypertrophy. (Friedman HH: Diagnostic Electrocardiography and Vectorcardiography. © 1977 McGraw-Hill, New York. Reproduced with permission.)

when they approach 95 percent specificity.[5] The simplest and oldest criterion for LVH is that described by Sokolow and Lyon.[6] It requires that the sum of the S wave in lead V_1 and the tallest R wave either in V_5 or V_6 be greater than 35 mm. Table 3–5 shows Estes's scoring system for LVH.[7] A total of four points indicates probable LVH, while five or more points indicates definite LVH. Scott's criteria for LVH, based solely on voltage, are shown in Table 3–6.[8–11] All these criteria can be summarized by saying that definite LVH is diagnosed in the presence of indisputable and preferably multiple voltage abnormalities accompanied by ST-segment and T-wave changes typical for LV strain in the presence of left atrial enlargement or left axis deviation. Further evidence for LVH comes from the delayed onset of the intrinsicoid deflection in the left precordial leads.[1]

Table 3–4. Conditions Found in Association with Left Ventricular Hypertrophy

Systemic hypertension
Aortic valve disease
Cardiomyopathy
Congenital heart disease
Aortic stenosis
Coarctation of the aorta
Ventricular septal defect
Patent ductus arteriosus
Tricuspid atresia
Left ventricular outflow tract obstruction

The presence of other ECG abnormalities can complicate the diagnosis of LVH. The following clarifications may be useful[1]:

1. In the presence of incomplete left bundle branch block (LBBB), LVH can be diagnosed by the usual voltage criteria. An example of combined LVH and incomplete LBBB is shown in Figure 3–17A.
2. In the presence of complete LBBB, there are no acceptable criteria for recognizing LVH; thus, the diagnosis for LVH should not be made.
3. In the presence of right bundle branch block (RBBB), LVH should be suspected if voltage criteria for LVH are fulfilled or if the R wave in lead V_5 or V_6 is larger than 22 mm.

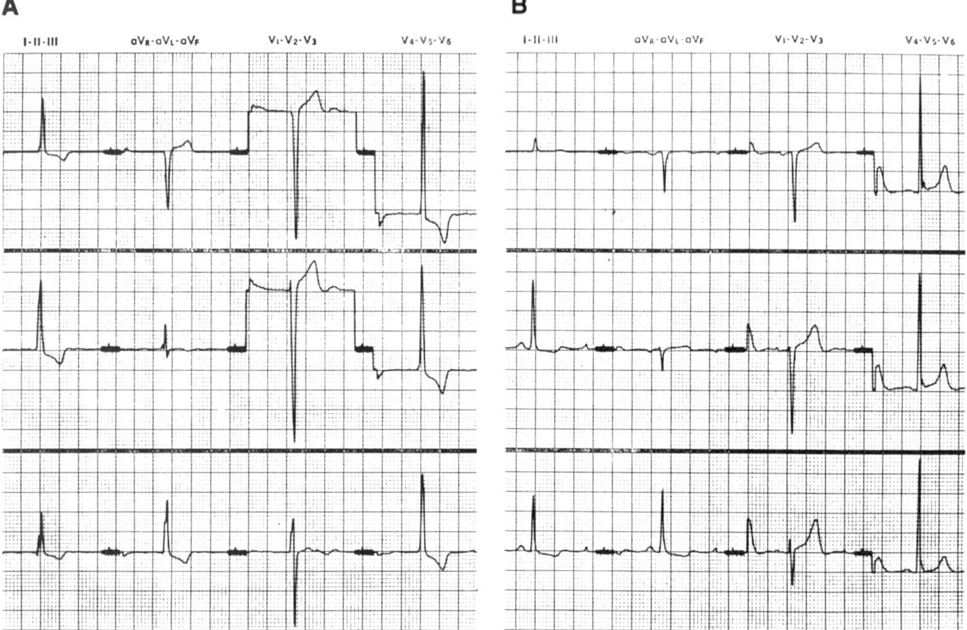

Fig. 3–15 (**A**) Left ventricular hypertrophy (LVH) in a 82-year-old patient with hypertension. The tracing demonstrates an LV strain pattern in the lateral chest leads. (**B**) Tracing demonstrating LVH and LV strain in the inferior limb leads. The QRS axis is about 80 degrees, suggesting a vertically oriented heart.

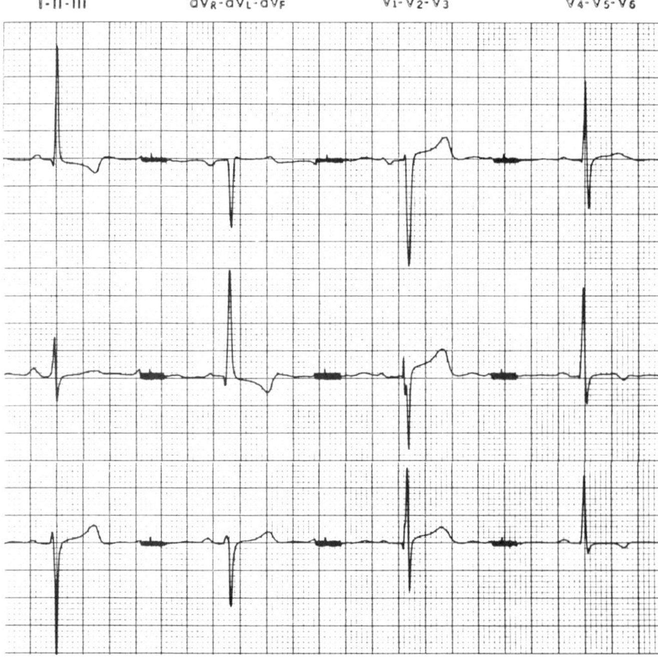

Fig. 3–16 Left ventricular hypertrophy (LVH) with secondary LV strain in the lateral limb leads. The QRS axis is −15 degrees, suggesting a horizontally oriented heart.

Table 3–5. Estes's Scoring System for Left Ventricular Hypertrophy

1. R or S in limb lead (20 mm or more) S in V_1, V_2, or V_3 (25 mm or more) R in V_4, V_5, or V_6 (25 mm or more)	3
2. Any ST shift (without digitalis) Typical "strain" ST-T (with digitalis)	3 1
3. Left axis deviation: −15° or more	2
4. QRS interval: 0.09 sec or more	1
5. Intrinsicoid QRS deflection in V_5–V_6 0.04 seconds or more	1
6. P-terminal force in V_1 more than 0.04 mm-sec	3
Total (maximum total score) (5 = LVH; 4 = probable LVH)	13

4. In the presence of myocardial infarction, LVH may be diagnosed by the usual voltage criteria (Fig. 3–17B).

5. Primary T-wave abnormalities indicative of ischemia are differentiated from the strain pattern of LVH by noting that they inscribe inverted T waves in the inferior limb leads or the right precordial leads, or symmetric inverted T waves in leads I, aVL, and V_4 to V_6 (Fig. 3–17C).

In the literature, one occasionally finds reference to LVH with either diastolic or systolic overloading. Diastolic overloading is diagnosed when the ECG pattern of LVH occurs in association with some of the following additional findings:

1. Prominent Q waves in the leads facing the left side of the septum (leads, I, aVL, V_5, V_6) (The Q waves are usually 0.025 second or less in width, but deeper than 2 mm, and reciprocal prominent R waves are observed in leads V_1 and V_2, which face the right side of the septum.)

2. Large R waves in leads V_5 and V_6 with large S waves in leads V_1 and V_2

3. Tall and peaked P waves in leads V_5 and V_6

Table 3–6. Scott's Criteria for Left Ventricular Hypertrophy

Limb Leads	
R in 1 + S in 3:	>25 mm
R in aVL:	> 7.5 mm
R in aVF:	>20 mm
S in aVR:	>14 mm
Chest Leads	
S in V_1 or V_2 + R in V_5 or V_6:	>35 mm
R in V_5 or V_6:	>26 mm
R + S in any V lead:	>45 mm

Diastolic overloading of the LV associated with aortic insufficiency is demonstrated in Figure 3–18, with prominent Q waves in leads I, aVL, V_5, and V_6 and prominent R waves in leads V_1 and V_2. Diastolic overloading in mitral valve regurgitation is demonstrated in Figure 3–12, where large R waves in leads V_5 and V_6 are accompanied by P waves with a P-mitrale pattern. Although the criteria for the diagnosis of diastolic overloading by ECG are neither very specific nor very sensitive, Braunwald[2] found the concept of diastolic overloading useful, since it draws the clinician's attention to a number of lesions which can produce increased LV preload. Finally, systolic or pressure overloading is read on the ECG in the presence of LVH when large R waves in leads V_5 to V_6 and large S waves in leads V_1 to V_2 occur in association with the LV strain pattern (any Q waves that may be present in leads V_5 and V_6 must be smaller than 2 mm) (Fig. 3–15A). The concept of systolic overloading is seen in disorders associated with high resistance to LV outflow (e.g., aortic stenosis, coarctation, and essential hypertension) and is of limited diagnostic value.

RIGHT VENTRICULAR HYPERTROPHY

The ECG pattern is frequently normal in the presence of RVH (Table 3–7). In adults this occurs because most of the QRS voltage is generated by the more massive left ventricle; therefore, a large increase in RV muscle mass must occur before RV voltages can dominate the ECG and produce an abnormal record. In normal infants and children, the RV is more massive than the LV; therefore, RVH can only slightly increase the RV voltage preponderance. The

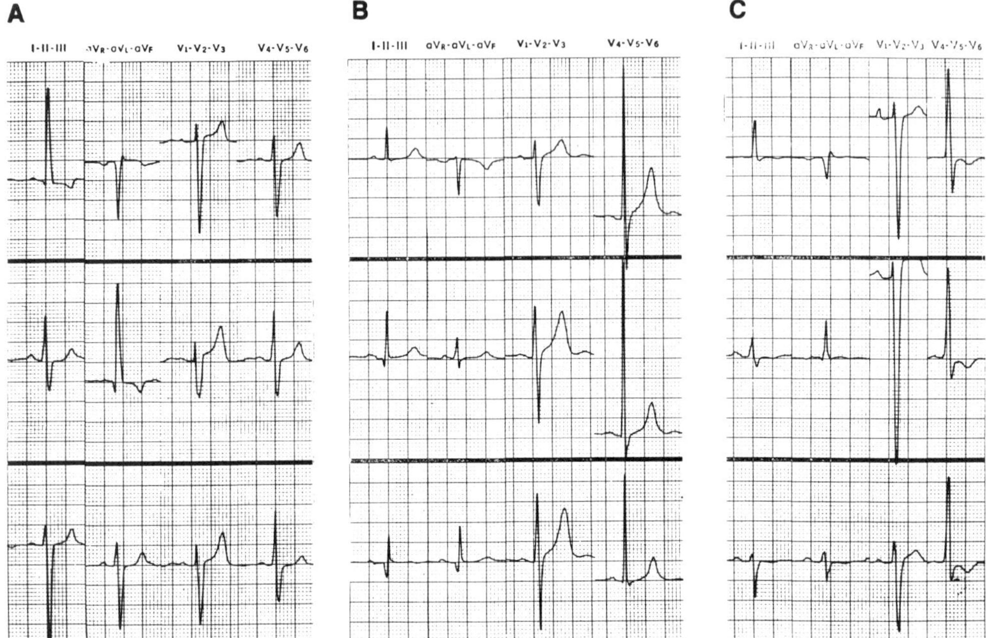

Fig. 3–17 **(A)** Left ventricular hypertrophy (LVH) and incomplete LBBB. QRS axis is −24 degrees, QRS duration is 116 msec, QRS voltages meet usual LVH criteria. ($R_1 + S_3 > 25$ mm, $R_L > 7.5$ mm, $S_{v1} + R_{v6} > 35$ mm). **(B)** LVH and probable inferior myocardial infarction. **(C)** LVH and lateral wall ischemia.

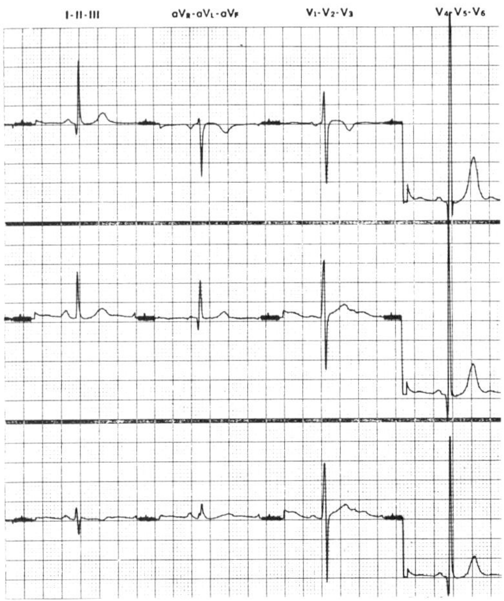

Fig. 3–18 Diastolic overloading in a patient with left ventricular hypertrophy (LVH) and aortic insufficiency.

Table 3–7. Conditions Associated with Right Ventricular Hypertrophy

Congenital heart disease
Tetralogy of Fallot
Pulmonic valve stenosis
Ventricular septal defect
Atrial septal defect
Anomalous pulmonary venous drainage
Tricuspid insufficiency
Pulmonary hypertension

result is a small change in the normal ECG pattern. When dominant S waves appear in all three standard leads (S_1, S_2, S_3 pattern) in children, RVH is most likely present (Fig. 3–19). The ECG pattern of an adult heart with moderate to marked RVH resembles that of a newborn. There is right axis deviation to >+90 degrees in the limb leads. Occasionally, prominent Q waves simulating inferior wall infarction appear in leads II, III, and aVF (Fig. 3–20). In the

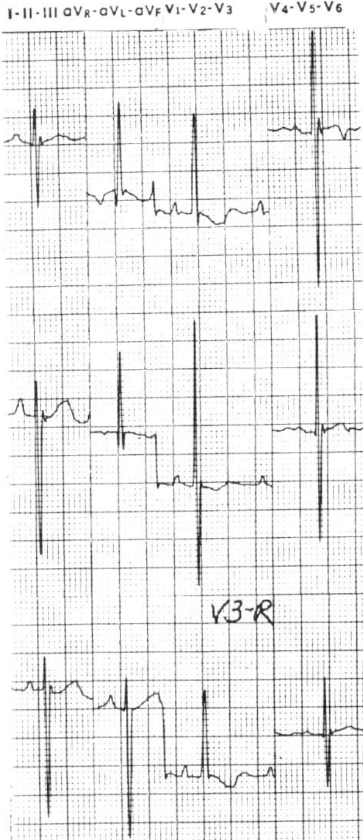

Fig. 3–19 Right ventricular hypertrophy (RVH) and right atrial hypertrophy (RAH) in a 3-year-old child with AV canal lesion. QRS axis is −130 degrees. Note S_1, S_2, S_3 pattern of dominant S waves.

ECG evolution of RVH, as RV voltages begin to dominate the ECG, the right chest leads V_1 and V_2 will shift from rS to an RS pattern, then Rs, and finally to an R pattern. Occasionally, early RVH will show the rSr′ pattern of an incomplete right bundle branch block (RBBB) in leads V_1 and V_2, as shown in Figure 3–21. On lateral chest leads V_5 to V_6, RVH produces a shift from the normal Rs to an RS pattern. Emphysema can produce a precordial lead pattern consisting entirely of rS waves (Fig. 3–22). The reasons for these different ECG representations of RVH are covered elsewhere and are not discussed here.[1] The QRS complex does not widen in RVH because even an enlarged right ventricle is still activated in a shorter time than the normal, more massive left ventricle. However, in the enlarged right ventricle, depolarization is slower as compared with normal RV depolarization. The ST segments and T waves usually show little changes in RVH except when RVH is marked. Depressed ST segments and inverted T waves may be seen in the right precordial V_1, V_2, and V_3 (Fig. 3–6) and inferior limb leads II, III, and aVF (Fig. 3–22). These changes constitute the RV strain pattern.

As is the case with enlargement of the other

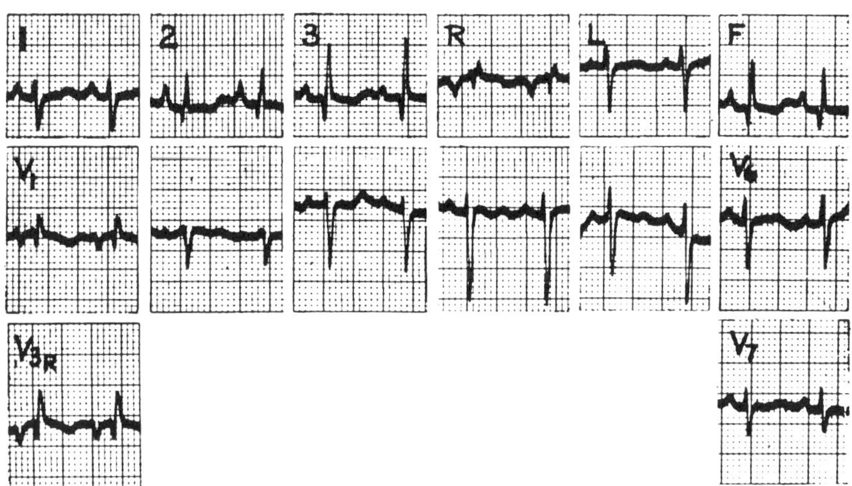

Fig. 3–20 Right ventricular hypertrophy (RVH) with Q waves simulating inferior myocardial infarction. Axis is +130 degrees, R : S ratio in V_1 is < 1.

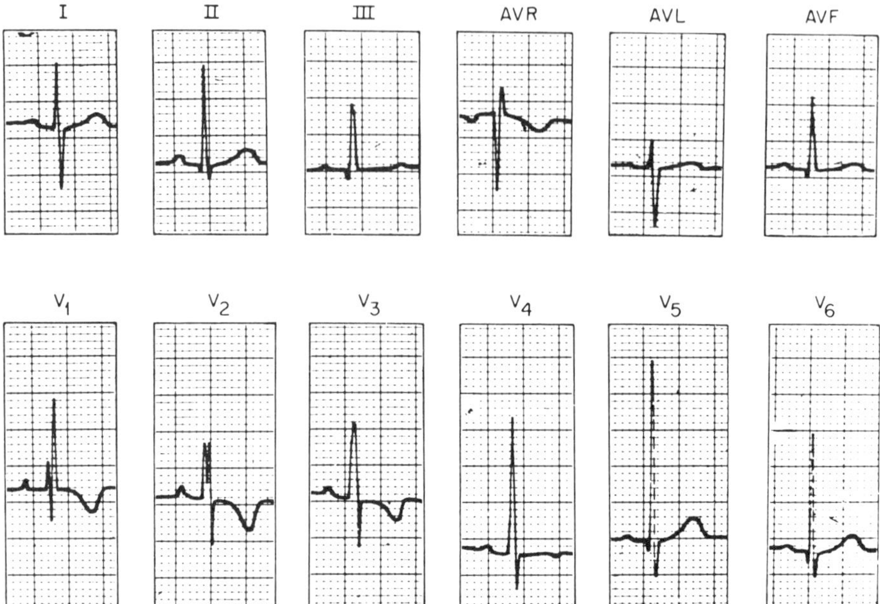

Fig. 3–21 Right ventricular hypertrophy (RVH) in a child with an ostium secundum type of atrial septal defect. The electrical axis is about +100 degrees. There is an rSR′ complex in lead V_1. The secondary R wave measures 12 mm. This is an example of diastolic overloading of the right ventricle. (Friedman HH: Diagnostic Electrocardiography and Vectorcardiography. © 1977 McGraw-Hill, New York. Reproduced with permission.)

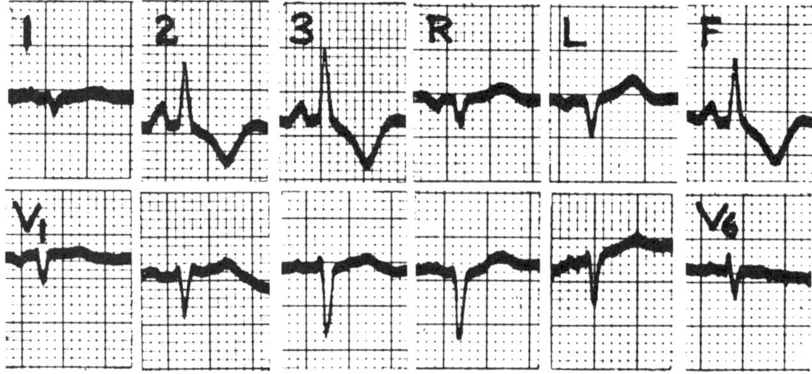

Fig. 3–22 ECG from a patient with emphysema. Note right axis deviation (+95 degrees) with rS complexes all across the precordium. The ST-T pattern of right ventricular strain is fully developed in leads I, III, and aVF. The P-wave pattern suggests P pulmonale with an axis of +80 degrees and pointed, though not very tall, P waves in II, III, and aVF. (Marriott HJL: Practical Electrocardiography. © 1983 The Williams & Wilkins Co., Baltimore.)

heart chambers, the sensitivity and specificity of the ECG in RVH are poor. The following criteria in adults help support the diagnosis of RVH.

1. Right axis deviation of +110 degrees or more in the absence of anterolateral or inferior MI, left posterior fascicular block, or RBBB
2. R/S ratio >1 in V_1
3. R wave in V_1 larger than 7 mm
4. S wave in V_1 smaller than 2 mm
5. QR pattern in V_1
6. The sum of the R wave in V_1 and the S wave in V_5 or V_6 greater than 10.5 mm
7. R/S ratio greater than 1 in V_5 or V_6
8. rSR′ pattern in V_1 with R′ greater than 10 mm

In children under 16 years of age, a qR or qRs pattern in lead V_1 is diagnostic of RVH regardless of the amplitude of the deflections, provided that preexcitation is ruled out. The above criteria are usually valid only when the QRS is less than 0.12 second in duration. Diagnosis of RVH should never be based solely on the observation of right axis deviation, unless such causes as emphysema or other clinical conditions (see criterion 1 above) have been ruled out.

Dilatation of the right ventricle may occur either together with RV hypertrophy or alone and acutely. The following ECG findings are suggestive of RV dilatation, especially if they are reversible[1]:

1. RV strain pattern
2. rS pattern in the right and sometimes also in the left precordial leads
3. A QR pattern in lead V_1 in conjunction with the above two findings
4. Complete or incomplete RBBB

Diastolic overloading of the right ventricle occurs in atrial septal defects, tricuspid insufficiency, and anomalous pulmonary venous drainage. The ECG usually shows right axis devia-

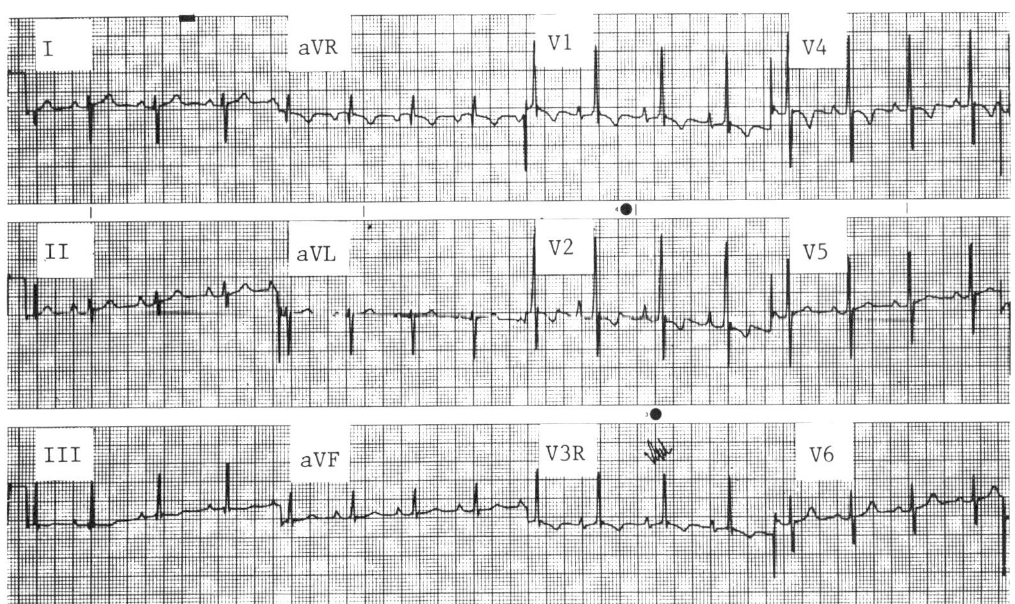

Fig. 3–23 A 3-year-old boy with tetralogy of Fallot demonstrating RVH with systolic overloading. QRS axis is +135 degrees, ST-T wave abnormalities in the precordial chest leads suggest RV strain, and V_1 has a prominent R wave.

tion, an rSr′ or rSR′ pattern in V_1, and a normal or slightly increased QRS duration. These changes are illustrated in the tracings of RVH in a child with an ostium secundum type of atrial septal defect, shown in Figure 3–21. Systolic overloading with RVH occurs in association with pulmonic stenosis (e.g., in tetralogy of Fallot) or pulmonary hypertension. Right axis deviation and a RV strain pattern are seen. The RS, Rs, qR, qRs, or rR′ pattern found in the V_1 lead has a large R wave. Figure 3–23 shows RVH with systolic overloading due to pulmonic stenosis in tetralogy of Fallot.

BIVENTRICULAR HYPERTROPHY

In biventricular enlargement, both the left and right ventricles are abnormal (Table 3–8). It is difficult to diagnose this entity by ECG because increased LV and RV forces may cancel each other, masking the changes produced by enlargement of either chamber. Thus an abnormal ECG, in the presence of marked cardiac enlargement demonstrated by other means, should suggest the diagnosis of biventricular enlargement, and by no means should a normal ECG rule it out. Enlargement of both ventricles is suggested by the following:

1. Voltage changes in the precordial leads diagnostic of both RVH and LVH
2. Definite ECG evidence of RVH plus
   a. An R wave in V_5–V_6 with an LV strain pattern in the same leads or an abnormal increase in the sum of R in V_5 or V_6 and S in V_1 or V_2
   b. Deep Q waves in the left precordial or inferior limb leads
   c. Large equiphasic QRS complexes in the mid-precordial and/or in two or more limb leads
3. Definite ECG evidence of LVH plus one or more of the following:
   a. A right-axis deviation
   b. Large R or R′ or an R/S or R′/S ratio larger than 1 in V_1
   c. An R larger than 5 mm with a Q/R ratio of less than 1 in aVR
   d. S waves in V_5 and/or V_6
4. A shallow S wave in V_1 followed by a strikingly deeper S wave in V_2, the shallow S-wave syndrome (Fig. 3–11A).

Table 3–8. Conditions Associated with Biventricular Hypertrophy

Ventricular septal defect with large left-to-right shunt and elevated pulmonary pressures
Patent ductus arteriosus with large left-to-right shunt
Persistent truncus arteriosus with large pulmonary arteries

A tracing demonstrating biventricular enlargement is shown in Figure 3–24. Combined ventricular enlargement may be seen in a VSD lesion with a large left-to-right shunt and elevated pulmonary artery pressures. In young children, the ECG manifestation of large equiphasic RS waves in the mid-precordial leads and two or

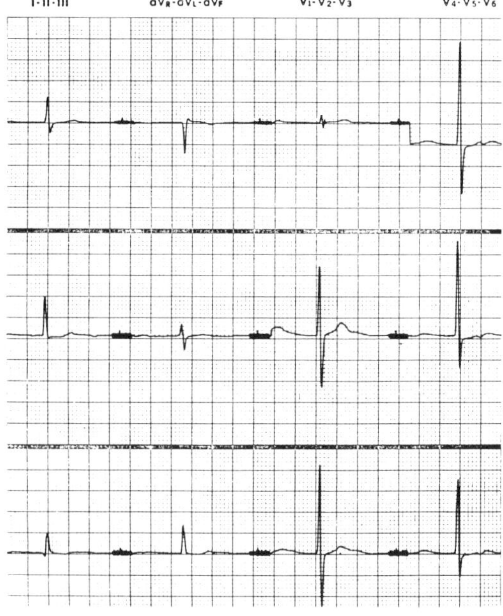

Fig. 3–24 ECG tracing from a 79-year-old man with biventricular enlargement. The rhythm is atrial fibrillation. $S_{v2} + R_{v5} = 35$ mm, V_1–V_3 show an RS pattern, $S_{v1} < S_{v2}$.

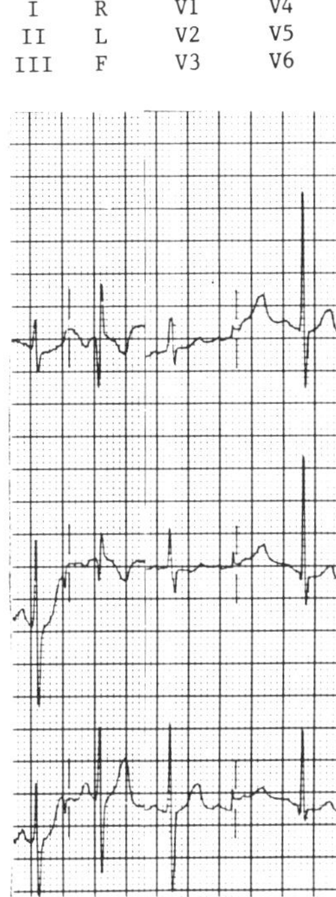

Fig. 3–25 Biventricular enlargement in an 18-month-old girl with a VSD defect. QRS axis is +95 degrees; large equiphasic QRS complexes are evident in the mid-precordial leads and leads II, III, aVR, and aVF.

more limb leads seen with biventricular enlargement has been named the Katz–Wachtel phenomenon. This ECG abnormality demonstrated in Figure 3–25 may also be seen in biventricular enlargement accompanying PDA lesions if they are associated with a large left-to-right shunt and pulmonary hypertension. Finally, a persistent truncus arteriosus abnormality with large pulmonary arteries generally shows all gradations of biventricular enlargement (and only rarely isolated chamber enlargement), RVH being dominant, and diastolic overloading of the LV becoming prominent with large pulmonary blood flow. When the persistent truncus arteriosus is associated with absent or hypoplastic pulmonary arteries, RVH is the predominant ECG feature.

HYPERTROPHIC OBSTRUCTIVE CARDIOMYOPATHY

Hypertrophic obstructive cardiomyopathy (HOCM), also known as asymmetric septal hypertrophy (ASH), hypertrophic cardiomyopathy (HCM), or commonly idiopathic hypertrophic

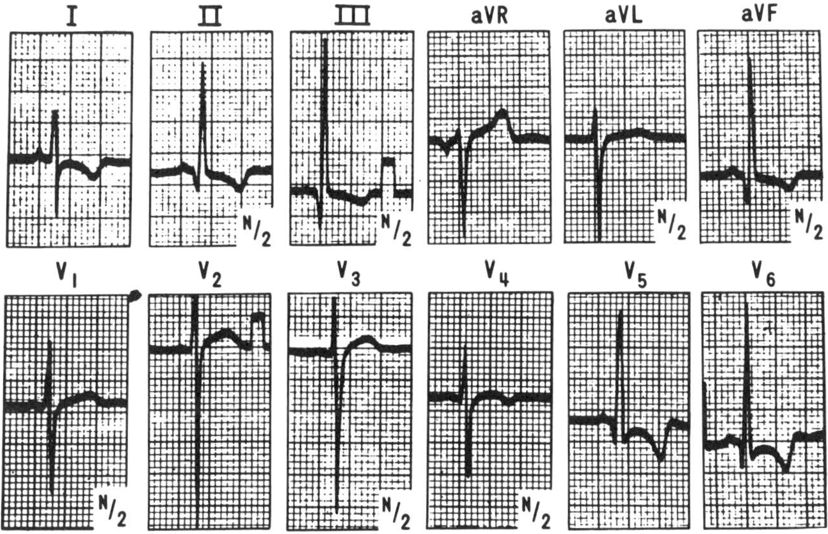

Fig. 3–26 Hypertrophic obstructive cardiomyopathy simulating inferior myocardial infarction by the presence of deep Q waves in leads II, III, and aVF. The Q waves are also prominent in leads V_5 and V_6. The QRS voltages and the strain pattern are diagnostic of left ventricular hypertrophy. (Marriott HJL: Practical Electrocardiography. © 1983 The Williams & Wilkins Co., Baltimore.)

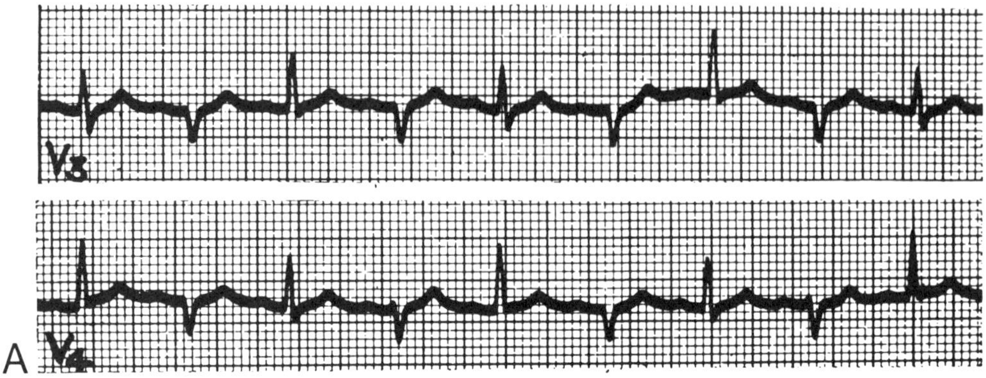

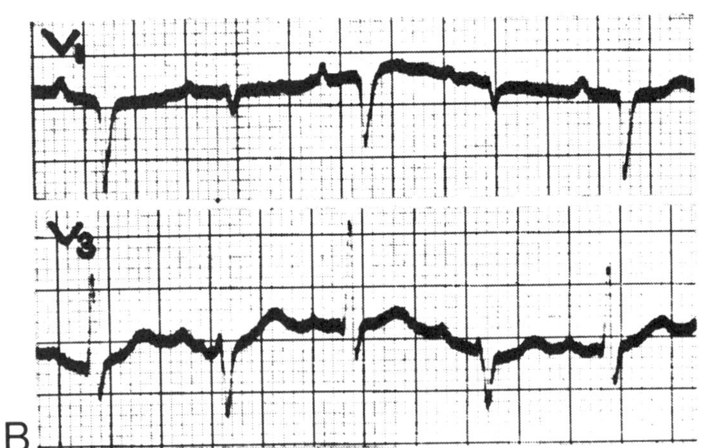

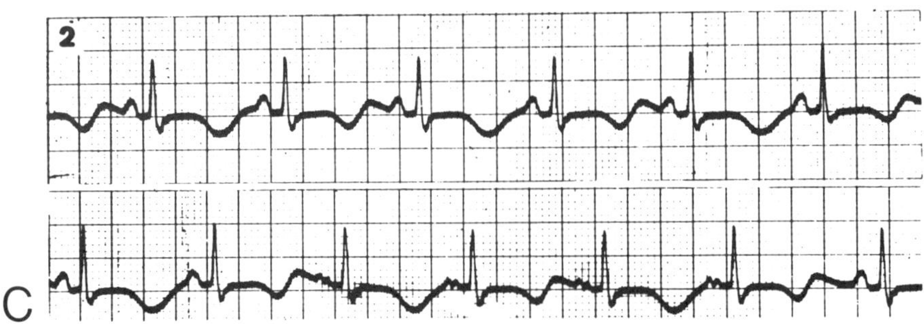

Fig. 3–27 Various forms of electrical alternans. (**A**) The common variety of electrical alternans. Note alternating direction of QRS complexes only. (**B**) Total alternans associated with a malignant pericardial effusion. Note alteration of P waves as well as QRS complexes. (**C**) Alternation of the T-U complex. Strips are continuous. Note shifting atrial pacemaker in bottom strip. (Marriott HJL: Practical Electrocardiography. © 1983 The Williams & Wilkins Co., Baltimore.)

subaortic stenosis (IHSS), is a condition in which there is localized enlargement of the left ventricle by hypertrophic muscle. In infants this can also be manifested by RVH. In the traditional form there is functional subaortic stenosis with mid- to late systolic obstruction of the LV outflow by the hypertrophied septum. The obstruction is variable and depends on heart rate, arterial pressure, contractility, and LV preload. There is an increased incidence of ventricular and supraventricular dysrhythmias.

Electrocardiographically, HOCM produces a normal ECG in more than 20 percent of individuals. In 20 to 50 percent of cases it produces pseudo-infarction Q waves, which are pathologic Q waves that simply do not look like Q waves of infarction. In Figure 3–26, the ECG in a patient with IHSS simulates inferior wall myocardial infarction with Q waves in leads II, III, aVF, V_5, and V_6 in addition to producing the pattern of LVH with strain. HOCM can also present an ECG picture of plain LVH, LVH with marked left axis deviation, or LVH with RAH and/or LAH. Figure 3–14 shows the ECG of a patient with IHSS with clear Q waves in leads V_5 and V_6, LVH by voltage changes, and either biatrial hypertrophy or LAH with a pseudo-P-pulmonale pattern.

PERICARDIAL EFFUSION

Pericardial effusions can decrease the size of all heart chambers by extrinsic compression of the epicardium. Not all pericardial effusions produce ECG changes, especially if small. The most consistent ECG abnormality with a pericardial effusion is a low QRS voltage. The triad of ECG findings of low voltage, ST-segment elevation, and electrical alternans is virtually diagnostic of a pericardial effusion. Electrical alternans refers to alternating amplitude of any component of the ECG in any or all leads. The most common alternans involves the QRS complexes, as shown in Figure 3–27A. Total electrical alternans refers to changing amplitude of both the QRS complex and the P waves. An example of total alternans is shown in Figure 3–27B. Total alternans is thought to be pathognomonic of either a large or malignant pericardial effusion, or both. Electrical alternans of either the T or U or both waves is usually described in association with electrolyte disturbances or terminal states (Fig. 3–27C).

The extreme example of a compromising pericardial fluid collection, the pericardial tamponade, may occur as an acute hemopericardium secondary to rupture of the heart or the aorta. The hemodynamic state of the patient quickly progresses to electromechanical dissociation. The accompanying ECG may show sinus bradycardia, junctional rhythm, electrical alternans, any type of ST-segment abnormalities, or T-wave inversion.

REFERENCES

1. Friedman HH: Diagnostic Electrocardiography and Vectorcardiography. McGraw-Hill, New York, 1977
2. Braunwald E: Heart Disease. WB Saunders, Philadelphia, 1984
3. Marriott HJL: Practical Electrocardiography. Williams & Wilkins, Baltimore, 1983
4. Chou T, Helm RA: The pseudo-P pulmonale. Circulation 32:96, 1965
5. Reicheck N, Devereux RB: Left ventricular hypertrophy: Relationship of anatomic, echocardiographic and electrocardiographic findings. Circulation 63:1391, 1981
6. Sokolow M, Lyon TP: The ventricular complex in left ventricular hypertrophy as obtained by unipolar precordial and limb leads. Am Heart J 37:161, 1979
7. Romhilt DW, Estes EH Jr: A point-score system for the ECG diagnosis of left ventricular hypertrophy. Am Heart J 75:752, 1968
8. Scott RC, et al: Left ventricular hypertrophy. A study of accuracy of current electrocardiographic criteria when compared with autopsy findings in one hundred cases. Circulation 11:89, 1955
9. Scott RC: The electrocardiographic diagnosis of left ventricular hypertrophy. Am Heart J 59:155, 1960
10. Scott RC: The correlation between the electrocardiographic patterns of ventricular hypertrophy and the anatomic findings. Circulation 21:256, 1960
11. Scott RC: Ventricular hypertrophy. Cardiovasc Clin 5(3):220, 1973

4

Conduction Defects

John Dolman, M.D.
Daniel M. Thys, M.D.

Optimal functioning of the heart as a pump relies on a normal conduction system. This system, consisting of a combination of pacemaker cells, other specialized nodal cells, and fiber bundles, is designed to transmit the pacemaker impulse in an orderly fashion throughout the atria and ventricles. In the atrioventricular (AV) node, conduction is slightly delayed to allow the atria to contract before the ventricles. Clinical evidence of disorders in the conduction system runs the gamut from no symptomatology to complete heart block, or even asystole; various conduction defects are associated with different risks of progression to complete heart block. The correct conduction abnormality must therefore be recognized and the electrocardiogram serves as the primary means of diagnosis (although the etiology of the abnormality cannot usually be discerned from the ECG.).[1]

Conduction defects may be broadly classified into AV conduction defects and intraventricular conduction defects, although recent information, obtained from His bundle ECGs, suggests that this distinction is not always absolute. AV blocks can generally be diagnosed by studying the relationship between the P waves (atrial depolarization) and QRS complexes (ventricular depolarization). The ECG tracing obtained in the operating room or intensive care unit (ICU) from a single monitoring lead is often sufficient to establish the diagnosis.

For intraventricular conduction defects, more than one ECG lead is usually required. Although intraventricular blocks may occasionally be observed as a new finding in the operating room, they are most commonly diagnosed during the preoperative period.

His bundle ECGs permit an appreciation of conduction through the bundle of His itself. They have greatly contributed to our understanding of some of the conduction defects described in this chapter and are occasionally referred to elsewhere in this volume. His bundle ECGs are obtained by insertion of a triple electrode across the tricuspid valve such that the first electrode detects low atrial depolarization, or the A wave; concurrent external ECG recording allows one to measure a PA interval, reflecting intraatrial conduction from the sinus node to the low right atrium. The second wave (H wave) records impulse conduction through the bundle of His, while the third (V wave) detects ventricular depolarization. Normal intervals are shown in Table 4–1 (Fig. 4–1).[2-4] HQ is also described, as is HS (ventricular conduction time).[5] The normal PR interval is composed of the PA, AH, and HV intervals.

Table 4–1. Normal His Bundle ECG Intervals

PA (intraatrial conduction) 20–45 msec
AH (approximately AV nodal conduction time) 60–130 msec
PH 80–140 msec
HV (His–Purkinje conduction time) 30–55 msec

ANATOMY OF THE CONDUCTION SYSTEM

The cardiac conduction system consists of the sinus node, internodal (or intraatrial) fibers, the AV node, the bundle of His, the right and left bundle branches, and the Purkinje fibers, which spread out over the ventricular walls (Fig. 4–2). The sinus node is located close to the epicardial surface at the junctions of the superior vena cava, right atrium, and right atrial appendage.[6]

Three internodal fiber pathways are involved in the spread of impulses from the sinus node throughout both atria, in addition to rapid conduction of the impulses to the (AV) node. The anterior internodal pathway, also known as Bachman's bundle, is considered the most important communication pathway, although the middle (Wenkebach) and posterior (Thorel) internodal pathways are also involved.[4,6]

The AV node is located on the subendocardial aspect of the right atrium adjacent to the coronary sinus and the tricuspid valve.[6] Fibers within the AV node converge into parallel pathways that leave as the bundle of His. This bundle, composed primarily of Purkinje cells, soon divides into right and left bundle branches. The right bundle branch traverses the right endocardial surface of the interventricular septum. It begins as a thin stalklike structure and then spreads out to cover the entire endocardial surface of the right ventricle. The left bundle branch divides into two main subdivisions and a smaller third division that lies between them. The latter supplies the upper aspect of the left surface of the interventricular septum: the anterior fascicle or division traverses the anterior and superior aspects of the interventricular septum and left ventricular subendocardium, while the larger posterior division runs along the posterior and inferior aspects of the same. The fascicles anastomose with each other in the periphery, and terminal portions spread out to cover the entire endocardial surface, as on the right side.[4] On both sides, the full thickness of ventricular mus-

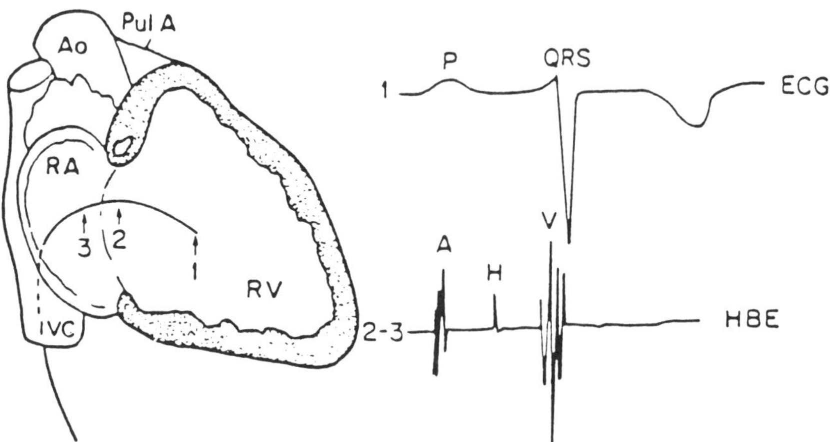

Fig. 4–1 An intracardiac electrocardiographic lead is shown coming up through the inferior vena cava, the right atrium and across the tricuspid valve with the tip in the right ventricle. Normal A, H, and V waves are demonstrated. (Akhtar M: Clinical use of His Bundle electrocardiography. Am Heart J 91:520, 1976.)

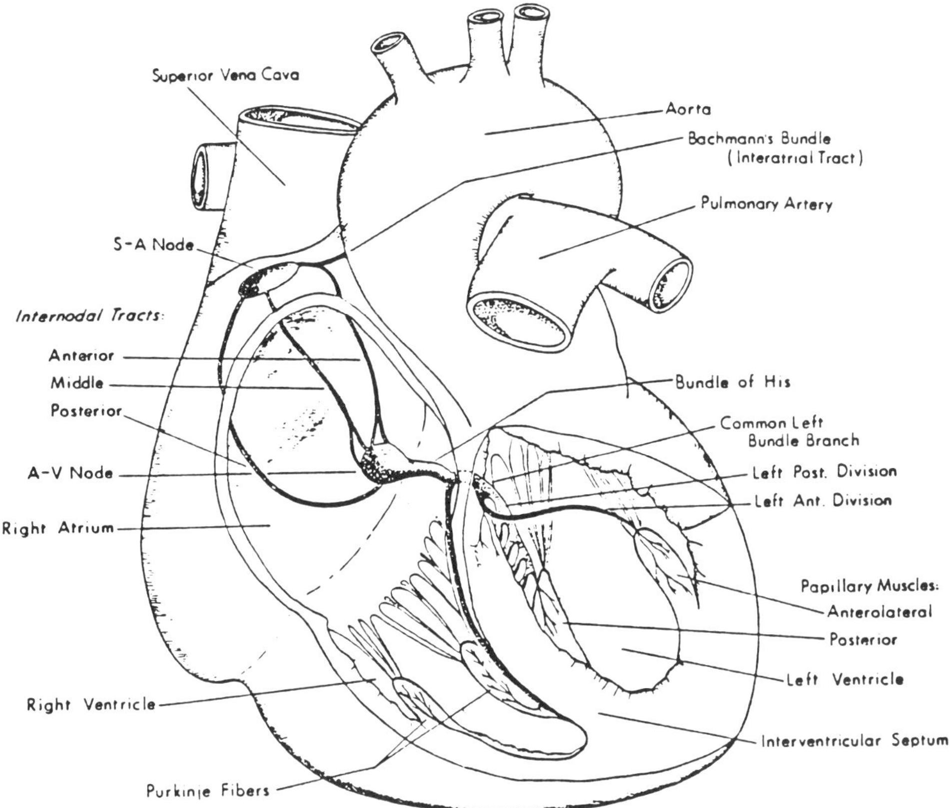

Fig. 4–2 Schematic representation of distribution of the specialized conductive tissues in the atria and ventricles, showing the impulse-forming and conducting system of the heart. (Lipman BS, Dunn M, Marsie E: Clinical Electrocardiography. 7th Ed. Copyright © 1984 by Year Book Medical Publishers, Inc., Chicago. Reproduced with permission.)

cle is depolarized from endocardial to epicardial surface.

BLOOD SUPPLY OF THE CONDUCTION SYSTEM

This is an important aspect in a consideration of conduction blocks, since the etiology of many conduction defects is localized myocardial ischemia or infarction. The sinus node is supplied by the sinus node artery, which arises directly from the right coronary artery in approximately 55 percent of cases and from the left coronary artery in the remaining 45 percent. Patterns of flow in the sinus node artery have been postulated as having a modulatory function on the rate of discharge of the pacemaker cells.[6]

The AV node is supplied by the AV nodal artery; this is a branch of the right coronary artery in roughly 90 percent of cases (right coronary dominance), arising from the left coronary circulation in 10 percent of cases (left coronary dominance).[6]

The remainder of the conduction system is supplied essentially by vessels that vascularize the adjacent myocardium. The left anterior descending coronary artery supplies the bundle of His, right bundle branch, and anterior division of the left bundle branch.[7] The posterior descending coronary artery, which may arise from either the right coronary artery or left circumflex coronary artery, supplies the posterior division of the left bundle branch.[8] Studies in which human hearts were studied by injecting a different colored gelatin into the three major coronary vessels[9] reveal that the bundle of His and the proximal bundle branches usually have a dual blood supply, consisting of the AV nodal artery and/or first septal branch of the left anterior descending coronary artery. Left coronary artery lesions, particularly those of the anterior descending branch, can result in serious blocks, such as irreversible bundle branch blocks or high-grade second-degree AV blocks; right coronary artery lesions usually carry less import, resulting in reversible AV blocks, such as the Wenckebach phenomenon.[10]

PHYSIOLOGY OF THE CONDUCTION SYSTEM

While all myocardial cells can undergo spontaneous depolarization, the pacemaker cells of the sinus node normally do so at the fastest rate. Various influences, mediated predominantly through the autonomic nervous system, govern the rate at which spontaneous depolarization occurs. Sinus node depolarization impulses are transmitted rapidly to the AV node via the internodal bundles. Conduction velocity is markedly decreased within the AV node (see Table 4–1), with the impulse normally being delayed about 0.04 second[6] to 0.07 second.[7] This allows time for the atrial muscle to depolarize and contract, before the impulse continues into the ventricles. It also protects the ventricles from a rapid volley of impulses (as may occur, for example, with atrial flutter of fibrillation).

From the AV node, the impulse travels down the bundle of His and then along both bundle branches and finally into ventricular muscle itself. The interventricular septum is depolarized in a left to right direction; the remainder of the ventricular muscle is depolarized from the endocardial surface outward to the epicardial surface. Conduction velocity is fastest in the Purkinje fibers of the bundle branches.

The PQRS of the normal ECG reflects the depolarization wave traveling through the heart. Depolarization of the sinus node itself is not visible on the ordinary ECG, but passage of the depolarization wave throughout the atrial muscle is manifested by the P wave. Impulse movement through the AV node and His bundle is also not visible on the ordinary ECG, although the delay in impulse travel is manifested as the PR interval. The QRS complex is caused by the depolarization wave traveling rapidly through the Purkinje fibers of the bundle branches.

PATHOLOGY OF THE CONDUCTION SYSTEM

The conduction system may be compromised anywhere along its length (see Table 4–2) by multiple pathologic entities,[5,11,12] both anatomic and physiologic.

Two of the most common classes of disease to affect conduction are primary degenerative diseases of the conduction system and ischemic heart disease. Degenerative diseases include Lev's and Lenegre's diseases.[5] Lev's disease

Table 4–2. Conduction Defects

A. Sinus node block
B. Atrioventricular conduction defects
  1. First degree
  2. Second degree
    a. Mobitz I
    b. Mobitz II
  3. Third degree (complete)
C. Intraventricular conduction defects
  1. Right bundle branch block (RBBB)
    a. Complete
    b. Incomplete
  2. Left bundle branch block (LBBB)
    a. Complete
    b. Incomplete
  3. Left fascicular block
    a. Left anterior hemiblock (LAHB)
    b. Left posterior hemiblock (LPHB)
  4. Bifascicular block
    a. RBBB + LAHB
    b. RBBB + LPHB
    c. Alternative LBBB/RBBB
    d. AV conduction defect + LBBB or RBBB
  5. Trifascicular block
  6. Indeterminate (bizarre conduction defect, not possible to allocate to above categories)

is due to invasion of the conduction system (especially the proximal His bundle) by spreading fibrosis or calcification from adjacent fibrous structures, such as the annuli of the AV valves or membranous portion of the interventricular septum; this may cause various combinations of blocks, comprising right and left bundle branch blocks (RBBB and LBBB) and left fascicular hemiblocks. Fibrous involvement of the intraatrial conduction system can also occur, resulting in sick sinus syndrome. Lenegre's disease is a sclerodegenerative process involving only the terminal portions of fascicles of the conduction system that tends to progress to complete heart block within several years; it is a common cause of a RBBB with left anterior hemiblock in patients over the age of 50 years.

Coronary artery disease, resulting in either ischemia or infarction, is an important cause of conduction defects. Acute abnormalities may be secondary to ischemia, but chronic blocks can result from the long-term effects of ischemia, including fibrosis and calcification.[13]

SINUS NODE BLOCK

Sinus node block, a relatively uncommon entity, involves failure of the sinus node to depolarize or failure of conduction of impulses from the sinus node to the atria.[12,14] It may be seen during anesthesia due to vagal reflexes. It may also occur secondary to drug therapy with agents such as digoxin, quinidine, or phenylephrine,[15] myocardial ischemia or infarction, and inflammatory diseases. An ectopic beat conducted in a retrograde fashion, leading to premature discharge and depression of the sinus node, may induce a temporary form of sinus node block. Dysfunction of the sinus node may occur as part of a normal aging process apparently rather different from that of atrial muscle.[16] Acute coronary insufficiency may induce a reversible sinus node dysfunction (due to a vagal reflex) or permanent (related to ischemia-induced fibrotic changes of the sinus node); the latter may be unresponsive to atropine and may require pacemaker insertion.[17]

The ECG[16] shows an absent P wave, and often an absent QRST as well, unless a lower pacemaker intervenes (Fig. 4–3). The interval between P waves may or may not bear a simple relationship to the previous sinus rhythm interval. Progressive lengthening of the interval between actual sinus node firing and atrial depolarization can occur. Manifested by a gradual shortening of the P-P interval preceding the long pause, this may be confused with a normal sinus dysrhythmia, but in the latter there is a cyclical variation in P-P intervals, in conjunction with the respiratory cycle.

Sick sinus syndrome is a term used for a conglomeration of disorders that involve degenerative changes in the cardiac conduction system, resulting in sinus node dysfunction[16] and possibly AV blocks as well.[20] The etiology[16,21] includes myocardial ischemia or infarction, cardiomyopathies, hypertension, electrolyte abnormalities, endocrine abnormalities, infiltrative diseases, inflammatory diseases, and drug effects.

Possible presentations include sinus node pauses or blocks, marked bradycardias, and bradycardias in conjunction with tachycardias. Ferrer[22] listed various criteria as manifestations of inadequacy of sinus node function (Table 4–3).

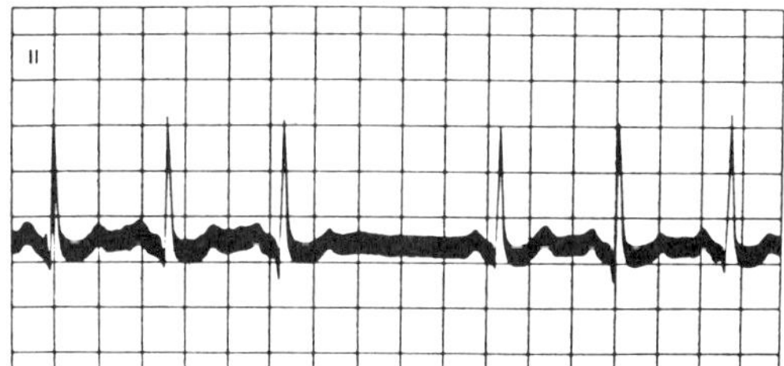

Fig. 4–3 Sinus node block. The ECG shows a period of sinus arrest after the first three beats indicated by the absence of the next sinus beat at the expected time. The P interval between the third and fourth P waves equals five large squares for a rate of 60 beats/min (300: 5=60). The interval between the other P waves is 2.6 large squares for a rate of 115 beats/min. (Ferrer I: The sick sinus syndrome. p 50. In Katz A, Selwyn A (eds): The Cardiac Arrhythmias. Hospital Practice, New York, 1983.)

Table 4–3. Diagnostic Criteria for Inadequacy of Sinus Node Function

1. Persistent severe and unexplained sinus bradycardia
2. Cessation of sinus rhythm for short intervals during which time no other escape rhythm arises
3. Long periods of sinus arrest without appearance of a new pacemaker, leading to total cardiac arrest
4. Chronic atrial fibrillation because the sinus node is permanently silent or repeated episodes of transitory atrial fibrillation due to total cessation of sinus rhythm at these times; atrial fibrillation often accompanied by slow ventricular rate (due to concurrent AV nodal disease)
5. Inability of the heart to resume sinus rhythm after cardioversion for atrial fibrillation (especially if ventricular response was slow)
6. Episodes of SA exit block, unrelated to drug therapy

The ECG may show bradycardias, intraatrial blocks, wandering pacemakers, sinus pauses or arrests, AV blocks, and tachycardias (especially paroxymal atrial tachycardia, flutter, or fibrillation). Pratila and Pratilas[19] claim a first-degree AV block and a left axis deviation to be the commonest abnormal finding. At times, the ECG may be perfectly normal, leading to delays in diagnosis.

ATRIOVENTRICULAR BLOCK

AV blocks are usually classified into three main degrees, as diagnosed by the routine surface ECG. A new classification[23] divides second- and third-degree AV blocks into type A (in which QRS duration is less or equal to 0.11 seconds) and type B (in which QRS duration is greater or equal to 0.12 seconds). In type A, the block lies above the bifurcation of the bundle of His, mostly in the AV node itself, or less commonly within the bundle of His. In type B, the block is below the bifurcation. The latter carries a poorer prognosis.

First-Degree AV Block

First-degree AV block is diagnosed from the ECG by a prolonged PR interval; the conduction disturbance, however, need not be limited to the AV node, but may also occur in the internodal pathway, bundle of His, and intraventricular conduction system.[4] Balanced disease in both the right and left bundle branches may produce a first-degree AV block but a normal QRS complex.[22] Premature His bundle depolarizations, not visible themselves, may lengthen the refractory period of the conduction system, causing a prolonged PR interval. One should note, however, that a prolonged PR interval may be found in perfectly healthy people as well.

Electrocardiographically, a first-degree AV block is diagnosed by a PR interval of greater than 200 msec, with a regular rhythm in which all atrial beats are conducted through the ventricles (Fig. 4–4). His bundle ECGs may demonstrate either an increased AH interval or increased HV interval, or both, the former being more common, however.[23–25] These ECGs have also been known to show abnormalities within the conduction system, while the standard ECG had a normal PR interval.[26]

Second-Degree AV Block

Second-degree AV block occurs where a proportion of the atrial impulses are not conducted to the ventricles. It is usually subdivided into two classes, depending on whether the conduction block occurs within the AV node (Mobitz type I or Wenckebach) or bundle of His (Mobitz type II). The original classification into type I and II block was based on ECG characteristics, although it is now known that these distinctions are not absolute; that is, type I block can be due to abnormalities anywhere in the conduction system, and type II block can occur due to abnormalities within the AV node.[22] The so-called Wenckebach phenomenon seen in Mobitz type I block involves a gradually increasing PR interval that eventally gives rise to a P wave that is not conducted through the ventricles. Mobitz type II block involves an intermittent block in conduction of the P wave into the ventricles, but the PR interval in surrounding beats remains unaltered.

Second-degree AV block (Mobitz type I) may

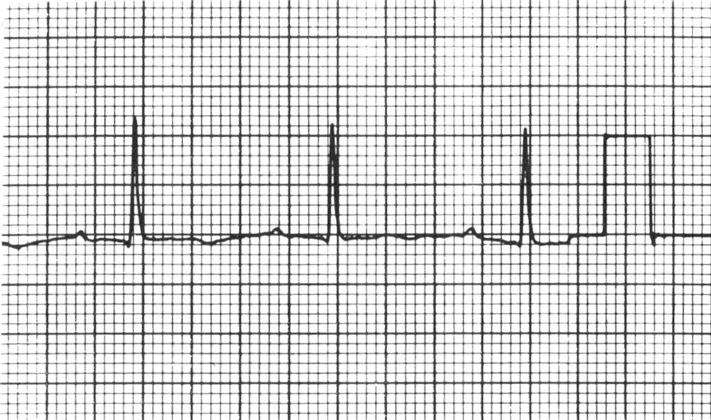

Fig. 4–4 First-degree AV block with prolonged P-R interval.

be seen in normal people with a strong vagal tone (such as athletes), but organic etiologies are more frequent. Ischemic heart disease is an especially common cause of these blocks. Mobitz type I block may be caused by right coronary artery occlusion yielding inferior wall infarctions; the block is thought to result from reversible AV nodal ischemia and is associated with a good prognosis. Anterior wall infarctions may result in a Mobitz type II block, involving a conduction defect distal to the bundle of His, often in association with a bundle branch block (effectively producing a bilateral bundle branch block); these blocks are generally permanent and carry a greater risk of progressing to complete heart block.[4]

The electrocardiographic diagnosis[4,23] of Mobitz type I block depends on a gradually lengthening PR interval, until a P wave occurs that is not succeeded by a QRST complex. The increment in PR lengthening is greater with the second beat of the cycle (a cycle resuming after the dropped beat) than with succeeding beats. The number of beats in each cycle may vary from case to case, and even from cycle to cycle in the same subject (Fig 4–5). Mobitz type II block is characterized by a constant PR interval (which may in itself be prolonged), but the ventricular response is not always present. The dropped QRS may occur after a regular or variable number of normal cycles (Fig. 4–6). If the block occurs in a constant 2:1 ratio, it becomes impossible to distinguish between Mobitz type I and II blocks, and one must resort to His bundle ECGs to make a definitive separation.

In Mobitz type I block, the His bundle ECG shows P waves intermittently not followed by

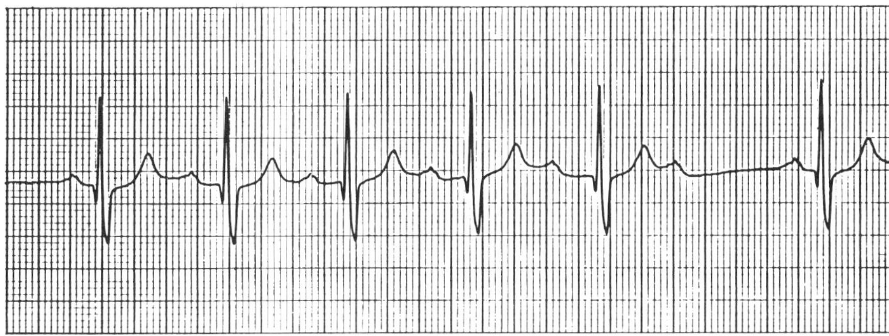

Fig. 4–5 Second-degree AV block (Mobitz type I). Note that the PR interval gradually lengthens and that the shortest PR interval follows the pause of the missing QRS complex.

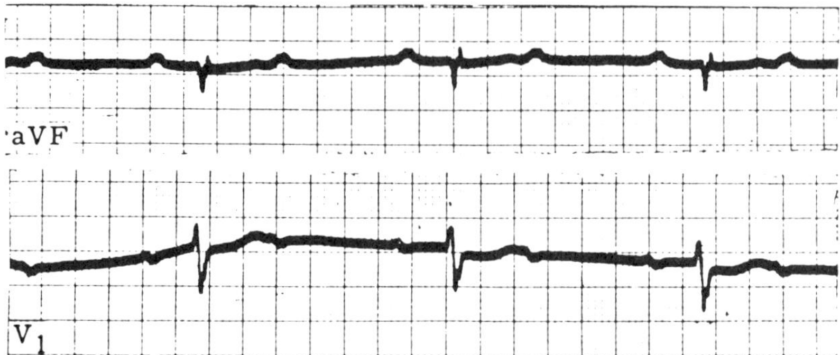

Fig. 4–6 Second-degree AV block (Mobitz type II). Note that the atrial rhythm is regular and that every other P wave is followed by a QRS. (Reproduced, with permission, from Goldman MJ: Principles of Clinical Electrocardiography, 12th ed. Copyright 1986 by Lange Medical Publications, Los Altos, CA)

H spikes, suggesting defective conduction in the AV node. Progressively longer AH or PH intervals with normal HV intervals may be seen in other beats, correlating with an increasing PR interval. In Mobitz type II block, H spikes are seen after each P wave, including nonconducted ones; HV intervals are prolonged, signifying a conduction defect below the bundle of His. Mobitz type II blocks may occur due to bilateral bundle branch block as well as bundle of His lesions.[29]

Third-Degree AV Block

Third-degree (or complete) AV block exhibits total disruption in conduction between the atria and ventricles. The atria continue to beat at the rate set by the sinus node pacemakers or may be in various tachycardic rhythms, including flutter and fibrillation; the ventricles beat at a much slower rate, as determined by an intrinsic ventricular pacemaker, which can be situated high in the conduction system (e.g., AV node or bundle of His) or which can be low, lying within the ventricular muscle itself.

The etiology of third-degree AV block includes all those disease states previously discussed. There is also a recent anecdotal record of complete AV block associated with cimetidine therapy.[28]

Complete heart block may also occur congenitally, sometimes in conjunction with other diseases. It takes two forms.[29] In the more common forms, the pacemaker is situated above the bundle of His, and the QRS is normal in shape and duration; these patients are usually entirely asymptomatic. A less frequent variety involves an infranodal block, with a low-lying pacemaker resulting in wide QRS complexes and a slower rate; these patients frequently experience Stokes–Adams attacks or heart failure. Congenital complete heart block may diagnosed prenatally by a fetal heart rate of less than 100 beats/min. It usually responds appropriately to atropine and may accelerate spontaneously during labor. During childhood, the intrinsic ventricular rate may be less than 50 beats/min, with response to atropine due to an increase in ventricular pacemaker firing.[30]

Although complete congenital heart block is usually thought to be benign, there are reports of sudden loss of consciousness or even death associated with the syndrome.[31]

The ECG in third-degree AV block shows a complete disruption in conduction between atria and ventricles (Fig. 4–7). Pacemakers situated in the AV node or His bundle generally result in normal conduction through the bundle branches and ventricular muscle, thereby generating a QRS complex of normal width. Pacemakers in either ventricle cause a wide abnor-

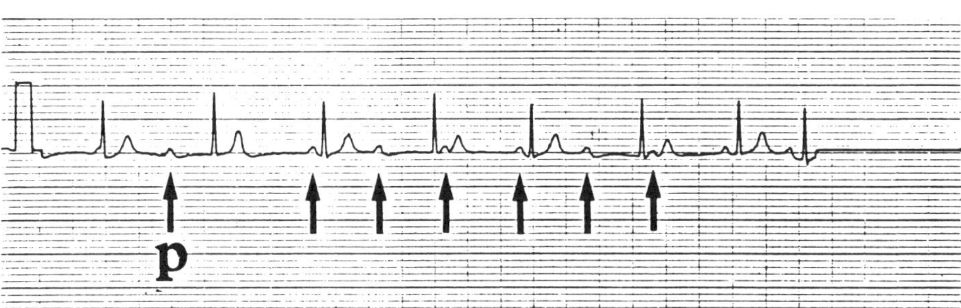

Fig. 4–7 Third-degree AV block. Note the complete disruption between the P wave and the QRS and the normal morphology of the QRS complex. (Tracing obtained at 12.5 mm/sec. Ventricular rate is 36 beats/min.)

mally shaped QRS complex, resembling a premature ventricular contraction.[4]

His bundle recordings can pinpoint the site of the pacemaker more definitively: if H spikes are consistently present, the pacemaker must be at the level of the bundle of His or higher; conversely, if these spikes are not present, the pacemaker must originate from below the bundle of His.[24]

It has been suggested that many cases of complete AV block may in fact represent a bilateral bundle branch block (e.g., a 2:1 block in one branch and a constant conduction prolongation in the other[32]). In this case, the form of the QRS complex is determined by the bundle branch with a greater degree of block, while the conduction delay in the other branch determine the PR interval. Lopez[33] reviewed ECG findings in 57 patients with a complete heart block and found that 45 of these had bilateral bundle branch disease. It was concluded that three stages are commonly passed through on progression to complete AV block: stage 1 involves a single bundle branch block; stage 2 involves a single bundle branch block with either a first- or second-degree AV block, or both, while stage 3 involves a bilateral bundle branch block and an autonomous ventricular pacemaker.

A ventriculophasic sinus dysrhythmia has been described with a third-degree AV block,[23] in which P-P intervals containing a QRS complex are shorter than those that do not. This has been thought to be due to (1) baroreceptor stimulation from a ventricular ejection-pulse-wave inducing a vagal reflex or altering blood flow through the sinus node artery or (2) traction exerted by ventricular contraction on the right atrium.

Clinical Significance

The main concern with these conduction blocks is that they can progress to higher-grade blocks and result in dangerous reductions of cardiac output.

Sinus node block occurs in a wide range of disorders. Some of these, such as acute infectious diseases or drug and electrolyte effects, are acute and reversible. Others, such as sick sinus syndrome, yield permanent dysfunction and, if the patient presents with symptomatic bradycardias, pacemaker insertion is warranted. Although ventricular pacing is the usual treatment, single-chamber atrial pacing has also been shown to be effective for long-term management of sinus node dysfunction, even though AV nodal conduction disease is also often present.[34]

First-degree AV block alone does not warrant pacemaker insertion, nor does Mobitz type I second-degree AV block. However, this does not mean that problems will not develop intraoperatively. A case was reported[35] in which a patient with a 32-year history of first-degree AV block with rare occurrences of Wenckebach blockade abruptly developed a third-degree AV block with a profound bradycardia during general anesthesia. Subsequent investigations demonstrated that the primary conduction disturbance was in the AV node, and the authors postulated that the sudden intraoperative event was due to vagal stimulation (Fig. 4–8). First-degree AV block in combination with bundle branch blocks and an axis deviation may indicate distal conduction system disease[36] and thus a greater risk of progression to complete heart block.

The presence of a Mobitz type II AV block, particularly if related to an acute myocardial infarction or associated with a wide QRS, indicates a serious consideration for a pacemaker insertion.[37] Dhingra et al.[38] considered that patients with second-degree AV blocks (with the block distal to bundle of His) should receive pacemakers, even if asymptomatic, because of the risk of progression to a higher-grade block. Second-degree AV block (types I and II) in combination with a bundle branch block carry a high risk of progression to a high-grade block.[39]

Patients with third-degree AV block obviously warrant pacemakers, but the recommendations are not as well defined for those with congenital complete heart block in which the intrinsic ventricular rate is considerably faster; these patients are frequently asymptomatic. A history of symptoms is probably a better indication for pacemaker insertion than the actual conduction abnormality. Table 4–4 summarizes indications for prophylactic preoperative transvenous pacing in children with complete congenital heart block.[29,30]

Table 4–4. Indication for Prophylactic Preoperative Transvenous Pacing in Children with Complete Congenital Heart Block

History of Stokes–Adams attacks
No chronotropic response to atropine
QRS interval greater than 0.10 seconds
Exercise intolerance
History of congestive heart failure
Other cardiac lesions

AV block associated with inferior myocardial infarcts have variable ramifications. Early AV block with myocardial infarction (during hyperacute ECG changes) is associated with high morbidity and mortality, whereas a later AV block is less dangerous.[31]

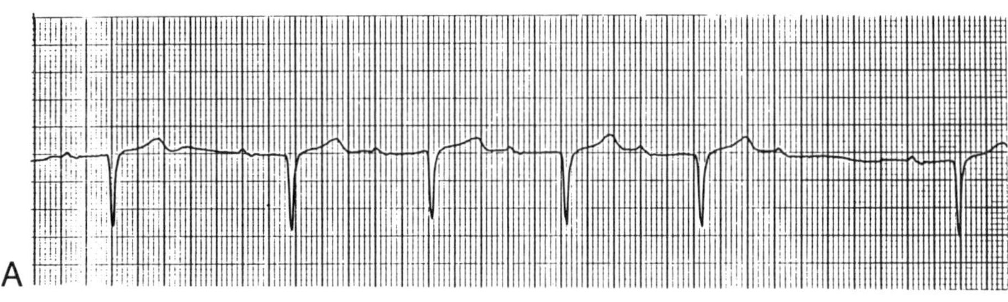

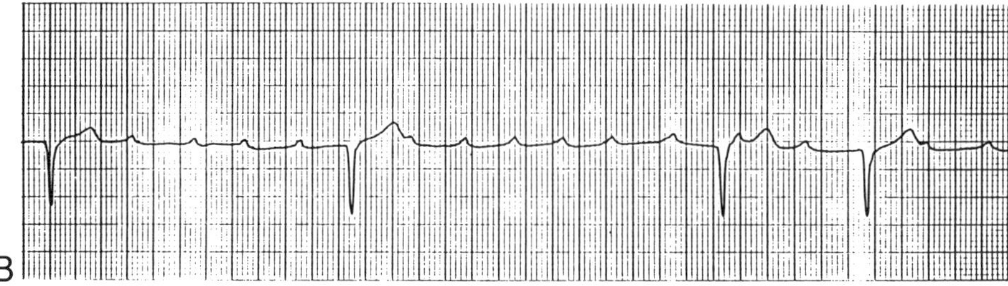

Fig. 4–8 (**A**) Second-degree AV block (Mobitz type I) which 1 hour later has progressed to a (**B**) third degree AV block.

BUNDLE BRANCH BLOCK

Bundle branch blocks may involve complete or incomplete blocks of the right bundle branch, left anterior or posterior fascicles, entire left bundle branch, or various combinations of these. The diagnosis is generally made by ECG and may be difficult because it relies essentially on the morphology of the QRS complex, which is subject to alterations by conditions other than bundle branch blocks. Other diagnostic modalities include His bundle recordings and vectorcardiography.

Right Bundle Branch Block

Right bundle branch block (RBBB) occurs more frequently in asymptomatic subjects than any other type of intraventricular conduction disturbance. Pathologic entities that are especially noted to be associated with a RBBB include[4,40] pulmonary hypertension and cor pulmonale, systemic hypertension, right ventricular hypertrophy, (RVH), congenital heart defects (especially atrial septal defects), surgery (especially closure of septal defects), coronary artery disease, and various cardiomyopathies and infections.

The septum and left ventricle are depolarized in a normal fashion in this condition, but RV activation is delayed. The RV itself is depolarized by an impulse that travels directly in the myocardium from the LV myocardium (see Fig. 4–9). The ECG findings reflect this abnormal ventricular activation. Thus, right-sided leads (e.g., aVR or V_1) would have a small initial positive deflection (an r wave), resulting from septal depolarization in the normal left to right manner, followed by a negative S wave, resulting from LV depolarization, and finally, a slurred positive R wave reflecting late RV depolarization (Fig. 4–10). The slurred quality of this last wave is indicative of the prolonged time required for an impulse to travel through the cardiac muscle as opposed to via Purkinje fibers. RV activation time, measured from the Q wave to the peak of this R′ wave, is thus prolonged.[4]

This above description essentially yields the classic rSR′ appearance of a RBBB, but other described variants include a small or even absent S wave, resulting in an rsR′ or rR′ type of pattern (Fig. 4–11). An rSr′ is occasionally seen in V_1 as a normal finding, but for this to be true, the r′ should be narrow, and the entire QRS duration should be within normal limits.[4]

Left-sided leads (e.g., I, aVL, V_6) may show

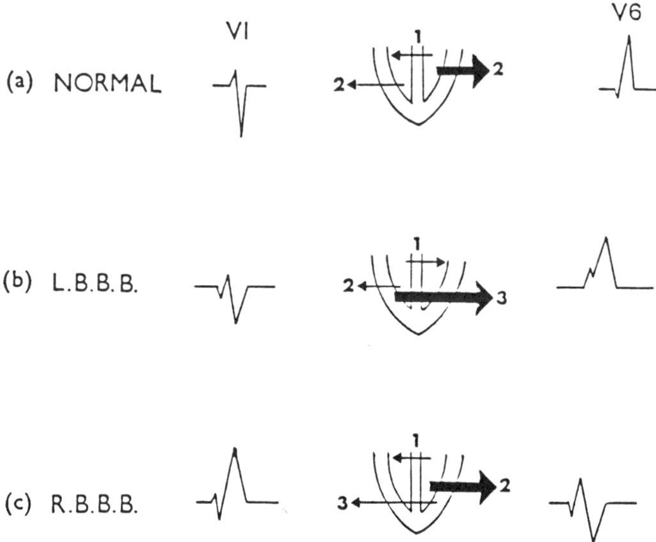

Fig. 4–9 Diagrammatic representation of ventricular depolarization in (a) normal and in (b) left and (c) right bundle branch block (LBBB, RBBB). The asynchronous depolarizaton (2 and 3) of the two ventricles should be noted. (Fleming PR: Electrocardiography. p. 196. In Scurr C, Feldman S (eds): Scientific Foundations in Anesthesia. 2nd Ed. William Heinermann, London, 1972.)

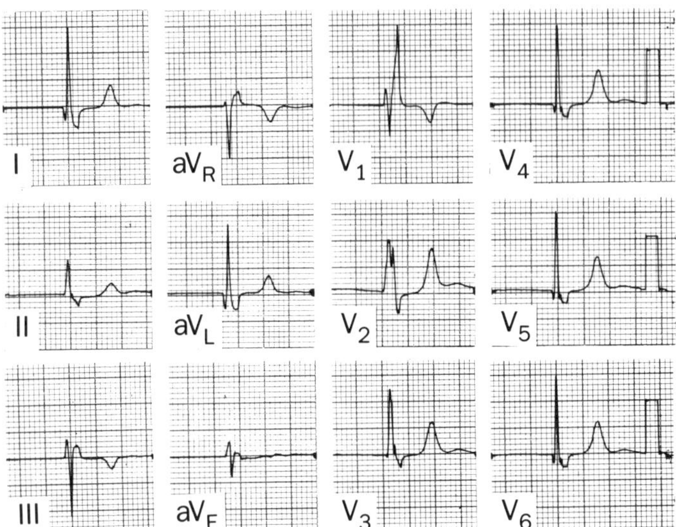

Fig. 4–10 Right bundle branch block. Note the rSR′ pattern in V_1 with slurring of R′ reflecting late right ventricular depolarization.

a small q wave, representative of septal depolarization, followed by an R wave from LV depolarization, and finally a slurred S wave from delayed RV depolarization. As compared with the right-sided leads, left-sided leads demonstrate an upright T wave. QRS appearance of inferior leads (II, III, aVF) may vary, depending on the orientation of the late force depolarization vector.

Along with these morphologic changes, an important aspect in the diagnosis of bundle branch blocks (both right and left) is an overall prolongation of the QRS complex duration to greater or equal to 0.12 second. Incomplete RBBBs may have similar morphologic abnormalities, but the QRS duration is shorter—between 0.10 to 0.12 seconds[4] (Fig. 4–12).

Intermittent RBBB also occurs: the right bundle branch conducts normally until a certain heart rate is achieved, at which point the conduction system becomes refractory, resulting in a rate-dependent block.[4]

The diagnosis of other concurrent ventricular abnormalities, such as RVH, may be difficult

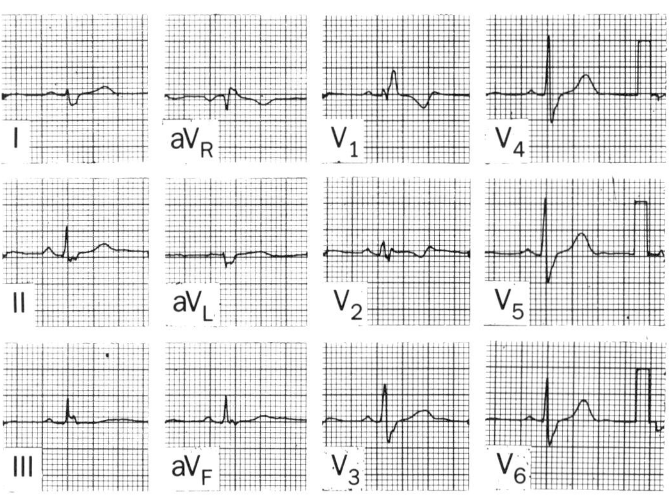

Fig. 4–11 Right bundle branch block. Variant pattern with small S-wave in V_1.

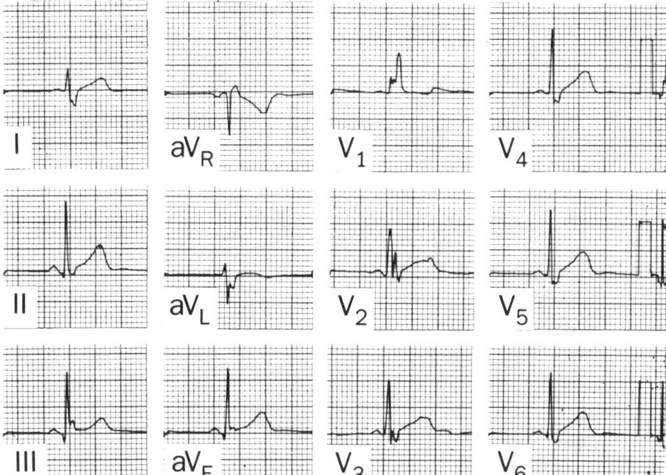

Fig. 4–12 Incomplete right bundle branch block. Note the rR′ pattern in V_1, and the duration of the QRS, which is 0.112 seconds.

in the presence of a RBBB. A concurrent myocardial infarction may or may not be diagnosable; an anterior myocardial infarction will result in a QR′ complex, with the initial positive r deflection being lost; a posterior myocardial infarction, however, may be difficult to diagnose in the presence of a RBBB—one may have an unusually tall R wave in addition to an R′ or a tall slurred R wave.[4]

Left Bundle Branch Block

Left bundle branch block is virtually always indicative of organic heart disease. The etiology includes coronary artery disease in particular, but also LVH, systemic hypertension, aortic valve disease, cardiomyopathies and infections, congestive heart failure, drug toxicities, and congenital heart defects (including congenital lesions of the left bundle branch.)[4,12]

In this case, the septum does not undergo its usual depolarization from left to right, since the left bundle branch, which normally depolarizes the septum, is refractory. The septum is now depolarized by the right bundle branch and the LV myocardium activated by a depolarization wave that originates from the right ventricular myocardium (see Fig. 4–9). The ECG reflects this abnormal conduction pathway as in the case of RBBB. In right-sided leads, a small q wave from septal depolarization is observed, followed by a small r wave due to the RV activation, finally followed by a wide prominent S wave, representing late activation of the left ventricle. Variants of this pattern include an rS (no initial q) or QS (no initial r). The T wave is of a normal configuration. In left-sided leads, a small initial r wave resulting from septal depolarization is followed by an S wave due to RV depolarization and finally by a slurred R wave resulting from the depolarization wave activating the left ventricle via the RV myocardium. This yields an rSR′ configuration or, if the S wave is minimally in evidence, a notched wide R′ wave. The T wave may be inverted and the ST segements may be depressed[15] (Fig. 4–13). The inferior leads may show R, RS, or rS configurations, depending on the main QRS vector axis.[23] Again, the total QRS duration must be greater or equal to 0.12 second and the LV activation time prolonged, in order to make the diagnosis of a LBBB. Incomplete LBBB may have a similar pattern, but the QRS duration is less than 0.12 second.[15] As with right-sided lesions, a LBBB may also be rate related.[4]

LVH is difficult to diagnose when present with a LBBB; an increased QRS voltage may be observed but may be related to aberrant conduction through the left ventricle rather than

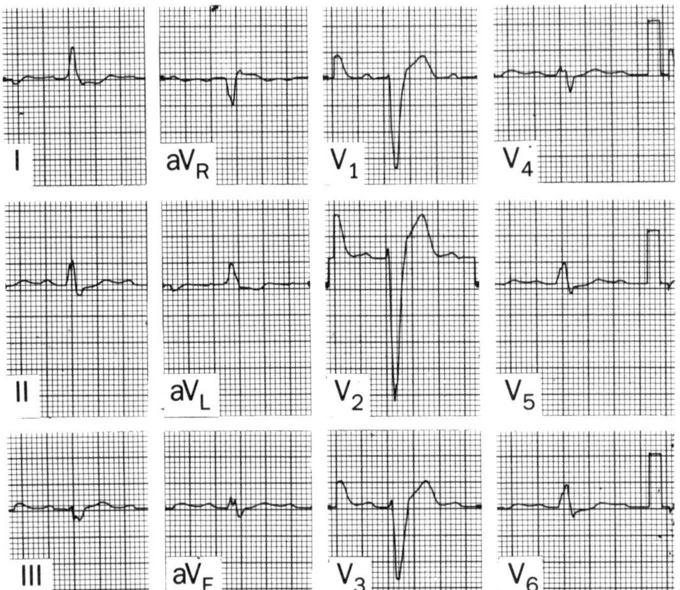

Fig. 4–13 Left bundle branch block. Note the rS pattern in V_1 and the notched rR′ pattern in V_6. In V_5 and V_6 a moderate depression of the ST segment is noted.

the thickness of the LV wall[23] (Fig. 4–14). Myocardial infarctions are notoriously difficult to diagnose[41] electrocardiographically in the presence of this block. Exceptions may be an infarction of the inferior wall (resulting in Q waves in the inferior leads) or lateral wall, evidenced by negative deflections—a q or S wave—in the lateral leads. LBBB is ruled out by a q wave in lead I or the lateral chest leads.

HEMIBLOCKS

Soon after its origin from the bundle of His, the left bundle branch divides into two fascicles, each of which may develop conduction impairment independently of the other. Conduction delays in either fascicle may alter the direction of the LV QRS depolarization vector but, as long as the other fascicle conducts normally, the overall time for LV depolarization is not prolonged; therefore, the QRS duration remains within normal limits.

Left Anterior Hemiblock

Left anterior hemiblock involves an impedence to conduction along the anterior fascicle. The LV depolarization vector is initially directed along the left posterior fascicle, in an inferior and rightward direction, resulting in r waves in inferior leads (II, III, and aVF), and q waves in lateral leads (I, aVL, and V_5–V_6. The anterior fascicle is activated later, distal to the site of the block, and the electrical force is now directed superiorly and leftward, causing a terminal S wave in inferior leads, and a terminal R in lateral leads.[4,23] The mean QRS axis is more negative than −30 degrees (some suggest even −45 degrees[5]) with left anterior hemiblock, causing a left axis deviation (Fig. 4–15).

Other recent suggestions of ECG criteria of a left anterior hemiblock include terminal R waves in both aVR and aVL, with the peak of the terminal R in aVR occurring later than that for aVL.[42]

A coexisting inferior myocardial infarction with a left anterior hemiblock can be diagnosed by observing a concurrent Q wave and a deep terminal S wave in lead II, and a terminal R wave in aVR[43,44] (Fig. 4–16).

Left anterior hemiblocks are commonly caused by fibrocalcific degeneration of the ventricular conduction system[45] and coronary artery disease[23] (especially anterior myocardial infarctions). Left axis deviations (possibly without actual conduction abnormalities) may also be

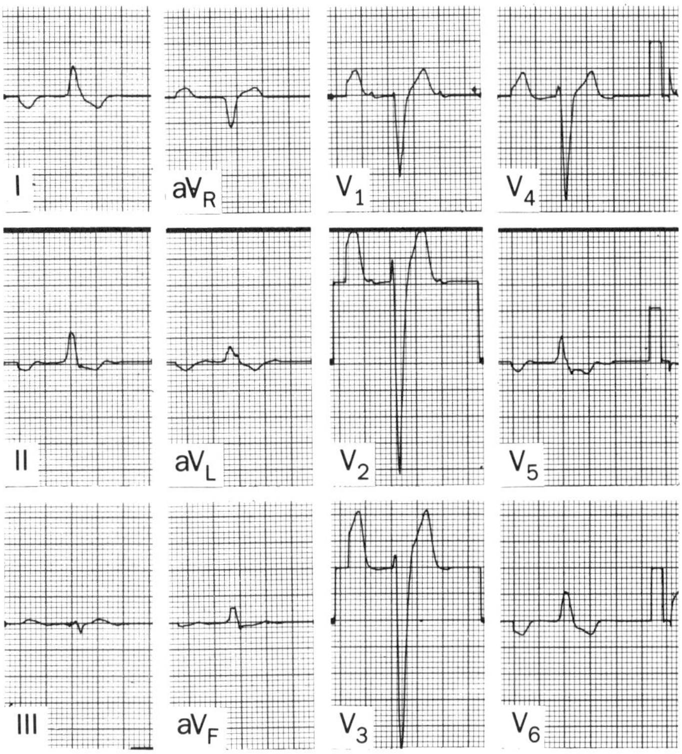

Fig. 4–14 Left bundle branch block (LBBB) with increased QRS voltage and negative T waves I, II, aVL, and V_5-V_6. This ECG illustrates the difficulties one encounters in the diagnosis of myocardial infarctions or left ventricular hypertrophy in the presence of a LBBB.

seen with LVH, hypertension, cardiomyopathies, pulmonary emphysema, congenital heart defects, connective tissue disease, infiltrative diseases such as amyloidosis or hemochromatosis, hyperkalemia, and preexcitation syndromes.[46] A left axis deviation may also occur in the presence of a LBBB; although the mechanism of the left axis deviation is not clear, there

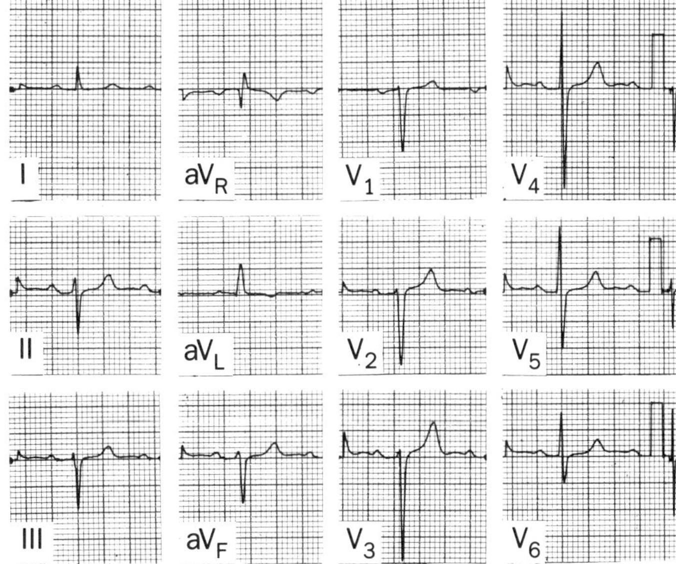

Fig. 4–15 Left anterior hemiblock. Note the left axis deviation and the terminal S in the inferior leads.

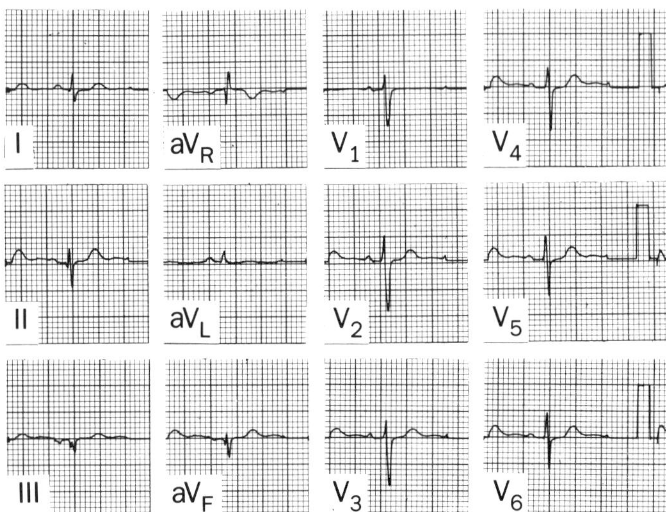

Fig. 4–16 Left anterior hemiblock with inferior myocardial infarction. Note the Q wave and deep terminal S in II and the terminal R in aVR.

is a higher incidence of myocardial dysfunction and conduction disease than with a normal axis.[46]

Left Posterior Hemiblock

Left posterior hemiblock involves compromised conduction along the posterior fascicle. Again, the most common cause of this block is fibrocalcific degeneration of the ventricular conduction system,[45] but it may also be seen with posterior myocardial infarctions, hypertension, or cardiomyopathies.[23]

The initial QRS vector is oriented in a leftward and superior direction, along the path of the anterior fascicle; this yields initial positive deflections in lateral leads and negative deflections in inferior leads. Later activation of the posterior fascicle causes the vector to move ultimately in a rightward and inferoposterior direction, resulting in final negative deflections in lateral and anterior leads, and positive deflections in inferior leads (Fig. 4–17).

The mean QRS electrical axis is shifted in a rightward direction to greater than +110 degrees. The presence of an anterolateral myocardial infarction, pulmonary emphysema, or RV hypertrophy should be excluded as possible causes of a right axis deviation.[15,45]

Septal Fascicular Block

Septal fascicular block is thought to be rare,[23] and it has an unknown clinical significance. ECG findings include abnormal Q waves in anterior precordial leads, similar to those in an anteroseptal myocardial infarction.

COMBINATIONS OF CONDUCTION BLOCKS

These most commonly involve combinations of various intraventricular conduction disturbances, although AV blocks may also be involved. They are of concern because more extensive compromise of the conduction system entails a greater risk of progression to complete heart block or even asystole.

RBBB with Left Anterior Hemiblock

A RBBB with left anterior hemiblcok is diagnosed from the ECG by the presence of criteria for both conduction abnormalities, the salient features of which include[4] (1) a wide S in lateral leads, and a wide R or R′ in right-sided precordial leads; and (2) a mean initial QRS vector of greater than −30 degrees (Fig. 4–18). His bundle recordings have shown that many patients with this combination of block also have

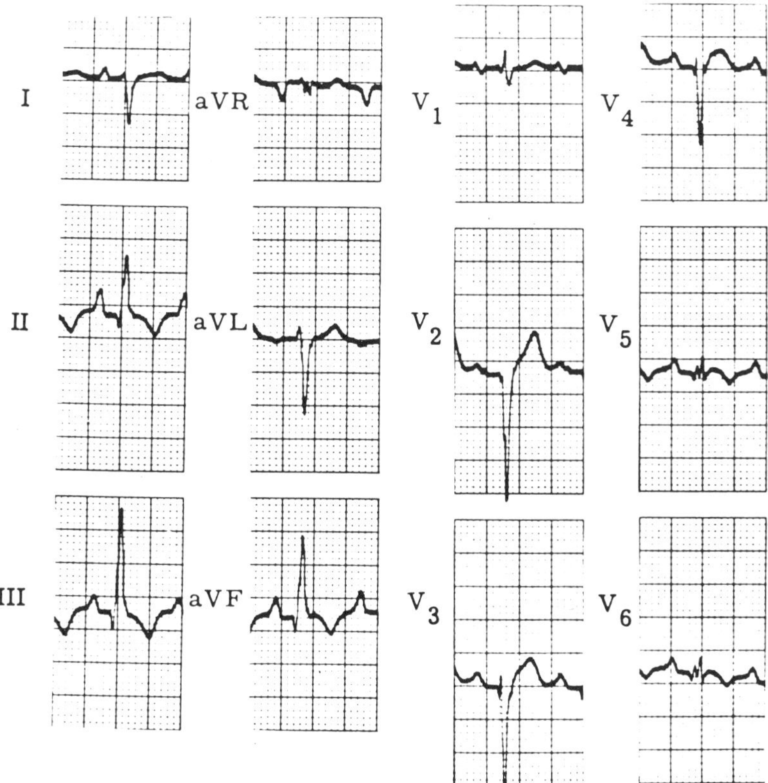

Fig. 4–17 Left posterior hemiblock. The axis of QRS vector is +110 degrees. The QRS interval is 100 msec. The P-waves are tall in II, III, and VF. (Reproduced, with permission, from Goldman MJ: Principles of Clinical Electrocardiography, 12th ed. Copyright 1986 by Lange Medical Publications, Los Altos, CA)

impaired conduction through the His-Purkinje system, thus actually resulting in a partial bilateral bundle branch block (BBBB) or even a trifascicular block. The actual site of the AV block may be above the bundle of His,[47] or within the His Bundle and in the latter, there is a higher associated incidence of cardiac complications and mortality.[48–50]

Serial ECG studies of patients with this combined block have demonstrated that in the usual sequence of events, the left axis deviation precedes the development of the right bundle branch block by days to months.[51]

RBBB with Left Posterior Hemiblock

A RBBB with left posterior hemiblock is also diagnosed from the ECG by the presence of criteria for both blocks, which includes[4] (1) a wide S in lateral leads, and a wide R or R′ in right-sided precordial leads; and (2) a mean initial QRS vector of greater or equal to +110 degrees (Fig. 4–19). In this case, as with left posterior hemiblock alone, RVH must be excluded first.[23]

Alternating RBBB–LBBB

An alternating RBBB and LBBB occasionally occurs and is recognized on the ECG by alternating patterns of both blocks.[4] Drug toxicities are implicated causes of this abnormality, as are cardiomyopathies and hypertension.

Bifascicular blocks may also include RBBB or LBBB in association with prolonged AV conduction. His bundle recordings have demonstrated that the AV conduction abnormality may lie above, within, or even beyond the bundle

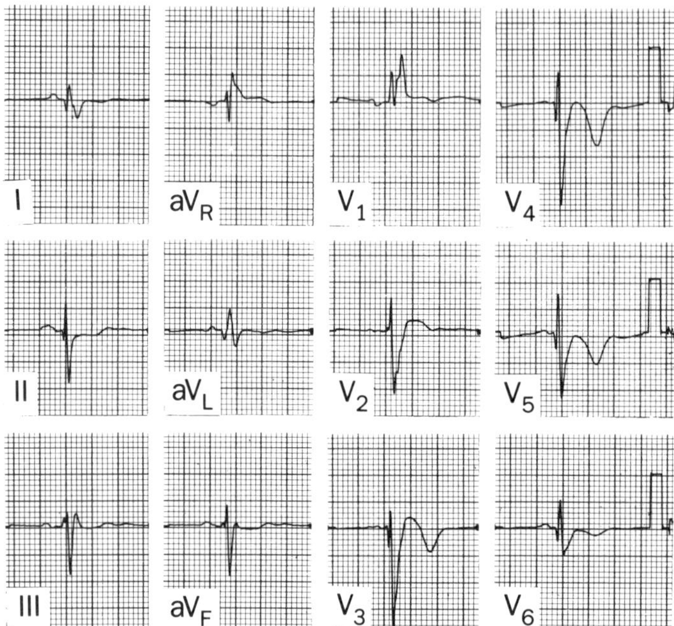

Fig. 4–18 Right bundle branch block with left anterior hemiblock. Note the RsR′ pattern in V_1 and the wide S in the lateral leads. The axis of the initial QRS vector is −88 degrees.

of His, thus representing an incomplete bundle branch block on the opposite side to the complete bundle branch block.[4]

Trifascicular Block

Trifascicular blocks are usually said to consist of one of the above BBBB (i.e. RBBB plus a left fascicular block) in addition to a prolonged PR interval (Fig. 4–20). As above, His bundle electrograms would be necessary to determine whether the atrioventricular conduction disturbance was in fact localized in the AV node, or whether it was distal, possibly representing an incomplete fascicular block in the last remaining fascicle.[4]

Clinical Significance

Perhaps the most important consideration in an analysis of the preoperative electrocardiogram for conduction abnormalities is to assess the risk of a particular conduction block to progress to a complete heart block, thus indicating the need for prophylactic pacemaker insertion, particularly during the preoperative period.

Patients with an isolated RBBB usually do not require pacing and indeed are frequently free of organic cardiac disease. Similarly, patients with a LBBB alone should not require pacing, unless the block is associated with an acute myocardial infarction.

Bilateral bundle branch blocks carry variable risks of progression to complete heart block. The indications for pacemaker insertion in these various lesions is quite controversial. A RBBB with a left anterior hemiblock is generally not considered an indication for preoperative pacemaker insertion, particularly if the patient has been asymptomatic; it has been suggested that this may be true even with a prolonged PR interval.[56] A prospective study of patients undergoing surgery and general anesthesia (using varied techniques) with a RBBB and a marked left axis deviation was done by Rooney et al.[53]; the only problems encountered were bradycardias (treatable with atropine) and premature ventricular contractions (treatable with an increased inspired oxygen concentration), and their conclusion was that routine preoperative pacemaker

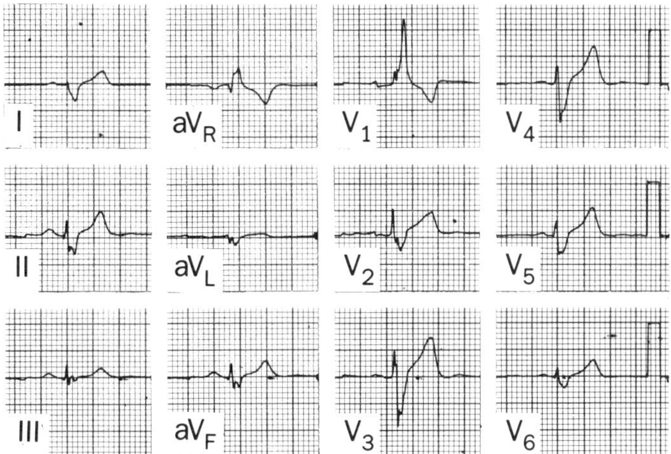

Fig. 4–19 Right bundle branch block with left posterior hemiblock. Note the wide S in the lateral leads and the rR′ pattern in V_1. The axis of the initial QRS vector is +166 degrees.

insertion was unnecessary. Another prospective study involving 44 surgical patients with the same conduction lesion was carried out by Pastore et al.[54]; these patients were given a variety of anesthetics, including general, spinal, and local anesthesia; temporary pacemakers were inserted in six patients because of a concurrent prolonged PR interval in the ECG. Only one episode of transient complete heart block occurred, while in two patients with the temporary pacemakers, significant pacemaker-related ventricular irritability occurred; again, the conclusion was that temporary pacing was rarely required. On the other hand, Falkoff et al.[55] describe a patient with apparently uncomplicated RBBB and left anterior hemiblock who developed a second-degree AV block (Mobitz type II) during anesthesia; these workers warn

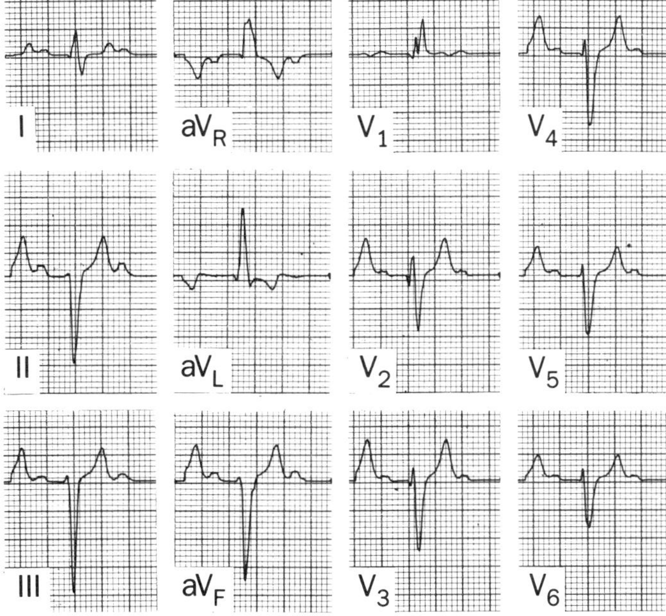

Fig. 4–20 Trifascular block. The PR interval is 232 msec and a right bundle branch block is noted. The axis of the QRS vector is −85 degrees, indicating a left anterior hemiblock.

that this bifascicular block is thus not always benign, and continuous monitoring is essential as well as the ability to institute emergency temporary pacing. Lack of symptoms with a chronic conduction impairment does not provide a guarantee that the block will not increase with provocation or under general anesthesia; thus, if possible, an accurate preoperative siting of the block and an assessment of the effectiveness of atropine are useful measures.[56] When this conduction deficit is associated with an acute myocardial infarction, pacemaker insertion is recommended.[22]

A RBBB in combination with a left posterior hemiblock is considered a more dangerous lesion in terms of risk of progression to complete heart block, although clinical reviews suggest that the clinical course is generally benign.[57]

The use of His bundle electrograms may be useful in helping decide whether a pacemaker is necessary. Bellocci et al.[50] studied HV intervals (His–Purkinje conduction time) in surgical patients with bifascicular blocks; those patients with a prolongd HV interval had a significantly greater incidence of organic heart disease and cardiac symptoms and also had a higher incidence of intra- and postoperative complications; although none developed complete heart block, ventricular fibrillation did occur on occasion. The HV interval has thus been postulated to be a much more accurate predictor of major complications than the findings on a surface ECG, but only in those patients with symptomatic heart disease, and these patients do not present a diagnostic problem.

Ventricular fibrillation has also been described by others as being a frequent mechanism of sudden death in patients with chronic bifascicular block (RBBB with either a left anterior or posterior hemiblock, or a complete LBBB), but while the group of patients experiencing sudden death had been more symptomatic (in terms of angina, congestive symptoms, or arrhythmias), there were no differences in AH (approximately AV nodal conduction time) or HV intervals.[56]

In another study,[58] involving a series of 217 patients with bi- and trifascicular blocks (47 percent of whom had associated coronary artery disease and 23 percent had primary conduction system disease), sudden death occurred in 27 patients; 17 of these deaths were not due to bradyarrhythmias and nothing had identified these patients as being at risk. This suggests again that preoperative pacemaker insertion should be reserved only for those with symptomatic bradyarrhythmias.

Postoperative bifascicular block is an indication for prophylactic pacemaker insertion since the incidence of subsequent complete heart block is high.[59]

Most patients with a bundle branch block and a second-degree AV block will require permanent pacemaker insertion, particularly if the block is in the distal bundle of His. When the AV block is in the proximal bundle of His and the patient is asymptomatic, careful observation may be adequate management.[60]

A trifascicular block (first-degree AV block and complete LBBB or RBBB with a left hemiblock) has been considered a criterion for prophylactic pacemaker insertion, but again, this may not be necessary if the patient has been asymptomatic.[61]

Thus, in summary, it would appear that unless the block is associated with an acute myocardial infarction or has occurred acutely in the postoperative period, the indication for preoperative pacemaker insertion depends primarily on a history of symptoms. Even His bundle recordings are not foolproof. Those patients with lesions considered to be of high risk do have a higher incidence of complications, but these are usually not of a nature deemed preventable by prior insertion of a transvenous pacemaker. Needless to say, any anesthesiologist involved with these patients should be aware of the relative risks associated with these lesions and should be capable and prepared to insert a pacemaker if necessary.

Occasionally bundle branch blocks may suddenly develop intraoperatively. Intermittent LBBB may occur as a heart rate and/or blood pressure-related phenomenon. Recently the appearance of a transient LBBB was reported during an episode of hypertension in a patient undergoing a cholecystectomy. This observation suggests that transient ischemia or stretch of Purkinje fibers secondary to the hypertension may be causative factors.[62] Intermittent LBBB has also been seen without changes in rate or blood pressure.[63]

Bundle branch blocks may also occur when the ventricular conducting tissue is refractory to rapid impulses. A clinical report of patients undergoing oral surgery illustrates this point. A number of patients responded to oral stimulation with a rapid heart rate from an ectopic pacemaker, firing in the AV node or bundle of His, but the peripheral conducting tissues were unable to respond, and an intermittent bundle branch block pattern resulted. In these cases, halothane was thought to have possibly contributed to the appearances of the blocks by impeding conduction through the AV node.[64]

REFERENCES

1. Chatterie K, Harris A, Patrick J, et al: The electrocardiogram in chronic heart block. Am Heart J 80:47, 1970
2. Rosen KA: The contribution of His Bundle recording to the understanding of cardiac conduction in man. Circulation 43:961, 1973
3. Gallagher JJ, Wallace AG: His bundle recordings: Methods clinical value, and indication. p. 354. In Hurst JW (ed): The Heart. McGraw-Hill, New York, 1979
4. Goldman MJ: Principles of Clinical Electrocardiography. 10th Ed. Appleton & Lange, East Norwalk, Connecticut, 1979
5. Wynands JE: Anesthesia for patients with heart block and artificial cardiac pacemakers. Anesth Analg 55:626, 1976
6. James TN: Anatomy of the conduction system of the heart. p. 47. Hurst JW (ed): The Heart. McGraw-Hill, New York, 1978
7. Lipman BS, Dunn M, Massie E: Clinical Electrocardiography. Year Book Medical Publishers, Chicago, 1984
8. Lev M: Anatomic basis for atrioventricular block. Am J Med 37:742, 1964
9. Frink RJ, James TN: Normal blood supply to the human His bundle and proximal bundle branches. Circulation 47:8, 1973
10. Rosen KM, Loeb HS, Chuquimia R, et al: Site of heart block in acute myocardial infarction. Circulation 42:925, 1970
11. Rossi L: Histopathologic Features of Cardiac Arrhythmias. Casa Editrice Ambrosiana, 1969
12. Cosby RS, Bilitch M: Heart Block. McGraw-Hill, New York, 1972
13. Lev M, Kinare SG, Pick A: The pathogenesis of atrioventricular block in coronary disease. Circulation 42:409, 1970
14. Marriott HJL, Myerburg RJ: Recognition and treatment of cardiac arrhythmias and conduction disturbances. p. 637. In Hurst JW (ed): The Heart. McGraw-Hill, New York, 1978
15. Corday E, Irving DW: Disturbances of Heart Rate, Rhythm and Conduction. WB Saunders, Philadelphia, 1961
16. Lev M: Aging changes in the human sinoatrial node. J Gerontol 9:1, 1954
17. Maor N, Keidar S, Palant A: Sinus node dysfunction in acute myocardial infarction and acute coronary insufficiency. Isr J Med Sci 20:63, 1984
18. Kaplan BM, Langendof R, Lev M, Pick A: Tachycardia–bradycardia syndrome (so-called "sick sinus syndrome"). Pathology, mechanisms and treatment. Am J Cardiol 31:497, 1973
19. Pratila MG, Pratilas V: Sick-sinus syndrome manifested during anesthesia. Anesthesiology 44:433, 1976
20. Ferrer MI: The sick sinus syndrome. Circulation 47:635, 1973
21. Watanabe Y, Dreifuss LS: AV block: Basic concepts. p. 406. In Mandel WJ: Cardiac Arrhythmias. JB Lippincott, Philadelphia, 1980
22. Pick A, Scheinman MJ: Are His bundle recordings being overutilized in the evaluation of patients with arrhythmias and conduction disturbances? p 633. In Current Controversies in Cardiovascular Disease. WB Saunders, Philadelphia, 1980
23. Cooksey JD, Dunn M, Massie E: Clinical Vectrocardiography and Electrocardiography. 2nd Ed. Year Book Medical Publishers, Chicago, 1977
24. Damato AN, Lau SH, Helfant R, et al: A study of heart block in man using His Bundle recordings. Circulation 39:297, 1969
25. Narula OS, Cohen LS, Samet P, et al: Localization of AV conduction defects in man by recording of the His bundle electrogram. Am J Cardiol 25:228, 1970
26. Narula OS, Scherlag BJ, Samet P, Javier RP:

Atrioventricular block. Localization and classification of His Bundle recordings. Am J Med 50:146, 1971
27. Narula OS, Samet P: Wenckebach and Mobitz type II AV block within the His bundle and bundle branches. Circulation 41:947, 1970
28. Tordiman T, Korzet A, Kotas R, et al: Complete atrioventricular block and long-term cimetidine therapy. Arch Intern Med 144:861, 1984
29. O'Gara JP, Edelman JD: Anesthesia and the patient with complete congenital heart block. Anesth Analg 60:906, 1981
30. Diaz JH, Friesen RH: Anesthetic management of congenital complete heart block in childhood. Anesth Analg 58:334, 1979
31. Camm AJ, Bexton RS: Congenital complete heart block. Eur Heart J 5 (suppl A): 115, 1984
32. Rosenbaum MB, Lepeschkin E: Bilateral bundle branch block. Am Heart J 50:38, 1955
33. Lopez JF: Electrocardiographic findings in patients with complete atrioventricular block. Br Heart J 30:20, 1968
34. Hayes BL, Furman S: Stability of AV conduction in sick sinus syndrome patients with implanted atrial pacemakers. Am Heart J 107:644, 1984
35. Hayward R, Domanic N, Enderby GEH, McDonald L: Anaesthesia in first degree atrioventricular block. Anaesthesia 37:1190, 1982
36. Bexton RS, Camm AJ: First degree atrioventricular block. Eur Heart J 5 (suppl A):107, 1984
37. Logue RB, Kaplan JA: The cardiac patient and noncardiac surgery. Curr Probl Cardiol 7(2):1, 1982
38. Dhingra KRC, Denes P, Wu KD, et al: The significance of second degree atrioventricular block and bundle branch block. Observations regarding site and type of block. Circulation 49:638, 1974
39. Bexton RS, Camm AJ: Second degree atrioventricular block. Eur Heart J 5 (suppl A):111, 1984
40. Mulcahy R, Kickey N, Maurer B: Aetiology of bundle-branch block. Br Heart J 30:34, 1968
41. Horan LG, Flowers NC, Telleson WJ, Thomas JR: The significance of diagnostic Q waves in the presence of bundle branch block. Chest 58:214, 1970
42. Warner RA, Hill NE, Mookheriee S, Smulyan H: Improved electrocardiographic criteria for the diagnosis of left anterior hemiblock. Am J Cardiol 51:723, 1983
43. Fisher ML, Mugmon MA, Carliner NH, et al: Left anterior fascicular block: Electrocardiographic criteria for its recognition in the presence of inferior myocardial infarction. Am J Cardiol 44:645, 1979
44. Warner RA, Hill NE, Mookheriee S, Smulyan H: Electrocardiographic criteria for the diagnosis of combined inferior myocardial infarction and left anterior hemiblock. Am J Cardiol 51:723, 1983
45. Pryor R: Fascicular blocks and the bilateral bundle branch block syndrome. Am Heart J 83:441, 1972
46. Dhingra R, Cummings J, Deedwania P, et al: The clinical significanc of left axis deviation in patients with left bundle branch block. Clin Res 25:217A, 1977
47. Schuilenburg RM, Durner D: Observations on atrioventricular conduction in patients with bilateral bundle branch block. Circulation 41:967, 1970
48. Denes P, Dhingra RC, Wu D, et al: H-V interval in patients with bifascicular block (right bundle branch block and left anterior hemiblock). Clinical, electrocardiographic and electrophysiologic correlations. Am J Cardiol 35:23, 1975
49. Narula OS, Gann D, Samet P. Prognostic value of H-V interval in patients with right bundle branch block (RBBB) and left axis deviation (LAD): follow-up observations from one to six years. Circulation (suppl III) 50:56, 1974 (abst)
50. Bellocci F, Santarelli P, DiGennaro M, et al: The risk of cardiac comolication in surgical patients with bifascicular block. Chest 77:343, 1980
51. Watt TB, Pruitt RD. Character, cause, and consequence of combined left axis deviation and right bundle branch block in human electrocardiograms. Am Heart J 77:460, 1969
52. Venkataraman K, Madias JE, Hood WB: Indications for prophylactic preoperative insertion of pacemakers in patients with right bundle branch block and left anterior hemiblock. Chest 68:502, 1975
53. Rooney S-M, Goldiner PL, Mun E: Relationship of right bundle-branch block and marked left axis deviation to complete heart block during general anesthesia. Anesthesiology 44:64, 1976
54. Pastore JO, Yurchak PM, Janis KM, et al: The risk of advanced hearth block in surgical patients with right bundle branch block and left axis deviation. Circulation 44:64, 1976
55. Falkoff M, Stowe S, Ong LS, et al:. Unusual complication of bifascicular block during surgery

under general anesthesia. PACE 1:260, 1978
56. Hayward R, Domanii N, Enderby GEH, McDonald L: Anaesthesia in first degree atrioventricular block. Anaesthesia 37:1190, 1982
57. Dhingra RC, Denes P, Wu D, et al: Chronic right bundle branch block and left posterior hemiblock. Clinical, electrophysiologic and prognostic observations. Am J Cardiol 36:867, 1975
58. McAnulty JH, Rahimtoola SH, Murphy ES, et al: A prospective study of sudden death in "high-risk" bundle-branch block. N Engl J Med 299:209, 1978
59. Perlroth MG, Hultgren HN: The cardiac patient and general surgery. JAMA 233:1279, 1975
60. Dhingra RC, Denes P, Wu D, et al: The significance of second degree atrioventricular block and bundle branch block. Observations regarding site and type of block. Circulation 49:638, 1975.
61. Ford BM, Weich HFH, Coetzee AR: Pre-operative assessment of cardiac patients for non-cardiac surgery. South Am Med J 65:235, 1984
62. Pratila MG, Pratilas V: Transient left-bundle-branch block during anesthesia. Anesthesiology 51:461, 1979
63. Edelman JD, Hurlbert BJ: Intermittent left bundle branch block during anesthesia. Anesth Analg 59:628, 1980
64. Alexander JP, Murtagh JG: Arrhythmia during oral surgery. Fascicular blocks in the cardiac conduction system. Br J Anaesth 51:149, 1979

5

Dysrhythmias

Ivan Dimich, M.D.
Vasilios Pratilas, M.D.
Daniel M. Thys, M.D.

Any patient with a history of dysrhythmias who requires anesthesia presents a considerable challenge to the anesthesiologist. Not only can the rhythm disturbance compromise hemodynamic stability but, in addition, numerous interactions are likely among the anesthetic agents and the antiarrhythmic medications. The aim of this chapter is to familiarize the clinician with some of the basic mechanisms of rhythm disturbances. Techniques used in their diagnosis are briefly reviewed and ECG characteristics of some of the more common dysrhythmias are discussed. A more detailed discussion of basic electrophysiology is presented in Chapter 7, and further information on specific dysrhythmias can be found in Chapter 10.

MECHANISMS OF DYSRHYTHMIAS

The normal electrical activity of the heart can be disturbed in many ways. For practical purposes it is convenient to divide the mechanisms leading to dysrhythmias into two major groups. Some dysrhythmias find their origin in abnormalities of impulse formation; while others are due to abnormalities in impulse conduction.[1]

Impulse Formation

Normal impulse formation depends on the ability of certain cardiac cells to depolarize spontaneously until they reach a threshold, at which point an action potential ensues. This property of initiating an action potential in the absence of external stimuli is called automaticity. Under normal circumstances, only a few cell types have the capacity to depolarize spontaneously. These cells are located in the sinus node and atria, the distal atrioventricular (AV) node, the bundle of His, the bundle branches, and the Purkinje fibers.[2]

Dysrhythmias can occur when automaticity is altered through either a reduction in the sinus node automaticity or enhancement of the automaticity in cells outside the sinus node. Examples of these dysrhythmias can be found in a number of supraventricular and nodal rhythms.[3]

ABNORMAL AUTOMATICITY

In addition to the dysrhythmias generated by increased or decreased activity of the normal automatic mechanisms, rhythm disturbances can be the result of abnormal automatic mechanisms.

Diseased cardiac cells can develop a variety of depolarization or repolarization abnormalities (e.g., during myocardial ischemia). As a result of these disturbances, cells that normally lack the capacity for automaticity (e.g., myocardial cells) can generate impulses and produce dysrhythmias.[2]

Triggered activity is one example of such an abnormal impulse formation. It is a rhythmic activity, occurring in cells in which normal repolarization at the end of the action potential has been interrupted or delayed, resulting in an afterpotential. An external stimulus during the afterpotential can produce a new action potential and trigger a run of repetitive responses.

Impulse Conduction

Abnormal properties of cardiac cells can produce AV conduction delays or blocks, which predispose to cardiac dysrhythmias. Decremental conduction occurs when a normal action potential encounters a region of myocardium with decreased conduction velocity and the impulse propagation is hindered or arrested. Decremental conduction is a normal property of the AV node, but it can be observed in other cells, such as Purkinje fibers, as a result of hypoxia and ischemia. One type of block, the unidirectional block, deserves particular emphasis, since it underlies most varieties of reentrant dysrhythmias. As the name implies, a unidirectional block permits impulse conduction in one direction but not in the other.

REENTRY

Under certain circumstances, in the presence of a unidirectional block, a tachyarrhythmia can develop by the mechanism of reentry. Reentry is defined as reexcitation caused by continuous propagation of the same impulse for one or more cycles (see Fig. 5–1). The requirements for a reentry phenomenon are a closed loop, a conduction delay, and a unidirectional block. The closed loop itself may be formed by anatomic or functional elements in normal cardiac structures or by accessory pathways.[4] Dysrhythmias due to reentry along accessory pathways are discussed under the preexcitation syndromes.

DIAGNOSIS

As in any disease state, the first approach to the patient with dysrhythmias consists of a complete history and physical examination. The history will facilitate assessment of the patient's perception of the dysrhythmias and will help determine whether any specific factors trigger the onset or end of the dysrhythmias. In addition, the functional consequences of the dysrhythmias can be evaluated. The physical examination will provide important clues about the dysrhythmia through study of the heart sounds as well as the arterial and venous pulses.

Although a precise diagnosis of the dysrhythmia can often be obtained by analysis of a rhythm strip, it is important to examine a complete 12-lead ECG as well. The critical information that the 12-lead ECG can provide concerns the contour and duration of both the P wave and the QRS complex in all standard leads. On the rhythm strip, each P wave and QRS complex must be identified, and the rate and regularity of P-P and R-R intervals must be ascertained. Analysis of the rhythm strip is facilitated by the construction of laddergrams.

When properly employed, laddergrams not only promote a better understanding of dysrhythmias but may also be indispensible in elucidating the mechanisms of complex dysrhythmias.[5] The laddergram for normal sinus rhythm shown in Figure 5–2 demonstrates its basic form.

Each laddergram is divided into three vertical sections corresponding to activity in the atrium, AV junction, and ventricle (levels A, AV, and V). Vertical distance is arbitrary, in contrast to the horizontal distance, which corresponds exactly to the time the impulse takes to enter and leave the atria, AV junction, or ventricle. The only direct information available from the

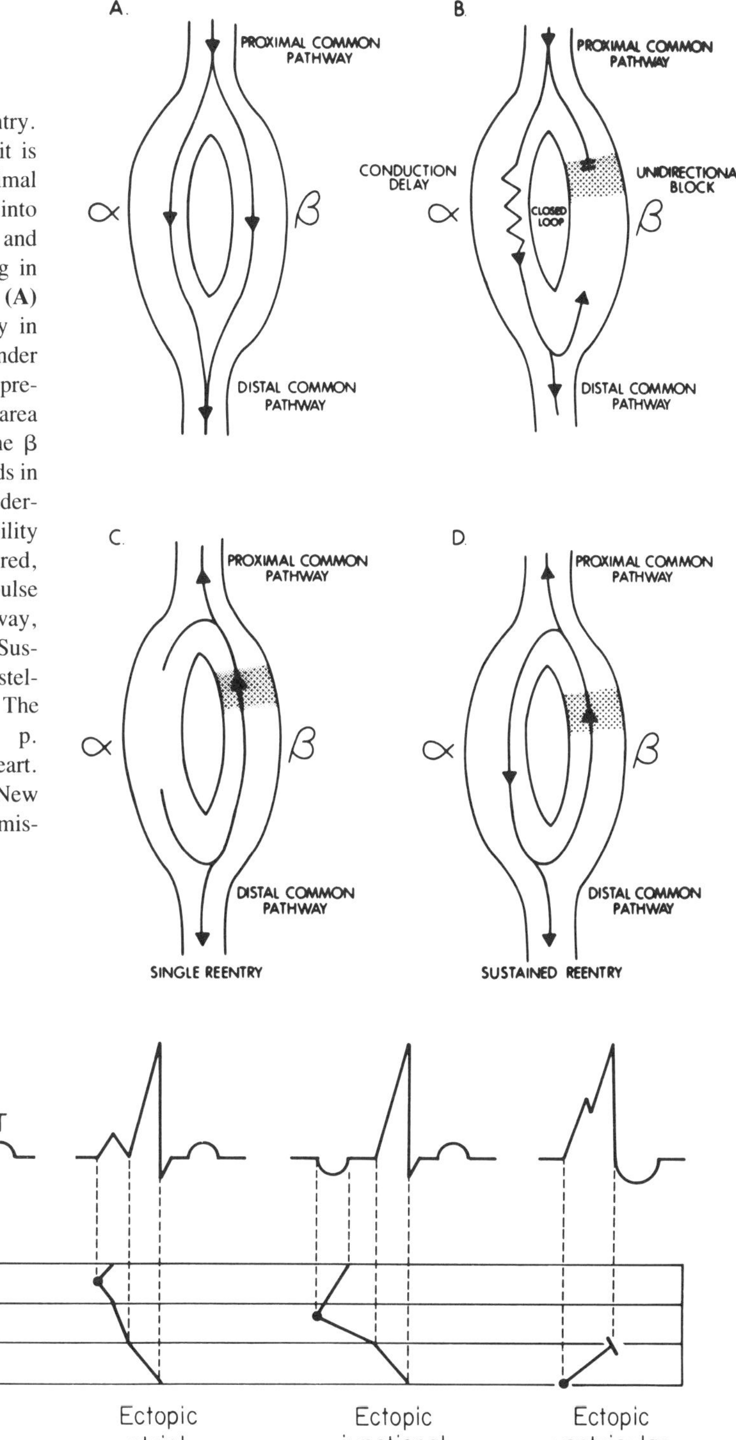

Fig. 5–1 Mechanism of reentry. A hypothetical reentry circuit is demonstrated in which a proximal common pathway divides into two divergent paths, the α and β pathways, before reuniting in the distal common pathway. **(A)** Conduction proceeds equally in both the α and β pathways under normal circumstances. **(B)** A premature beat encounters an area of unidirectional block in the β pathway. Conduction succeeds in the α pathway, but with considerable delay. **(C)** The excitability of the β pathway has recovered, allowing passage of the impulse traveling down the α pathway, resulting in reentry. **(D)** Sustained reentry is present. (Castellanos A, Myerburg RJ, et al: The resting electrocardiogram. p. 257. In Hurst W (ed): The Heart. © 1982 McGraw-Hill, New York. Reproduced with permission.)

Fig. 5–2 Construction of laddergrams for a normal sinus complex and for various beats.

ECG is the timing of P waves and QRS complexes; while the other electrical events (AV conduction) are inferred from the relationship between the P waves and the QRS complexes.[6]

The electrical activity of each beat is expressed in a laddergram by using a sloping line for each zone of conduction. The line begins at the point at which the cardiac cycle is initiated (i.e., the pacemaker). If the P wave is normal in configuration, as in sinus rhythm, the line will start directly under the beginning of the P wave, at the top of the A level, and slope downward and to the right, ending at the cessation of the P wave, at the bottom of the A level (Fig. 5–2). A similar procedure is followed at the V (ventricular) level with respect to the QRS complex. The AV level that represents AV conduction is not depicted directly on the ECG. It is constructed by connecting the bottom of the atrial line with the top of the ventricular line when conduction is antegrade and in reverse fashion when conduction is retrograde.[7]

Certain symbols are employed to designate special events. A dot is used to depict the site of impulse formation and a horizontal short line to mark a conduction block.

Another common technique used in the diagnosis of dysrhythmias is Holter monitoring.[8] A Holter ECG is an ECG tape recorded during activity (dynamic electrocardiography), which can be used to detect either dysrhythmias or myocardial ischemia (see Chapter 6).[1,9] It provides a continuous magnetic tape recording of the ECG and permits recordings of up to 24 hours duration. It has been documented that less than ten hours of monitoring are insufficient for the detection of some of the most serious dysrhythmias.[10] The advantages of Holter monitoring over a standard ECG are that it may detect dysrhythmias that are transient in nature or precipitated by different activities (i.e., anxiety, effort).

Holter monitoring may be indicated preoperatively in (1) patients presenting with syncope, dizziness, or palpitations whose routine ECG fails to explain their symptoms; and (2) patients who present with severe sinus bradycardia (rate less than 50 beats/min) or with ECG findings of an occasional sinus pause. In this last group of patients, sick sinus syndrome must be excluded before surgery. Holter monitoring may also be used to screen patients who have conditions that may predispose to dysrhythmias, such as mitral valve prolapse, severe coronary arteriosclerosis, prolonged QT interval syndrome, Wolff–Parkinson–White syndrome, or cardiomyopathies, as well as in the evaluation of antiarrhythmic drug therapy or pacemaker function.

ELECTROPHYSIOLOGIC DIAGNOSIS

Intracardiac Recording of His Bundle Activity

The introduction of His bundle recording by Berber et al.[11] in 1974 ushered in the modern era of intracardiac electrophysiology. Recording of His bundle electrocardiograms (HBE) has enabled the clinician to better understand AV conduction disturbances and the etiology of a variety of dysrhythmias. Intracardiac electrophysiologic studies provide the bridge between microelectrode studies in isolated tissue and the surface ECG, since the conventional ECG displays only atrial and ventricular depolarization. The depolarization amplitudes are low in the conduction system (sinus node, AV node, His Purkinje system) and are not visible on a regular ECG tracing. The advantage of the intracardiac recordings is that they augment the amplitude of these deflections and divide the PR interval into three visible segments (Fig. 5–3)[12,13]:

1. The PA interval corresponds to the intra-atrial conduction time from the SA node through the atria. It is measured from the onset of the P wave on the surface ECG to the low intracardiac atrial deflection. The normal value is 20 to 45 msec.
2. The AH interval represents the AV nodal conduction time. It is measured from the beginning of the low atrial wave to the onset of the His bundle potential. The range of normal values is 60 to 130 msec.
3. The HV interval represents conduction

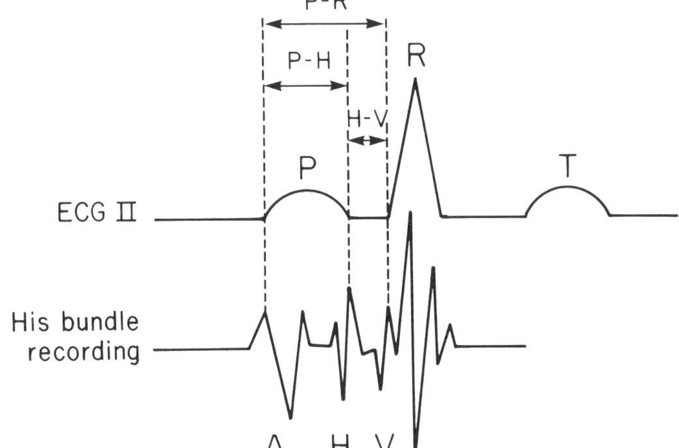

Fig. 5–3 Simultaneous recordings of the surface electrocardiogram and His bundle electrocardiogram. See text for explanation of PA, AH, and HV intervals.

through the ventricular myocardium near the atrioventricular ring and His–Purkinje system and is measured from the onset of the His bundle potential to the ventricular wave on HBE. The normal range is 30 to 55 msec.[14]

Recordings of HBE are obtained by passing an electrode catheter from the femoral vein into the right heart, so that at least two of the poles straddle the tricuspid valve. Regular ECG leads are recorded simultaneously as a reference. Results from HBE recordings can be of considerable help in the preoperative evaluation of patients with AV conduction disturbances or recurrent dysrhythmias. For instance, patients with a conduction delay during the AH interval have a much better prognosis than do those with a delay in the His bundle or below it. Recordings from HBE may also help identify patients who would benefit from implantation of a permanent pacemaker prior to surgery. In the preoperative diagnostic evaluation of sick sinus syndrome, HBE is also helpful since it can be used to measure the sinoatrial (SA) conduction time, recovery time, and response of the sinus node to premature atrial stimulation. Delays in conduction are diagnostic of sick sinus syndrome.[15]

In patients with Wolff–Parkinson–White syndrome, HBE is used for mapping the electrical conduction in the heart. Abnormal conduction pathways can be recognized, and patients can be evaluated for possible surgical interruption of the abnormal bundle.

Electrical Stimulation

During complete clinical electrophysiologic studies, dysrhythmias are evaluated by the combined application of His bundle electrocardiography, incremental pacing, and programmed electrical stimulation. The purpose of these electrophysiologic techniques is: (1) to evaluate the function of the cardiac conduction system, (2) to analyze the mechanisms responsible for the onset and termination of dysrhythmias, and (3) to assess the effects of medical therapy or electrical interventions in the treatment of the dysrhythmias.[16]

Stimulations are performed by applying single or multiple electrical stimuli of varying amplitude and duration to different areas of the heart including the sinus node, atria, AV conduction system, and ventricles. A 12-lead ECG is recorded during the stimulation to compare the stimulated dysrhythmias with those occurring spontaneously. Using these techniques it is possible to differentiate supraventricular tachycardias from ventricular tachycardias and to determine whether a tachycardia is due to reentry or abnormal automaticity.

Intraoperative Cardiac Mapping

Mapping is another technique that enables the cardiac surgeon and electrophysiologist: (1) to diagnose dysrhythmias, (2) to localize a dysrhythmic focus with accuracy, (3) to resect the focus, and (4) to evaluate the surgical therapy.[17] Bipolar electrodes and amplifiers are used to record potentials 1 mm apart. A filter eliminates deflections during the ST-, T- and P-wave segments of the cardiac cycle, so that only ventricular muscle activity between 50 and 500 Hz is recorded. Activation mapping is usually done after cannulation for cardiopulmonary bypass is completed and partial bypass has been initiated to maintain a good perfusion pressure. Programmed electrical stimulation initiates the ventricular tachycardia, and a bipolar electrogram records the selected epicardial sites. After the focus of the dysrhythmia is localized total cardiopulmonary bypass is instituted, and the dysrhythmic focus, ventricular aneurysm, or infarcted area is removed. If the ventricular tachycardia persists after surgical ablation of the focus, endocardial mapping is performed under direct vision for further evaluation and treatment of the dysrhythmia.

ECG DIAGNOSIS OF DYSRHYTHMIAS

Atrial Dysrhythmias

The term supraventricular dysrhythmia is used to describe a variety of dysrhythmias that originate in the atria or the atrioventricular (AV) node. The most common cause of these dysrhythmias appears to be reentry, while other mechanisms, such as abnormal automaticity and triggered activity, occur much less frequently (see Chapter 10).

SINUS TACHYCARDIA

Sinus tachycardia is characterized by a regular rate greater than 100 beats/min in adults and 120 to 140 beats/min in children. A narrow QRS is preceded by a normal P wave and PR interval (Fig. 5–4). When the heart rate is faster than 150 beats/min, sinus tachycardia must be differentiated from paroxysmal atrial tachycardia (PAT). A P-wave contour different from that of the normal sinus P-wave contour or an abnormal prolongation of the PR interval favor the diagnosis of PAT. Carotid massage will usually slow a sinus tachycardia, whereas in PAT it will either produce an abrupt break and reversal to sinus rhythm or it will not be effective. The causes of a sinus tachycardia during anesthesia include increased sympathetic activity produced by pain, hypoxia, hypercarbia, hypovolemia, fever, or drugs. Treatment should be directed at the underlying cause. Occasionally, if the clinical situation demands it (e.g., patient with coronary artery disease), propranolol can be useful.

REENTRANT SINUS TACHYCARDIA

The etiology of reentrant sinus tachycardia is unknown, but several suggestions have been made. One possibility is that there is an ectopic atrial focus very close to the sinus node. Another possibility is that there is an abnormality in phase 4 of the sinus node action potential itself. A characteristic of this tachycardia is that it appears in the absence of fever, anxiety, or hyperthyroidism. Reentrant atrial tachycardia usually causes visible P waves and shorter PR than R-P intervals. The rate is slower than in PAT, and the P waves are distinctly different from sinus P waves. This dysrhythmia begins and ends abruptly, and the rate is between 140 and 200 beats/min. Clinically, this type of dysrhythmia causes no particular disabilities.

PREMATURE ATRIAL CONTRACTIONS

Premature atrial contractions (PACs) are defined as premature P waves, different in contour from the sinus wave, which in general are followed by a normal QRS-T sequence. The interval following the premature beat is equal or

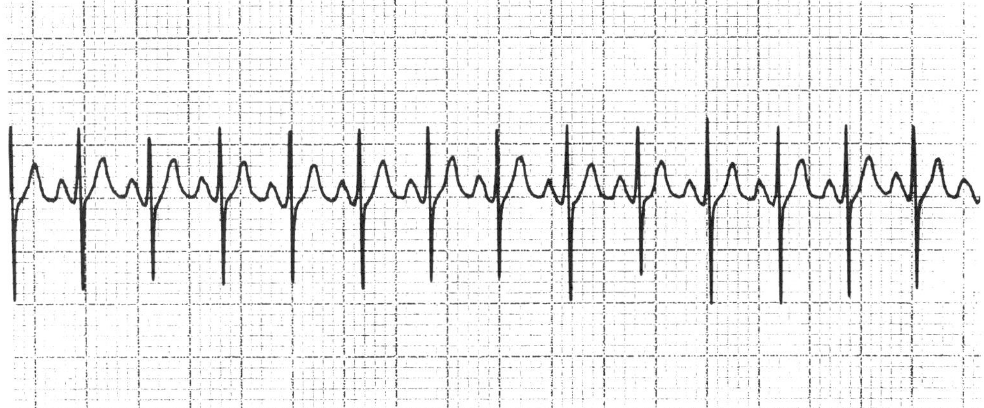

Fig. 5–4 Sinus tachycardia.

slightly longer than the normal sinus interval (Fig. 5–5).

PACs are not only very common during anesthesia and during the postoperative period, but they are often erroneously diagnosed as AV junctional premature beats, ventricular premature beats, or sinus arrest. The reasons for these errors are that (1) the premature P wave that defines the atrial premature beat is often superimposed on the preceding T wave; (2) atrial premature beats are often nonconducted or blocked, causing sudden lengthening of the PR interval; and (3) atrial premature beats are frequently associated with aberrant ventricular conduction simulating ventricular premature beats (Fig. 5–6). Simple identification of the premature P wave should avoid these diagnostic pitfalls. Other helpful points in distinguishing a PAC with aberrant conduction from a PVC include the observations that (1) the aberrant conduction is of a right bundle branch configuration, (2) there is an rSR^1 pattern in V_1, and (3) the initial vector force is identical to the one of the preceding beat, whereas it is usually in the opposite direction with a premature ventricular contraction (PVC).[18]

PAROXYSMAL ATRIAL TACHYCARDIA

Paroxysmal atrial tachycardia (PAT) is a reentrant supraventricular tachycardia that runs in paroxysms of rapidly repeating ectopic beats. Although it is seen in 5 percent of young adults without organic heart disease, it is usually associated with advanced heart disease, thyrotoxicosis, chronic lung disease, or Wolff–Parkinson–White syndrome. The sudden onset of this dys-

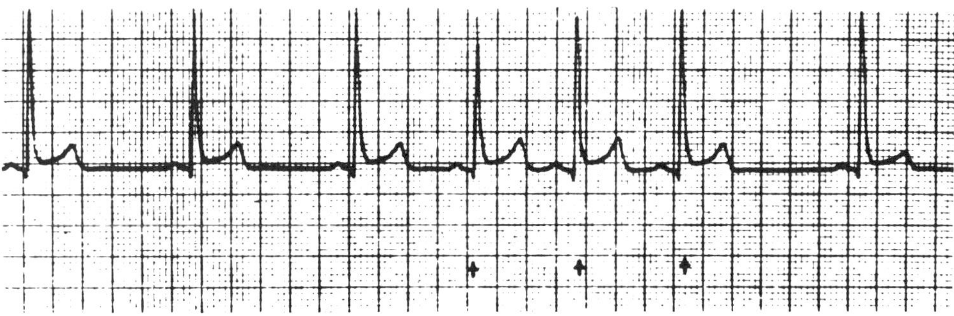

Fig. 5–5 Premature atrial contractions. (Kaplan J (ed): Cardiac Anesthesia. Grune & Stratton, Orlando, Florida, 1979, by permission.)

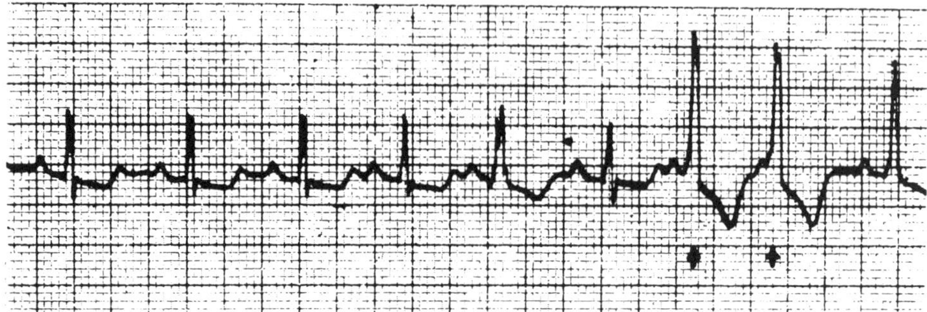

Fig. 5–6 Premature atrial contractions with aberrant conduction. (Kaplan J (ed): Cardiac Anesthesia. Grune & Stratton, Orlando, 1979, by permission.)

rhythmia during anesthesia may lead to serious hemodynamic deterioration, especially in cardiac patients.[19]

Electrocardiographic features of PAT include a rapid rate of 150 to 250 beats/min. The P waves may occur before, within, or after the QRS complex. Sometimes the P and T waves are superimposed, so that the P wave and PR interval cannot be seen. In this case, the P wave can be identified by slowing with carotid massage or by the use of an exploring lead V_{3R} or an esophageal lead. The QRS complexes are usually normal and regularly spaced. Frequently, depression of the ST segment and inversion of the T wave accompanies sustained paroxysms (Fig. 5–7). If there is ventricular aberration or bundle branch block, the QRS may be wide, resembling ventricular tachycardia.

PAT can be treated by a number of drugs, including verapamil, phenylephrine, and edrophonium. In the past, intravenous digoxin has been successfully used with propranolol. In an emergency, when PAT is accompanied by significant hemodynamic deterioration, electrical cardioversion is indicated (see Chapter 10).

PAROXYSMAL ATRIAL TACHYCARDIA WITH BLOCK

PAT with block is usually a result of digitalis intoxication and is often associated with hypokalemia. Sensitivity to the toxic effects of digitalis is markedly increased during anesthesia, particularly in the presence of alkalosis, hypoxia, potassium depletion, or decreased renal function. The ECG in this condition displays an atrial rate of 120 to 150 beats/min and is associated with some degree of AV block (Fig. 5–8).[20]

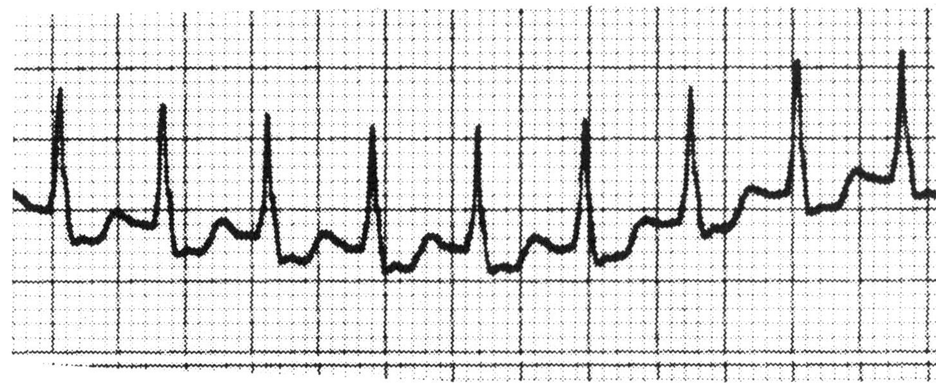

Fig. 5–7 Paroxysmal atrial tachycardia.

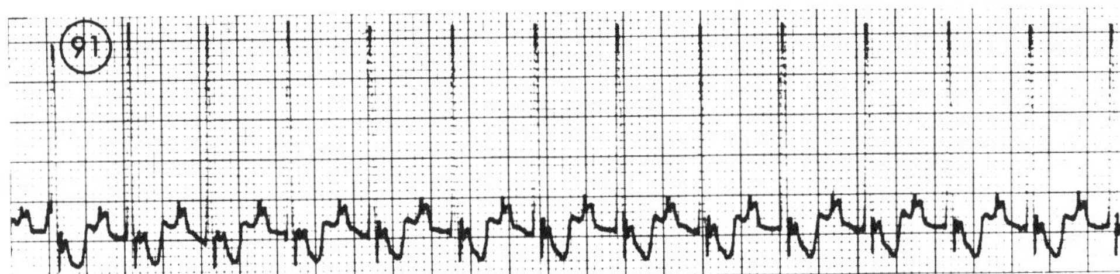

Fig. 5–8 Paroxysmal atrial tachycardia with block. (Reprinted with permission from Phillips R, Feeney M (eds): The Cardiac Rhythm. WB Saunders, Philadelphia, 1973.)

MULTIFOCAL ATRIAL TACHYCARDIA

Multifocal atrial tachycardia indicates diffuse atrial disease, including distention of the atria and/or sinus node degeneration. Frequently seen in patients with advanced chronic obstructive lung disease,[21] this dysrhythmia is characterized by multiple and multifocal atrial premature complexes and a heart rate of 100 to 200 beats/min (Fig. 5–9). The rate is irregularly irregular. This rhythm may lead to marked impairment of atrial and ventricular filling, resulting in hemodynamic deterioration. It has been reported that the rhythm returns to normal when acute pulmonary problems such as pulmonary infection subside.

ATRIAL FLUTTER

Atrial flutter usually results from a reentrant circuit located totally within the atrial wall. It is rarely seen in patients without heart disease but can be seen in association with most forms of heart disease, especially rheumatic heart disease involving the mitral valve (e.g., mitral stenosis).

The ECG features include an atrial rate between 250 and 350 beats/min, with a sawtooth appearance (F waves) best seen in leads II, III, aVF, and V_1 (Fig. 5–10). Although 2:1 AV block is common, the degree of AV block is variable and can change quite rapidly. Symptomatology will depend on the cardiac status of the patient and the AV conduction rate. Rapid rates with 1:1 conduction to the ventricle may lead to a reduction in cardiac output and pulmonary edema.

Sudden onset of atrial flutter during the perioperative period should be treated with electrical cardioversion. Electrical conversion with 10 to 25 watt-sec can easily convert atrial flutter to a sinus rhythm. Digitalis is very effective in slowing the nodal conduction; while propranolol or verapamil slow the ventricular response considerably and sometimes revert the rhythm to normal sinus.

ATRIAL FIBRILLATION

Atrial fibrillation is thought to be caused by multiple microreentry circuits within the atrial muscle. It is usually associated with chronic

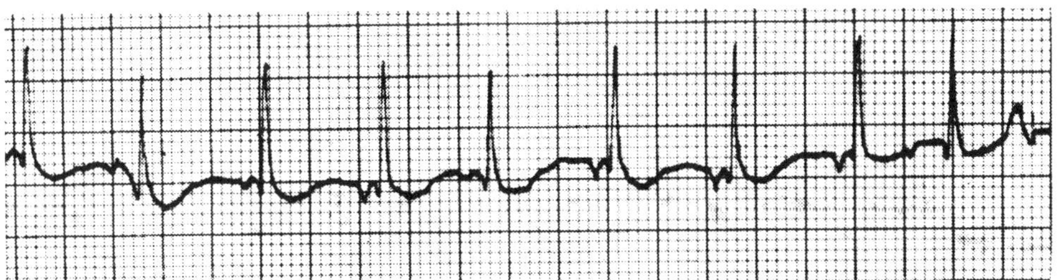

Fig. 5–9 Multifocal atrial tachycardia.

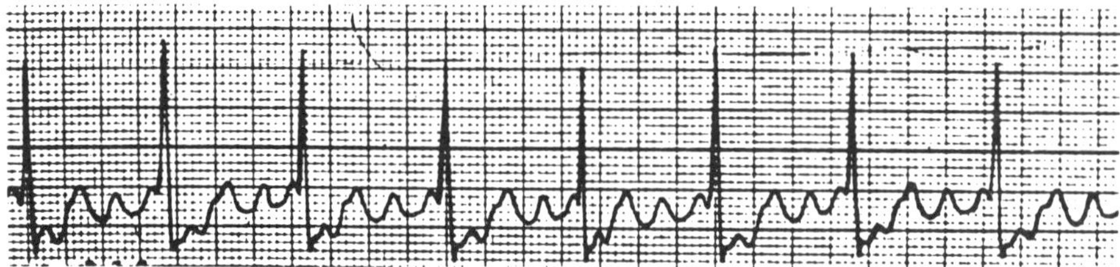

Fig. 5–10 Atrial flutter. (Kaplan J (ed): Cardiac Anesthesia. Grune & Stratton, Orlando, Florida, 1979, by permission.)

heart disease, either valvular, myocardial or pericardial. It is also seen in pulmonary embolism, chronic lung disease, or hyperthyroidism.[22] Atrial fibrillation is characterized by rapid irregular fibrillating atrial waves (f waves) at a rate of 300 to 600 beats/min, best seen in leads II, III, aVF, and V_1 (Fig. 5–11). A certain degree of AV block is always present. The ventricular response is irregularly irregular at a rate of 140 to 200 beats/min, except in patients with sick sinus syndrome, in whom it may be much slower.

In the presence of hemodynamic deterioration, emergency cardioversion is indicated, while in long-standing fibrillation, conversion to sinus rhythm is usually less successful. In patients with chronic fibrillation, digitalis is often administered to maintain a ventricular rate of less than 100 beats/min; digitalis is not indicated, however, in patients with Wolff–Parkinson–White syndrome. Patients on long-term digitalis therapy for treatment of atrial fibrillation should be carefully screened for digitalis intoxication preoperatively. The presence of PVCs or a slow ventricular rate suggests digitalis intoxication.

Junctional Dysrhythmias

JUNCTIONAL RHYTHM

Junctional rhythm may occur when the sinus rate is slowed or when the junctional pacemaker increases its rate of discharge. The normal rate of discharge of the junctional pacemaker is 40 to 60 beats/min. Junctional rhythms are common under anesthesia, especially with halogenated anesthetic agents, and may produce a decrease in blood pressure and cardiac output.[23] Depending on whether conduction from the pacemaker site is anterograde or retrograde, inverted P waves (in the inferior leads) may be seen preceding, following, or coinciding with the QRS complex. Because the pacemaker site is above the division of the bundle branches, the QRS com-

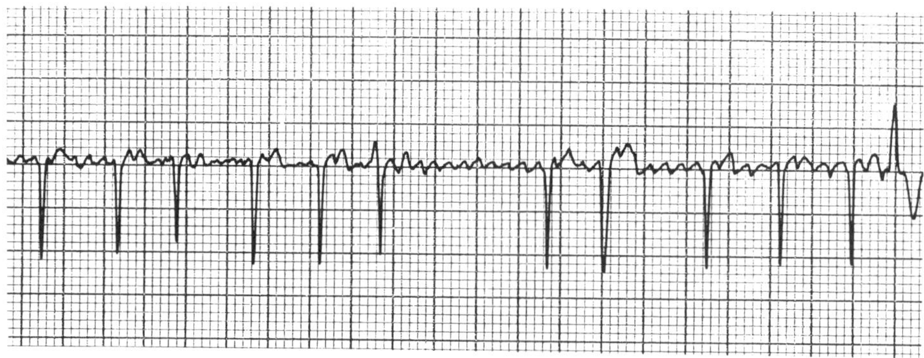

Fig. 5–11 Atrial fibrillation.

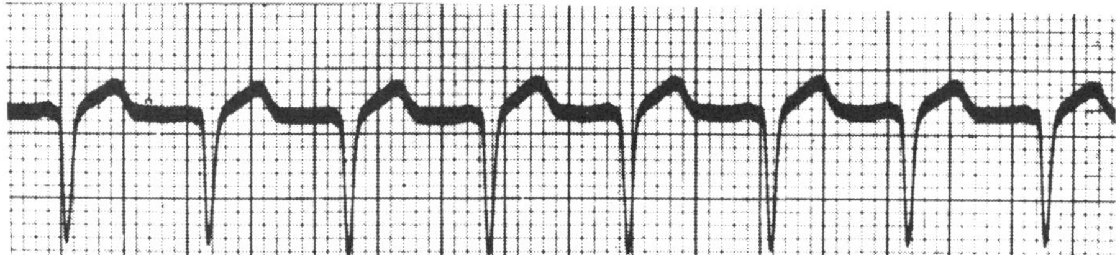

Fig. 5–12 AV nodal tachycardia. (Reprinted with permission from Phillips R, Feeney M (eds): The Cardiac Rhythms. WB Saunders, Philadelphia, 1973.)

plex is identical to that resulting from sinus conduction. In general, treatment is not necessary; if significant hypotension is present, however, atropine, ephedrine, or isoproterenol may be needed.[24]

AV NODAL TACHYCARDIA

Nodal tachycardia is manifested as a passive escape rhythm with a rate of 70 to 140 beats/min, or as a paroxysmal junctional tachycardia of 150 to 200 beats/min (see Fig. 5–12). The P waves may occur before, within, or after the QRS complexes, or they may be unrelated. The QRS complex is usually narrow, but in the presence of a bundle branch block it may be wide. This relatively common dysrhythmia is sometimes seen during halothane anesthesia or following pancuronium administration; it rarely requires treatment.[25] If indicated, propranolol can be useful to control the rate. In patients receiving digitalis, this dysrhythmia may represent digitalis intoxication.

Ventricular Dysrhythmias

PREMATURE VENTRICULAR CONTRACTION

A ventricular extrasystole is an impulse that originates prematurely in the ventricles and disturbs the prevailing rhythm. Premature ventricular contractions (PVCs) are frequently seen during anesthesia in normal individuals and those with cardiac disease. PVCs are more common in the elderly and in patients with ischemic heart disease, particularly following myocardial infarction.

The mechanism of PVCs may be either increased automaticity of ventricular foci or reentry. On the ECG, PVCs produce a premature wide, slurred, bizarre QRS complex followed by a T wave that is usually in the opposite direction to the main deflection of the QRS complex (Fig. 5–13). The QRS complex is not preceded by a premature P wave, but it may be preceded by a sinus P wave occurring at its expected time. Fully compensatory pauses usu-

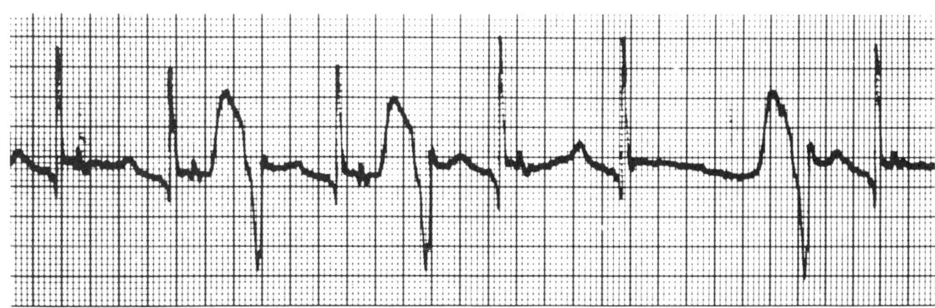

Fig. 5–13 Premature ventricular contractions. (Kaplan J (ed): Cardiac Anesthesia. Grune & Stratton, Orlando, Florida, 1979, by permission.)

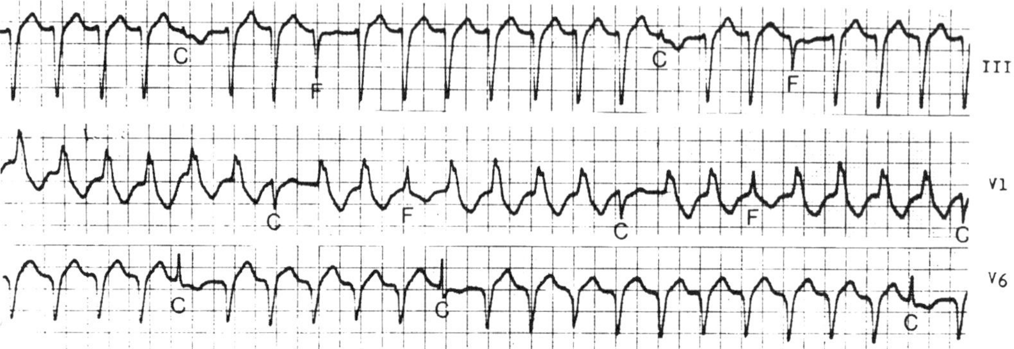

Fig. 5–14 Premature ventricular contractions (c) and fusion beats (F). (Reprinted by permission from Braunwald E (ed): Heart Disease. WB Saunders, Philadelphia, 1980.)

ally follow PVCs. Interference within the ventricle may result in ventricular fusion beats that may on occasion be narrower than the dominant beat. Fusion beats indicate activation of the ventricle from two different foci, one of supraventricular and the other of ventricular origin (Fig. 5–14). PVCs usually exhibit fixed or variable coupling, and the interval between the normal QRS complex and the PVC complex is usually relatively stable and constant.

The term bigeminy refers to the situation in which PVCs alternate with normal beats. This dysrhythmia is frequently seen in digitalis intoxication. Multifocal PVCs are characterized by at least two abnormal QRS complexes of different configurations and varying coupling intervals (Fig. 5–15). Certain types of PVCs are potentially dangerous and may lead to ventricular tachycardia. This is particularly true when PVCs occur in couplets or triplets, are multifocal, or with the occurrence of the R-on-T phenomenon (when the R wave of the PVC falls on the T wave of the previous beat).[25]

VENTRICULAR TACHYCARDIA

Ventricular tachycardia is defined as episodes of four or more consecutive PVCs. It arises in the specialized conduction system distal to the bifurcation of the His bundle.[26] The accepted mechanisms of ventricular tachycardia are abnormal automaticity or reentry. A characteristic ventricular tachycardia is uniform, consisting of a series of widened QRS complexes, usually regular or moderately irregular, with a rate ranging from 70 to 250 beats/min (Fig. 5–16). When evident, the hallmark of ventricular tachycardia is AV dissociation. The ECG distinction between supraventricular tachycardia with aberration and ventricular tachycardia is important, especially during anesthesia. The presence of fusion and capture beats, AV dissociation, left axis deviation, and compensatory pauses strongly suggest a diagnosis of ventricular tachycardia.[24] By contrast, the presence of P waves preceding the QRS, the onset of the dysrhythmia with a premature P wave, an RSR^{1}

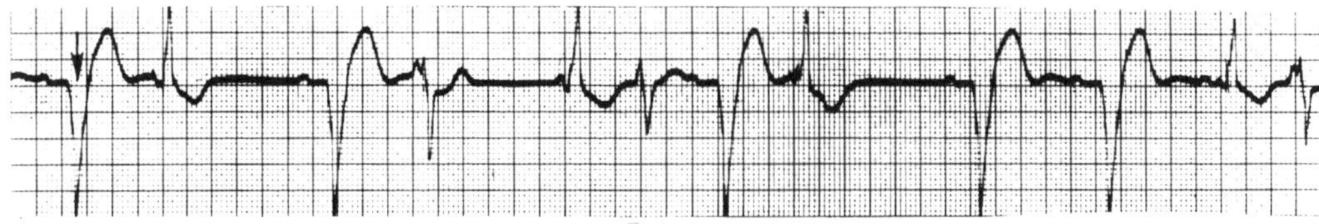

Fig. 5–15 Multifocal premature ventricular contractions. (Kaplan J (ed): Cardiac Anesthesia. Grune & Stratton, Orlando, Florida, 1979, by permission.)

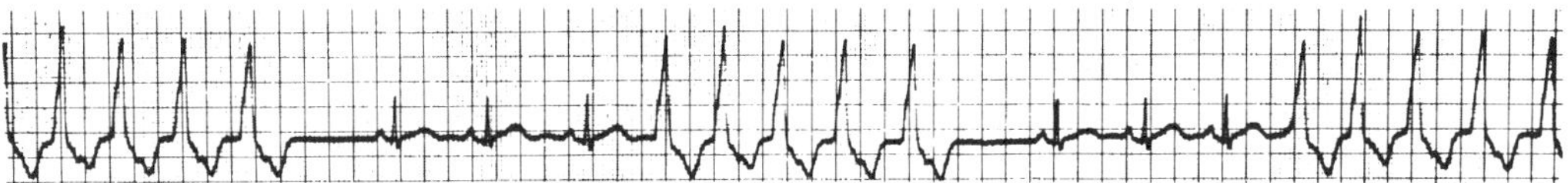

Fig. 5–16 Ventricular tachycardia. (Reprinted by permission from Braunwald E (ed): Heart Disease. WB Saunders, Philadelphia, 1980.)

pattern in V_1, and slowing or termination of the tachyarrhythmia by vagal stimulation indicate a supraventricular tachycardia with aberration.

The acute onset of ventricular tachycardia requires immediate treatment because it may lead to ventricular fibrillation. Lidocaine and procainamide can be used, but sustained ventricular tachycardia is best treated with synchronized cardioversion.

DYSRHYTHMIA SYNDROMES

Sick Sinus Syndrome

Sick sinus syndrome is generally associated with arteriosclerotic heart disease, although it is sometimes seen in rheumatic heart disease or other conditions. In the pediatric age group, sinus node dysfunction most commonly occurs in children with congenital heart disease following corrective cardiac surgery.[27]

The anatomic basis of sick sinus syndrome is fibrosis of the SA node, atrial muscle, AV node, and the conduction system. The most common clinical manifestations of sick sinus syndrome are syncope and chest pain,[28] which are associated with the following ECG findings:

1. Persistent spontaneous sinus bradycardia, not caused by drugs, and inappropriate for the physiologic circumstances (i.e., exercise, hypovolemia)
2. Sinus arrest with atrial or junctional escape rhythm
3. Paroxysmal supraventricular tachycardia, atrial fibrillation, or atrial flutter with episodes of alternating bradycardia and tachycardia (bradycardia–tachycardia syndrome); chronic atrial fibrillation with a slow ventricular response that is not drug induced
4. Combination of SA and AV conduction disturbances
5. Moderate or absent increases in heart rate in response to exercise or isoproterenol

More than one of these conditions can be recorded in the same patient on different occasions. Figure 5–17 represents a typical ECG finding in a patient with sick sinus syndrome.

The most important anesthetic consideration in sick sinus syndrome is the proper preoperative identification of the patient who has not been previously diagnosed. Any patient, especially an elderly patient, presenting with an unexplained sinus bradycardia and symptoms of syncope or chest pain should be evaluated before surgery. Long-term ECG monitoring, analysis of heart-rate response to stress testing or drugs, and detection of abnormal sinus node suppression by atrial pacing are most helpful diagnostically.

Permanent pacing is often required preopera-

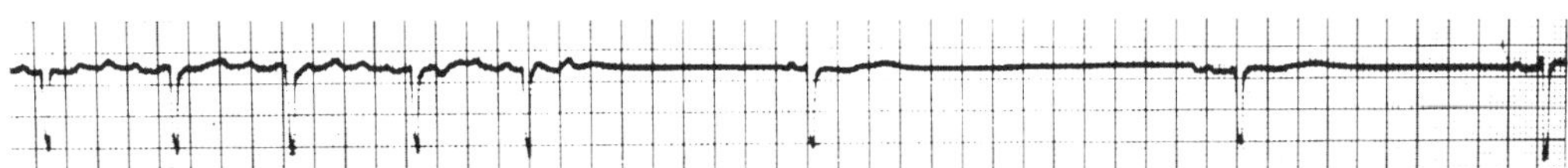

Fig. 5–17 Sick sinus syndrome. (Reprinted by permission from Phillips R, Feeney M (eds): The Cardiac Rhythms. WB Saunders, Philadelphia, 1973.)

tively to treat bradycardias and permit safe suppression of tachycardias with drugs such as digitalis and propranolol. If the condition presents itself intraoperatively in an undiagnosed patient, it may produce significant hemodynamic disturbance, requiring temporary transvenous or esophageal pacing.[29] Digitalis, β-adrenergic receptor blockers, and calcium channel blockers should be used cautiously in patients with the sick sinus syndrome.

PREEXCITATION

Preexcitation has been defined as a condition in which the ventricular myocardium is activated earlier than would be expected had the impulse reached the ventricle by way of the normal AV conduction system.[30] Early activation of the ventricle occurs because of a bypass tract from the atria to the ventricles. Three abnormal tracts have been defined anatomically and electrophysiologically: the bundle of Kent (most common), Mahain fibers, and James tract.[31]

Wolff–Parkinson–White (WPW) syndrome was first described in 1936. It has been documented that it is caused by a direct muscular connection between the atria and the ventricles via the bundle of Kent. This tract permits a very rapid depolarization rate, in the range of 300 beats/min, to be transmitted from the atria. In WPW syndrome, the ventricles are depolarized via two pathways: the accessory pathway and AV nodal pathway. During sinus rhythm, ventricular preexcitation may be permanently present or may alternate for varying periods of time with normal ventricular activation (normal conduction).

The ECG characteristics of the WPW syndrome include (1) a short PR interval of 0.11 seconds or less, (2) a wide QRS complex of greater than 0.10 seconds, (3) notching and slurring of the ascending limb of the QRS complex deflection (Δ waves), and (4) secondary changes in the ST segment and T waves (Fig. 5–18).

The PR interval is shortened because of rapid conduction through the anomalous pathway. The wide QRS complex is produced by the synchronous activation of the ventricle by an impulse passing through both the accessory pathway and the AV node (fusion beat). Most adults with WPW syndrome do not have associated heart disease. In the pediatric age group, however, one-third of those with WPW syndrome may have congenital heart disease (e.g., Ebstein's malformation or transposition of the great arteries). In contrast to WPW syndrome, patients with Mahain syndrome will show a normal PR interval and an abnormally wide QRS configuration. Patients with a James bundle will demonstrate a short PR interval and a normal QRS complex.

The WPW syndrome would be somewhat of an academic curiosity to the anesthesiologist if it were not for the accompanying high incidence of paroxysmal tachycardia (50 percent).[32] This type of paroxysmal tachycardia is almost invariably of supraventricular origin, with atrial and nodal tachycardias most commonly noted, followed by atrial fibrillation. Recurrent sustained supraventricular tachycardia over a long period may lead to congestive heart failure or myocardial ischemia. This is especially true of atrial fibrillation, which may be present with an unusually rapid ventricular rate.

Paroxysmal supraventricular tachycardia can be precipitated during anesthesia as a result of atrial ectopic beats (i.e., during intubation).[32] These ectopic beats are conducted downward through the AV node and returned to the atria through the accessory pathway, producing a paroxysmal tachycardia. Preexcitation may also be induced by vagal stimulation or by the administration of adrenergic drugs. In the presence of preexcitation, atropine or sympathomimetic drugs tend to enhance conductivity through the AV node. Therapy of supraventricular dysrhythmias in patients with WPW syndrome is directed to slowing the conduction through the bundle of Kent with drugs such as quinidine or procainamide. In a small percentage of patients, in whom the dysrhythmias are life threatening and cannot be controlled medically, surgical interruption of the anomalous pathways is warranted.

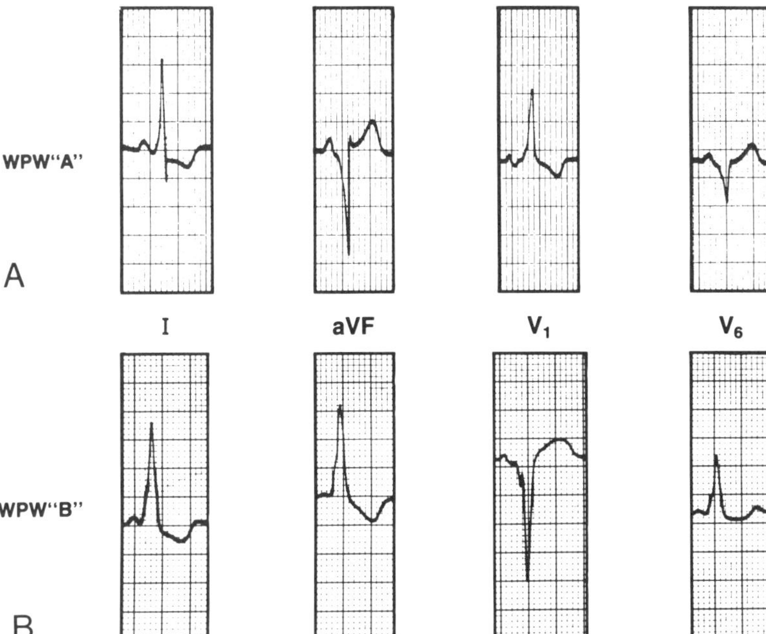

Fig. 5–18 Wolff–Parkinson–White syndrome. **(A)** Rosenbaum type A. R wave is the sole or largest deflection in V_1. **(B)** Rosenbaum type B. S or QS is the chief deflection in V_1. (Garson A Jr (ed): The Electrocardiogram in Infants and Children. Lea & Febiger, Philadelphia, 1983.)

LONG QT SYNDROME

The prolonged QT interval syndrome, also known as the Jervell–Lange–Neilson syndrome, consists of the triad of a prolonged QT interval, syncopal attacks due to ventricular fibrillation, and congenital deafness.[33] The otherwise identical condition without deafness is called the Romano Ward syndrome. Patients with a prolonged QT syndrome are at obvious risk of developing serious dysrhythmias during any period of stress or emotional disturbance, including surgery and anesthesia. Induction of anesthesia or the use of drugs such as epinephrine may precipitate ventricular tachycardia or fibrillation.[34]

Typical ECG findings include prolongation of the QT interval, which may be associated with abnormal or alternating T waves. The upper limit for the duration of the normal QT interval corrected for heart rate (QT_c) is 0.44 seconds. The main factor in the production of these dysrhythmias is a delay in ventricular repolarization, resulting in an increased vulnerability to the R-on-T phenomenon.

This syndrome should be differentiated from QT interval prolongation caused by (1) metabolic abnormalities such as hypocalcemia or hypokalemia; (2) drugs including quinidine, disopyramide, and phenothiazines; or (3) a prolapsed mitral valve or myocardial infarction.

Symptomatic patients with a prolonged QT syndrome are treated with β-adrenergic receptor blockers or phenytoin. For patients who do not respond to medical therapy, left-sided cervicothoracic sympathetic ganglionectomy has been proposed.[34]

REFERENCES

1. Moe GK, Mendes C: Physiologic basis of premature beats and sustained tachycardia. N Engl J Med 288:250, 1973
2. Chung EK: Principles of Cardiac Arrhythmias. Williams & Wilkins, Baltimore, 1977

3. Cranefield PF, Wit AL, Hoffman BF: Genesis of cardiac arrhythmias. Circulation 47:190, 1973
4. Rosen KM: A-V nodal reentrance: An unexpected mechanism of paroxysmal tachycardia in a patient with preexcitation. Circulation 47:1267, 1973
5. Friedman HC: Diagnostic Electrocardiography and Vectorcardiography. McGraw-Hill, New York, 1971
6. Lipman BS, Dunn M, Massie E: Clinical Electrocardiography. Year Book Medical Publishers, Chicago, 1981
7. Phillip P, Feen T: The Cardiac rhythms—Systematic Approach to Interpretation. WB Saunders, Philadelphia, 1980
8. Holter N: New method for heart studies. Science 134:1214, 1961
9. Harrison DC, Fitzgerald B, Winkle R: Contribution of ambulatory electrocardiogram monitoring to antiarrhythmic management. Am J Cardiol 41(6):996, 1978
10. Bleifer S, Bleifer D, Hausman D: Diagnosis of occult arrhythmias by Holter electrocardiography. Prog Cardiovasc Dis 16:569, 1974
11. Berber EG, Scherlag BM, El Sherif NI: The His Purkinje electrocardiograms in man. Circulation 54(2):219, 1974
12. Gillete P, Garson A: Pediatric Cardiac Dysrhythmia—Clinical Cardiology. Grune & Stratton, Orlando, Florida, 1986
13. Lipman BSS, Dunn M, Massie F: Clinical Electrocardiography. Year Book Medical Publishers, Chicago, 1984
14. Narula OS, Sherlag BJ: Atrioventricular block. Am J Med 40:141, 1971
15. Aichter M, Damaks AN, Carota HR: Clinical uses of His bundle electrocardiography. Am Heart J 91:660, 1976
16. Fisher YD: Role of electrophysiologic testing in the diagnosis and treatment of patients with known and suspected bradycardias and tachycardias. Prog Cardiovasc Dis 24:25, 1981
17. Waldo AL, Gawes NT: The cardiac conduction system. Electrophysiological studies during open heart surgery. Arch Intern Med 135:411, 1975
18. Kaplan JA (ed): Cardiac Anesthesia. Grune & Stratton, Orlando, Florida, 1979
19. Sprague DH, Mandel SD: Paroxysmal supraventricular tachycardia during anesthesia. Anesthesiology 46:75, 1977
20. Bellet SP: Essentials of Cardiac Arrhythmias. Diagnosis and Management. WB Saunders, Philadelphia, 1972
21. Hudron LD, Kurt TL, Petty TL, et al: Arrhythmias associated with acute respiratory failure in patients with chronic airway obstruction. Chest 63:661, 1973
22. Abildskov JA, Millar K, Burgeosi MJ: Atrial fibrillation. Am J Cardiol 28:263, 1971
23. Pratila MA, Pratilas V: Anesthetic agents and cardiac electromechanical activity. Anesthesiology 49:338, 1978
24. Ziper DP, Fish C: Premature AV junctional contractions. Arch Intern Med 128:663, 1971
25. Stevenson RL, Rogers MC: Electrocardiographic changes. Semin Anesth 1:207, 1982
26. Kartor JA, Horowitz LN, Harken AH, et al: Clinical electrophysiology of ventricular tachycardia. N Engl J Med 304:1004, 1981
27. Sobel B, Braunwald E: Cardiac Dysrhythmias. p. 432. In Harrison S, Thorn GW (eds.): Principles of Internal Medicine. McGraw-Hill, New York, 1977
28. Ziper D: Specific arrhythmias: Diagnosis and treatment. p. 683. In Braunwald E (ed): Heart Disease. WB Saunders, Philadelphia, 1984
29. Pratila M, Pratilas V: Sick sinus syndrome manifested during anesthesia. Anesthesiology 44:432, 1976
30. Durrer D, Schuilenberg S: Pre-excitation revisited. Am J Cardiol 25:690, 1976
31. Lipman BS, Dunn M, Massis E: Clinical Electrocardiography. Year Book Medical Publishers, Chicago, 1984
32. Sadowsui AR, Moyers JR: Anesthetic management of the Wolff–Parkinson–White syndrome. Anesthesiology 51:553, 1979
33. Schwartz PJ, Perith M, Mallan A: The long QT syndrome. Am Heart J 89:378, 1975
34. Owitz S, Pratilas V, Pratila M, Dimich I: Anesthetic considerations in the prolonged QT interval. Can Anaesth Soc 26:50, 1979

6

Preoperative Diagnosis of Myocardial Ischemia

Barry Feinberg, M.D.

Atherosclerotic coronary artery disease (CAD) produces a decrease in blood flow to cardiac tissue that can result in ischemia accompanied by derangements in depolarization and repolarization of the myocardium. The presence of recognizable signs and symptoms of ischemia depends on the myocardial oxygen demand, degree of coronary occlusion, collateral circulation of the myocardium, and preexisting disease. It is therefore possible for a patient to have significant CAD without demonstrating ECG changes.[1] Thus, it is always important to correlate the patient's clinical history and physical examination with interpretation of the ECG. It is the purpose of this chapter to guide the anesthesiologist in the preoperative detection of CAD through ECG analysis.

CORONARY ARTERY DISEASE

Discussions of the ECG diagnosis of CAD typically separate the changes seen into three categories which correlate with the severity of myocardial disease. In order of increasing severity, these changes are (1) ischemia, (2) injury, and (3) infarction, with infarction being the stage of irreversible damage to the myocardium.

The coronary arteries originate at the root of the aorta and divide into vessels supplying the epicardial surface of the heart (Fig. 6–1). Penetrating branches supply the inner myocardial cells and course through the thickness of the ventricle to form a plexus of vessels in the subendocardium. These vessels are often tortuous and offer less flow to the endocardium than to the epicardium. Coupled with the anatomic shortcomings of the endocardial circulation is the high intraventricular pressure that further impedes the flow of blood to the endocardium. Therefore, coronary insufficiency is usually first seen in the subendocardium.[2]

ISCHEMIA

Coronary insufficiency causes a delayed repolarization of ischemic cells. Normal repolarization is directed from the epicardium to the endocardium; thus, as cells in the endocardium become ischemic, there is an unopposed increase in magnitude of the forces of repolarization and resultant tall, upright T waves may be seen. With transmural ischemia (implying epicardial ischemia), there is reversal of the direction of repolarization and recovery will proceed from endocardium to epicardium in the area of injury. This causes an inversion of the T wave seen in the recordings of the corresponding electrodes (Figs. 6–2 and 6–3). In leads with upright QRS complexes, the T wave will be inverted; and in leads with inverted QRS complexes, the T waves will be upright. T-wave changes similar to those of ischemia have been

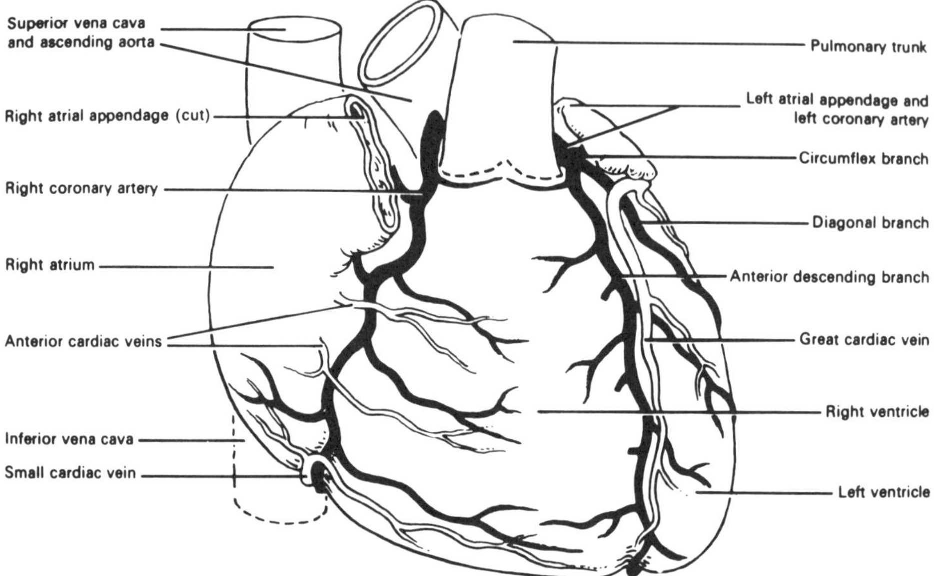

Fig. 6–1 Principal arteries and veins on the anterior surface of the heart. Part of the right atrial appendage has been resected to expose the origin of the right coronary artery from the right (anterior) coronary aortic sinus. The left coronary artery arises from the left (left posterior) coronary aortic sinus and appears on the anterior surface between the root of the pulmonary trunk and the left atrial appendage. In this case it terminates in three branches: the anterior descending (interventricular) and circumflex branches, which are constant, and one diagonal branch. (Walmsley R, Watson H: Clinical Anatomy of the Heart. Churchill Livingstone, Edinburgh, 1978.)

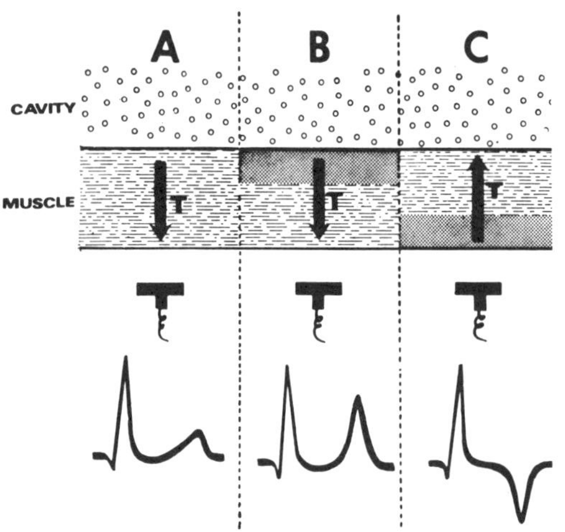

Fig. 6–2 Diagrammatic illustration of **(A)** the normal endocardial to epicardial T-wave vector, **(B)** the T-wave vector of subendocardial ischemia, **(C)** the T-wave vector of subepicardial ischemia. (Schamroth L: The ECG of Coronary Artery Disease. Blackwell, Oxford, 1984.)

described in other conditions, including healthy athletes.[3,4] The T wave is normally upright in leads I, II, and V_3 to V_6, inverted in aVR, and variable in the rest of the leads. The height of the T wave is normally up to 10 mm in the precordial leads and 5 mm in the standard limb leads. Alterations in T-wave morphology, especially in the precordial leads, can be seen with drug effects, ischemia, electrolyte disorders, and other situations (Table 6–1). Ischemia may also affect the shape of the T wave as well as its position and height. The normal T wave is asymetrical (Fig. 6–4), and ischemia may result in symmetry of the T wave.

MYOCARDIAL INJURY

The second degree of severity of coronary insufficiency is that of myocardial injury. There are two currents of injury: a diastolic current

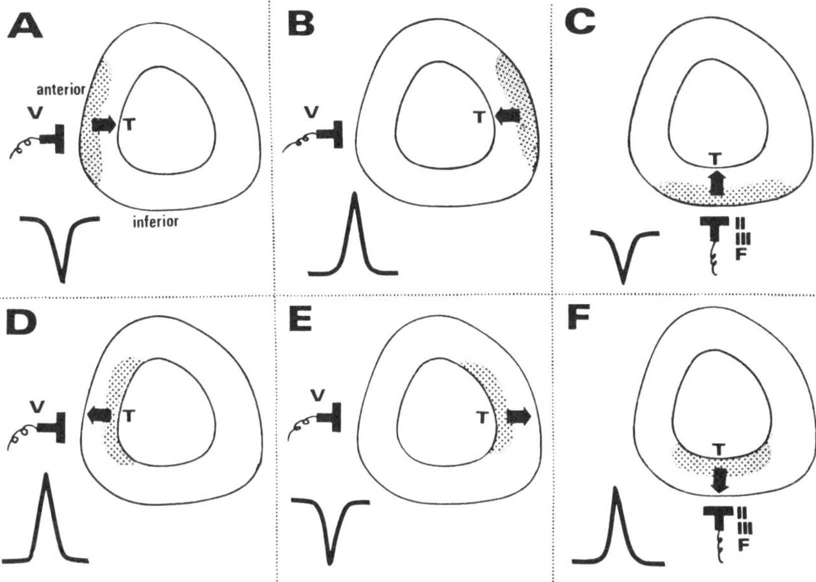

Fig. 6–3 Diagrams illustrating the theoretical direction of the T-wave vectors with **(A–C)** epicardial and **(D–F)** endocardial ischemia of the **(A,D)** anterior, **(C,F)** inferior, and **(B,E)** posterior wall of the heart. (Schamroth L: The ECG of Coronary Artery Disease. Blackwell, Oxford, 1984.)

and a systolic current. The diastolic current of injury is the flow of electricity between the tissue with normal resting potential and tissue with an altered resting potential. This current causes TP-segment changes, which are not detected by standard 12-lead ECGs. The systolic current of injury is caused by a flow of current toward the injured zone that leads to a shift of the ST segment that is impossible to distinguish from the oppositely directed TP segment shift seen with the diastolic current of injury.[5–8] When injury occurs in the subendocardium, there is a slight delay of depolarization and increase in the speed of repolarization.[9] This causes a relative positive charge of the subendocardium compared with the epicardium, as well as a flow of the systolic current of injury from epicardium to endocardium, resulting in ST-segment depression in the corresponding leads recorded from these areas. By contrast, with transmural or subepicardial injury, the flow of systolic current is from the endocardium to epicardium and the ST segment is elevated in the corresponding lead (Fig. 6–5). As ischemia progresses, calcium ions bind to injured cell membranes and prevent flux of potassium ions from the cell, thereby limiting the systolic current of injury which accounts for the disappearance of the ST segment changes with time.[10]

Table 6–1. Differential Diagnosis of Abnormal T Waves in Precordial Leads

Diagnosis	T-Wave Picture
Anterior wall subendocardial ischemia	Tall
Posterior wall subendocardial ischemia	Inverted
Posterior wall epicardial ischemia	Tall
Anterior wall epicardial ischemia	Inverted
Hyperkalemia	Tall
Acute pericarditis	Tall
Healthy athletic vagotonic patients	Tall
Disorders of left ventricular diastolic overload	Tall
CVA pattern (acute head injury)	Tall

CVA, cerebrovascular accident.

The ECG can be normal in the presence of CAD with myocardial ischemia or injury or appear to be abnormal with signs suggestive of ischemia when no coronary artery disease is present. The assumption that CAD is absent because of a normal ECG is as much an error as the misinterpretation of nonspecific ECG

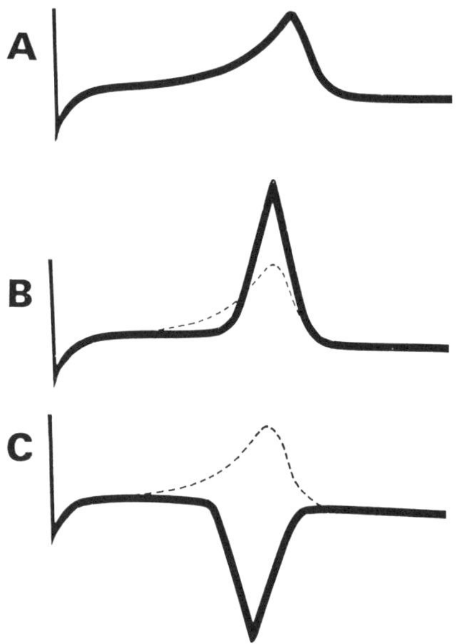

Fig. 6–4 Diagrams illustrating **(A)** the normal ST segment and T wave and **(B, C)** the T wave of myocardial ischemia. (Schamroth L: The ECG of Coronary Artery Disease. Blackwell, Oxford, 1984.)

changes to infer the presence of CAD. Fifty to 70 percent of patients with a history of stable angina pectoris will have a normal ECG if it is taken while they are not experiencing angina.[11] With a single normal ECG and the history of angina, it is possible to miss subtle changes in the electrical patterns of depolarization and/or repolarization. The use of serial ECGs and the availability of previous ECGs for comparison can prove valuable in making the diagnosis of myocardial ischemia or old injury.

When evaluating ST-segment depression, certain points should be considered. First, the magnitude of depression should be greater than 1 mm or 0.1 mV on a standard ECG recording. This value has been chosen as a compromise between the sensitivity in the criteria to detect ischemia and the specificity needed to avoid frequent false-positive indications of ischemia. Second, the angle of the ST-segment depression is important to consider in making the diagnosis

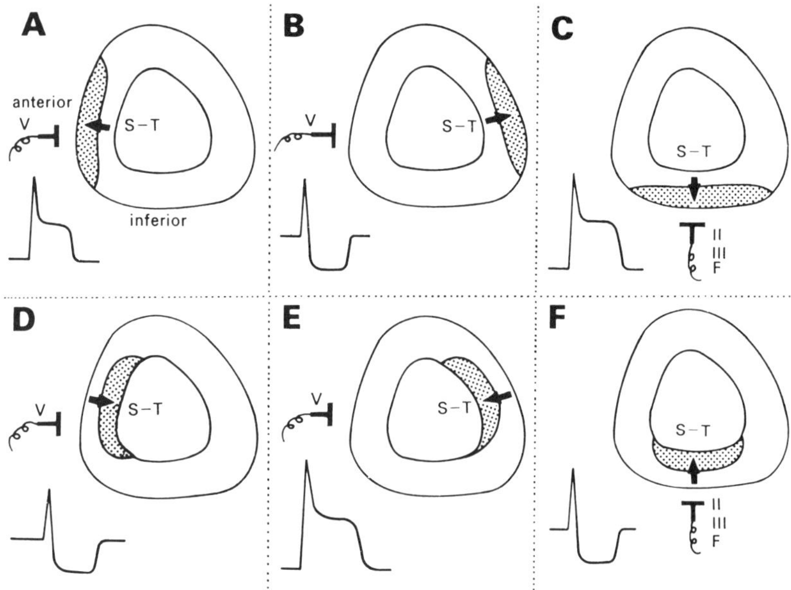

Fig. 6–5 Diagrams illustrating the theoretical direction of the ST-segment vectors with **(A–C)** subepicardial and **(D–F)** subendocardial injury of the **(A,D)** anterior, **(C,F)** inferior, and **(B,E)** posterior walls of the heart. (Schamroth L: The ECG of Coronary Artery Disease. Blackwell, Oxford, 1984.)

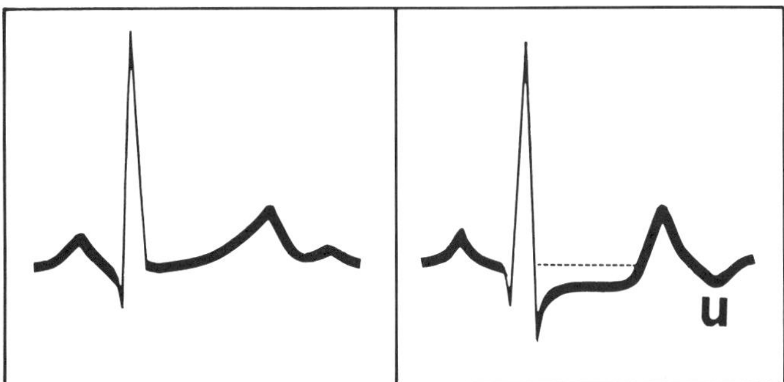

Fig. 6–6 Normal and ischemic ST segments.

of ischemia. The most common pattern of ST-segment depression with ischemia is called plane depression, a horizontal segment that merges sharply with the T wave (Fig. 6–6). ST depression can also be seen with other conditions including conduction defects, electrolyte disorders, and drug effects, thus emphasizing the need for clinical correlation.

MYOCARDIAL INFARCTION

Infarction of myocardial tissue is the third and most severe manifestation of CAD. The vast majority of infarcts are located in the left ventricle, although inferior and anteroseptal ones may involve portions of the right ventricle. Atrial infarctions and isolated right ventricular (RV) infarctions are considered relatively rare. The diagnosis of RV infarction is difficult because of the minimal contribution of the right ventricle to the electrical forces that comprise the ECG.

In making the diagnosis of a myocardial infarction from the ECG, three questions arise: Is there an infarction?, When did it occur?, and What is its general location? Determination of the age of an infarction is dependent on the availability of previous ECGs or association of electrical changes with a strong clinical history. In the absence of this information, the dating of an infarction is impossible unless the acute ST-T-wave changes of injury are observed.

The diagnosis of a myocardial infarction without the characteristic ECG sign of a pattern of injury in the ST segments is generally made by evaluation of QRS abnormalities (Fig. 6–7). The value of the Q wave in diagnosing a

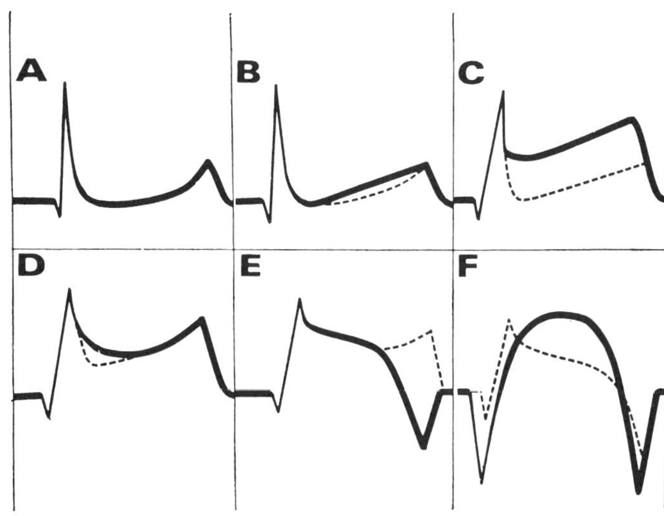

Fig. 6–7 Diagrams illustrating the evolution of the infarction pattern from normal **(A)**, through various stages of the hyperacute phase **(B–E)**, to the fully evolved phase **(F)**. (Schamroth L: The ECG of Coronary Artery Disease. Blackwell, Oxford, 1984.)

myocardial infarction continues to be an area of controversy. Bayley and LaDue,[12] in a classic experiment in 1944, occluded coronary arteries and induced new Q-wave formation. Subsequent studies confirmed this finding and also demonstrated the reversibility of the process. These findings suggest that an abnormal Q wave (defined as greater than 0.03 seconds in duration) is a reflection of myocardial ischemia, but is not synonymous with necrosis. Horan et al.[13] found that the presence of an abnormal Q wave (greater than 0.03 seconds) made the correct diagnosis of myocardial infarction, as verified by autopsy in 79 percent of their patients. This rate fell to 74 percent in the presence of a right bundle branch block (RBBB), 67 percent with complete left bundle branch block (LBBB), and 57 percent with incomplete LBBB.[14] Furthermore, it was found that (1) with normal conduction, abnormal Q waves that were isolated to either leads V_1–V_4 (anteroseptal) or leads II, III, and AVF (inferior) had a false-positive rate of 46 percent, and (2) with normal conduction, abnormal Q waves in leads V_5–V_6 (lateral) or Q waves found in a combination of more than one ECG zone had a false-positive rate of only 4 percent.

It is classically described that the presence of a QS deflection is the ''pattern of necrosis'' and a sign of irreversible damage (Fig. 6–8).[12,15] When an area of myocardium becomes necrotic, no electrical force is generated and no current flows toward the surface electrode, resulting in production of a negative deflection on the ECG over the distribution of the necrosis.

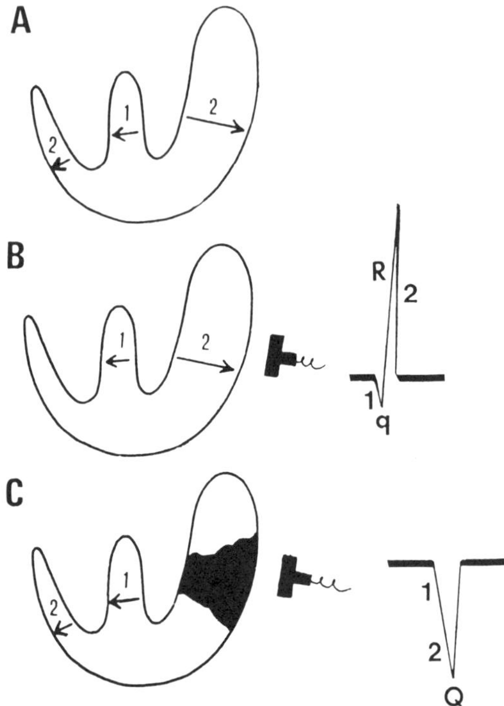

Fig. 6–8 Diagrammatic representation of normal ventricular activation **(A,B)** as reflected by a qR complex in a lead orientated to the left ventricle, and the ventricular activation associated with transmural necrosis, as reflected by a QS complex in a lead orientated to the left ventricle **(C)**. (Schamroth L: The ECG of Coronary Artery Disease. Blackwell, Oxford, 1984.)

The process of localizing myocardial infarctions by ECG analysis is imprecise, but it is possible to identify the principal area or areas of infarction.[15] Electrocardiographic changes indicating infarction are evident in the leads that face the injured zone of myocardium, while reciprocal changes are seen in leads opposite the injury. Thus, anteroseptal infarctions show QS deflections or abnormal Q waves in leads V_1,V_2, and occasionally V_3 (Fig. 6–9); anterior myocardial infarctions have QS deflections or abnormal Q waves in leads V_2, V_3, and V_4 (Fig. 6–10); and anterolateral infarctions have abnormal Q waves in leads I, II, V_5, and V_6 (Fig. 6–11). Extensive anterolateral infarctions may have abnormal Q waves in lead I and all the precordial leads. Inferior (diaphragmatic) infarctions have abnormal Q waves in leads II, III, and AVF (Fig. 6–12).

Posterior lateral infarctions have abnormally tall and/or wide R waves in lead V_1 and abnormal Q waves in leads I and V_6, while true posterior myocardial infarctions have low RR^1 deflections or RSR^1 deflections in leads V_1 and V_2 (Fig. 6–13). An inferior and lateral infarction with posterior extension is shown in Figure 6–14. Right ventricular infarctions characteristically show abnormal Q waves in leads II, III, and aVF and can be very hard to distinguish from

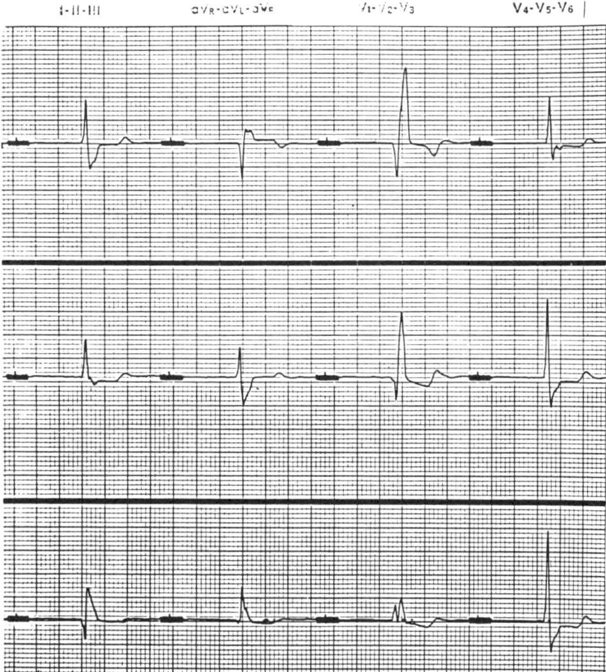

Fig. 6–9 Anteroseptal infarction with Q waves in V_1 and V_2. A right bundle branch block pattern is also present.

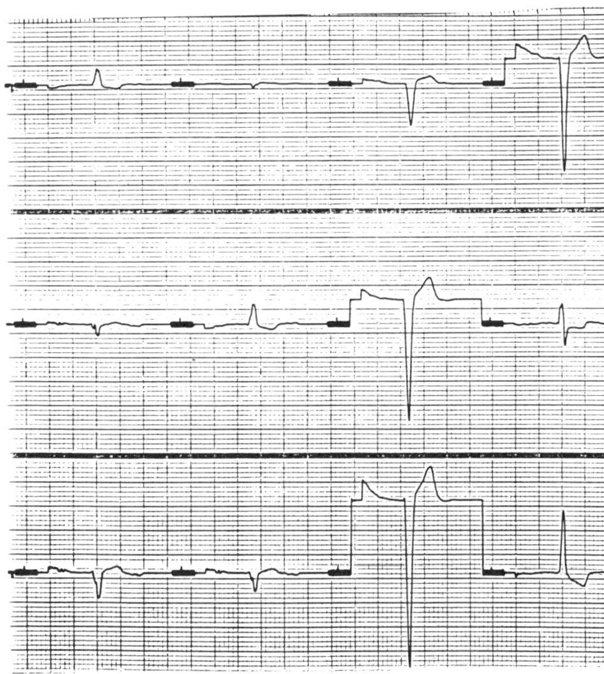

Fig. 6–10 Anteroseptal-to-anterior infarction with Q waves in V_1 to V_4 in a patient with atrial fibrillation and diffuse ST-segment abnormalities.

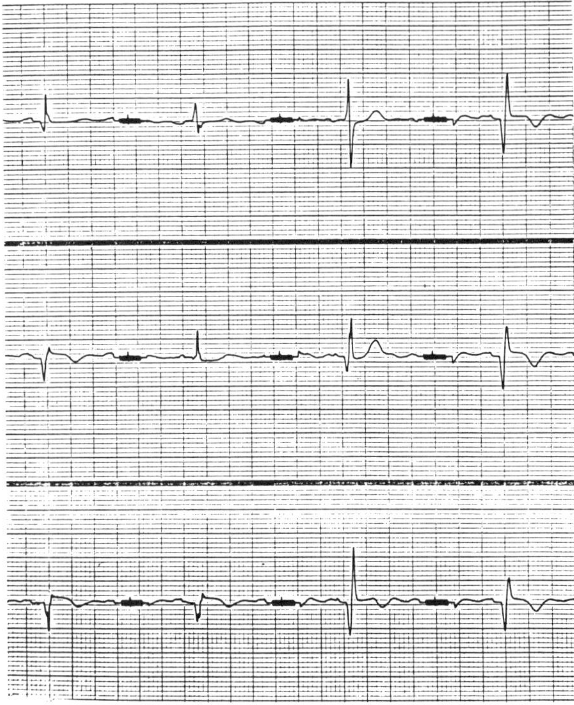

Fig. 6–11 Anterolateral and inferior myocardial infarction in the same patient with Q waves in I, V_5, and V_6 and II, III, and aVF.

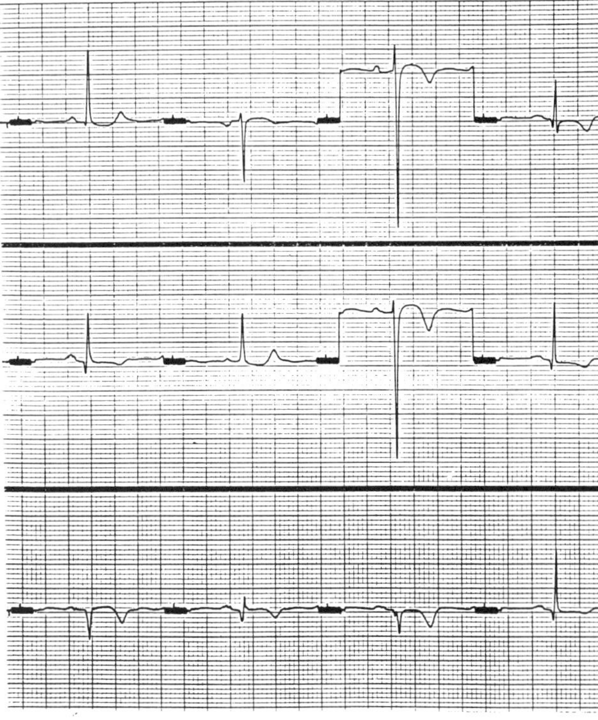

Fig. 6–12 Inferior wall myocardial infarction with Q waves in II, III, and aVF. Also anterior ischemia and possible infarction are seen in the precordial leads.

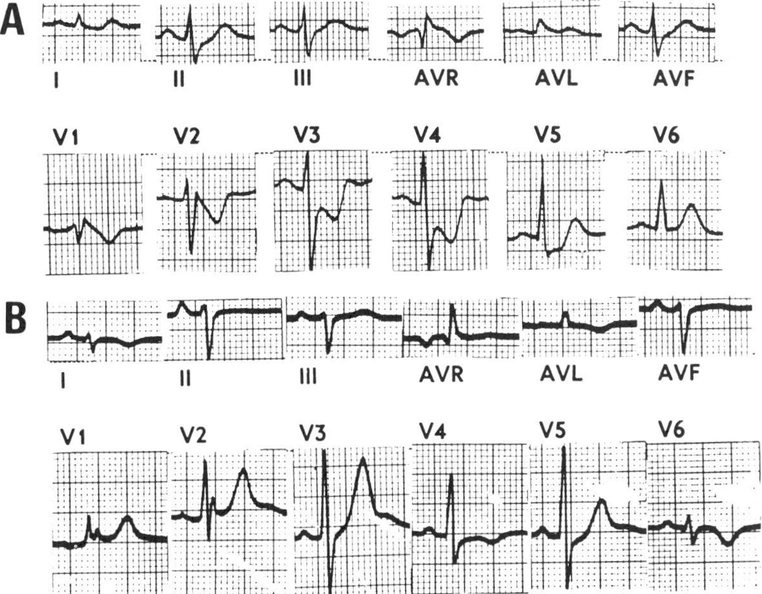

Fig. 6–13 Posterior wall infarction **(A)** during the hyperacute phase and **(B)** 24 hours later. (Schamroth L: The ECG of Coronary Artery Disease. Blackwell, Oxford, 1984.)

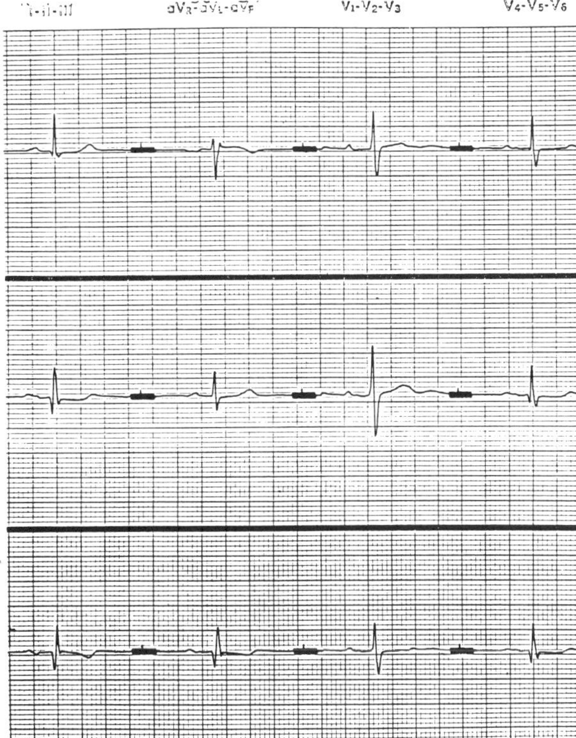

Fig. 6–14 Inferior and lateral infarction with posterior extension.

inferior myocardial infarctions. Atrial infarctions produce shifts in the PT segment, but this is generally obscured by the greater ventricular electrical forces that occur at the same time.

The ischemic cells may alter conduction, causing late activation of adjacent normal areas of myocardium. QRS complexes have been shown to be wider in most cases of myocardial infarction.[16,17] These delays in conduction associated with ischemia or infarction may predispose to reentrant dysrhythmias and markedly confuse the ECG diagnosis of ischemia. Septal infarction is most often associated with the development of bundle branch block (Fig. 6–9), but these conduction defects have been reported with infarcts of all ventricular zones.[18] Left bundle branch block is an ECG change that confounds the diagnosis of infarction; when trying to make the diagnosis of myocardial infarction in the presence of LBBB, previous ECGs are very helpful. The appearance of new Q waves in leads I, aVL, or V_6, notching of the S waves in V_3 or V_4, or decreased R-wave amplitude in the precordial leads are findings suggestive of myocardial infarction. In addition, the acute ST changes of a myocardial infarction are not disguised by the presence of a left bundle branch block.[19] In an uncomplicated LBBB, the ST segment and T wave are usually in the opposite direction from the QRS complex, while with acute infarction the current of injury will cause a rise in the ST segment that is diagnostic (Fig. 6–15). In the presence of RBBB, the basic deflections of the QRS complex remain unchanged; therefore, the diagnosis of a myocardial infarction should not be obscured by the RBBB pattern (Fig. 6–16). However, the development of a new RBBB may be an indication of myocardial ischemia. The ST- and T-wave vectors associated with RBBB are normally diverted opposite from the terminal QRS vector. Ischemic changes affecting these vectors will cause the development of symmetric T waves and a redirection of the ST-T-wave vector in the same direction as the terminal QRS vector.

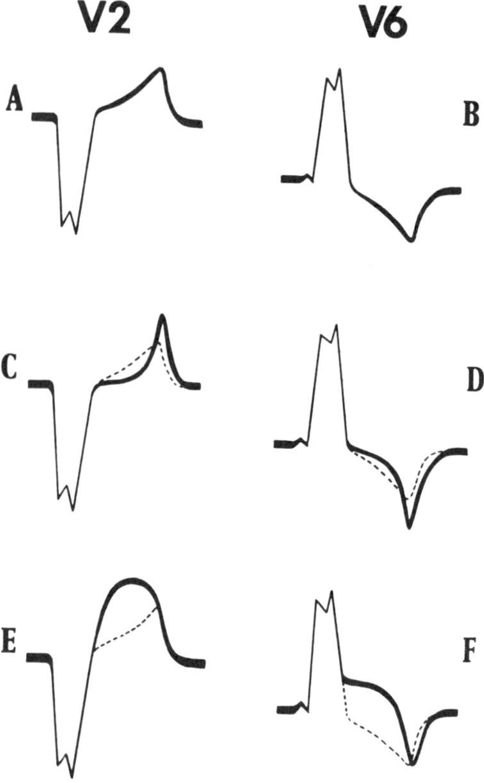

Fig. 6–15 **(A,B)** Normal QRST configuration in left bundle branch block. **(C,D)** Effect of myocardial ischemia on the ST segment and T wave in left bundle branch block. **(E,F)** Effect of anterior wall myocardial infarction on the ST segment and T wave in left bundle branch block. (Schamroth L: The ECG of Coronary Artery Disease. Blackwell, Oxford, 1984.)

AMBULATORY ELECTROCARDIOGRAM

The ambulatory ECG is a valuable clinical aid in the diagnosis and management of cardiac dysrhythmias. The use of the ambulatory ECG (i.e., Holter monitor) for detecting and monitoring of ischemia has historically been fraught with technical problems. Changes in the ST segment may occur with changes in body position, medications, or as a result of factors other than CAD. Different studies have reported various incidences of statistical false positive and false negative results, depending on the criteria

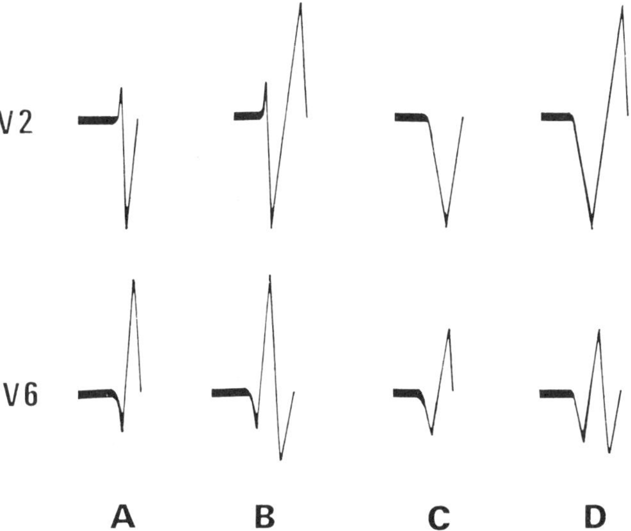

Fig. 6–16 Diagrams illustrating **(A)** normal QRS complexes in leads V_2 and V_6, **(B)** the effect of right bundle branch block, **(C)** the effect of anteroseptal myocardial infarction on normal intraventricular conduction, **(D)** the effect of anteroseptal myocardial infarction in the presence of right bundle branch block. (Schamroth L: The ECG of Coronary Artery Disease. Blackwell, Oxford, 1984.)

used for diagnosis of ischemia and upon the patient population studied.[20,21]

The continuous ambulatory ECG may prove useful in detection of myocardial ischemia in the future as the technology is improved, as its use in patients with CAD has demonstrated transient episodes of ST-segment changes that would have been missed.[22–26]

Figure 6–17 is a tracing of lead V_5 from an ambulatory ECG taken during an episode of chest pain and shows depression of the ST segment. The vast majority of ST changes during Holter monitoring are not associated with episodes of angina pectoris, but are electrically indistinguishable from ST-segment changes associated with angina.[24–26] These silent ST-segment changes have been shown to be associated with increases in left ventricular (LV) filling pressure and decreases in indices of myocardial contractility,[27,28] as well as to correlate with the severity of CAD.[29] The potential value of continuous ambulatory ECG monitoring of ischemic ST-segment and T-wave changes is obvious in the preoperative diagnosis of CAD, and new techniques such as computer analysis of Holter tracings will expand its role.[30]

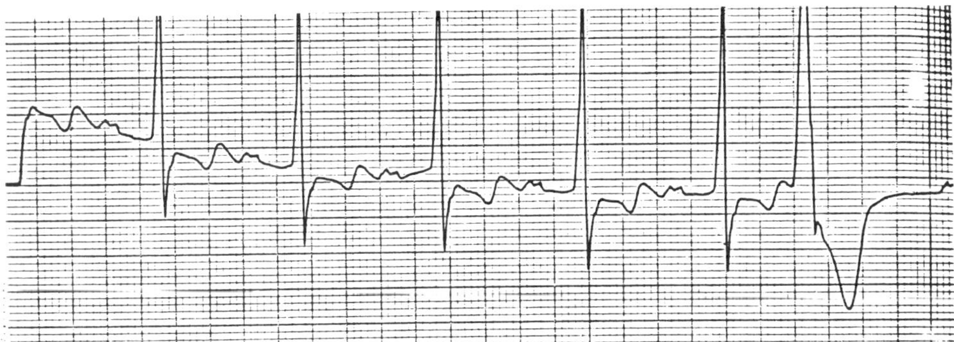

Fig. 6–17 ST-segment depression on lead V_5 of an ambulatory ECG during an episode of angina. Premature ventricular contractions (PVCs) are also seen.

THE EXERCISE ELECTROCARDIOGRAM

The diagnosis of ischemic heart disease is often difficult to make with the standard 12-lead ECG if the patient is not having an episode of angina at the time of the recording. The exercise ECG was introduced as a means of stimulating an episode of relative coronary insufficiency in order to determine the presence or absence of ischemia and as a means of quantitating the degree of ischemia by observing the stimulation necessary to provoke the ischemia.[31] Current indications for exercise stress testing are (1) to aid in predicting the presence of CAD, (2) to quantitate the severity of the disease, (3) to evaluate medical and surgical therapy, and (4) to assess the patient's ability to handle increased myocardial stress and various fitness programs.

The exercise ECG has been limited in its use due to numerous criticisms. As a screening test for CAD, its predictive value is determined by the prevalence of the disease in the population being studied, and there is a high incidence of false-positive results in asymptomatic patients. Exercise-induced ECG changes can also be seen in patients with hypertension, primary myocardial disease, valvular disease, hyperventilation, Wolff–Parkinson–White syndrome, digitalis, electrolyte disturbances, and anemia. When a population suffering from chest pain is studied, a higher prediction rate will result than in asymptomatic patients. A positive test in adult males who have a history of chest pain has a predictive value of 70 percent for CAD. This value increases with increasing severity of disease.[32,33] A positive response in women with similar histories has less of a predictive value than in men.[34]

Despite these limitations, the exercise stress test remains the primary means of noninvasive evaluation of patients for CAD. The low incidence of complications, ease of performance, low cost, and quality of data obtained have popularized its use. Contraindications of both a relative and absolute nature are listed in Table 6–2. Complications must be expected from a test that provokes coronary insufficiency; in a large study by Rochmis and Blackburn,[32] a morbidity rate of 0.01 percent and a mortality rate of 0.02 percent were reported.

Table 6–2. Contraindication to Exercise Testing

A. Absolute contraindications
  1. Severe acute disease, especially acute myocardial infarction (within the first 2 weeks), myocarditis, recent pulmonary or systemic embolus, thrombophlebitis
  2. Ventricular tachycardia and other dangerous arrhythmias (multifocal ventricular activity)
  3. Severe associated disease such as pulmonary or renal failure, orthopedic or neurologic impairment or a systemic infection
  4. Dissecting or enlarging aneurysm

B. Relative contraindications
  1. Rapidly increasing or unstable angina pectoris
  2. Uncontrolled or high-rate arrhythmias
  3. Repetitive or frequent ventricular ectopic activity
  4. Severe myocardial or valvular obstructive syndromes (aortic stenosis, mitral stenosis, tetralogy of Fallot, or hypertrophic subaortic stenosis)
  5. Circulatory insufficiency (congestive heart failure)
  6. Ventricular aneurysm
  7. Right-to-left shunts (Eisenmenger's complex, transposition of great vessels, truncus arteriosus, or tetralogy of Fallot)
  8. Untreated severe pulmonary or systemic hypertension
  9. Severe conduction disturbance (complete heart block or unstable AV conduction)
  10. Uncontrolled metabolic disease (diabetes, thyrotoxicosis, myxedema)

C. Not contraindications
  1. Stable angina pectoris
  2. Healed myocardial infarction (more than 2 weeks)
  3. Past history of supraventricular or ventricular arrhythmia
  4. Conduction disturbances such as chronic bundle branch block, left or right
  5. Most chronic valvular cardiac disease
  6. Left-to-right shunts
  7. Nonspecific abnormalities of the electrocardiographic T wave and/or S-T segment
  8. Clinical or ECG evidence of ventricular hypertrophy

(Rochmis P, Blackburn H: Exercise tests: A survey of procedures of safety, and litigation experience in approximately 170,000 tests. JAMA 217:1061, 1971. Copyright 1971 American Medical Association.)

Displacement of the ST segment with ischemia induced by exercise testing is of three major types (Fig. 6–18). In type I changes, with early ischemia, J-point depression and upsloping of the ST segment into the T wave is seen. As ischemia progresses, the J-point depression increases and the ST segment flattens or becomes downsloping. Termination of the exercise causes prompt improvement in the ST

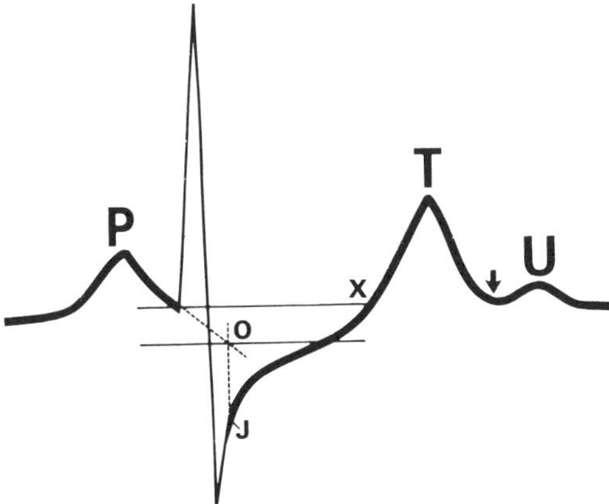

Fig. 6–18 Diagram illustrating methods of measuring (1) true and false ST-segment depression, and (2) the degree of horizontality of the ST segment. (1) The line of the sloping PR segment is continued until it meets, at point 0, a vertical line drawn from the junction of the QRS complex and ST segment. Distance O–J indicates the true amount of ST-segment depression. (2) A horizontal line drawn from the beginning of the QRS deflection is continued until it meets the T wave at point X. Distance Q–X is expressed as a percentage of the Q–T interval (measured from the beginning of the QRS complex to the end of the T wave at the arrow). Q–X is greater than 50 percent of Q–T in most true positive tests. (Schamroth L: The ECG of Coronary Artery Disease. Blackwell, Oxford, 1984.)

segments. In type II ST-segment changes, the progression of change is similar to type I, except that ischemic changes continue into the postexercise period, with a worsening of the ECG picture. The type III changes are ST-segment elevations caused by either Prinzmetal's spastic angina with resultant localized transmural ischemia or by severe transmural injury. J-point depression is seen in normal patients during exercise, although rarely more than 2 mm.[33–35] To differentiate these changes from true ischemia, the protocol of stress induction is continued to higher stages in order to elicit more diagnostic changes.

During the stress test, the patient's ECG, blood pressure, and physical appearance are continuously monitored. This monitoring should continue into the postexercise period for 5 to 10 minutes or until the heart rate returns to baseline.[36]

When evaluating the results of an exercise ECG, it is important to observe the time to onset of ST changes, persistence of ST changes at the cessation of exercise, blood pressure and heart rate at time of ischemia, ECG leads in which ischemia occurred, and the degree of ST-segment change. Significant information about the patient's cardiac reserve as well as information about which lead to monitor during surgery can be ascertained from careful evaluation of the stress ECG. A normal response of the blood pressure during exercise is an increase in systolic pressure as exercise intensity increases. Diastolic pressure falls in young patients, while in older patients it may rise or remain the same indicating that the fall in systemic vascular resistance does not compensate for the increase in cardiac output induced by stress.[35] Heart rate responds to exercise in a manner similar to blood pressure. With increased exercise, there is an increase in rate, since tachycardia is the principal means of increasing cardiac output during stress. Presuming that the patient is in sinus rhythm, a lower heart rate than expected is seen in patients taking medication, such as β-adrenergic blockers, and a higher rate in patients with poor cardiovascular performance. Rate-pressure product calculations, although not ideal, can provide a guide to the ischemic threshold and exercise capacity of the patient.[36]

REFERENCES

1. Martinez-Rios MA, Boto Da Costa BC, Cecena-Selender IA, Gensini GG: Normal electrocardiogram in the presence of severe coronary artery disease. Am J Cardiol 25:320, 1970
2. Elliot WC, Gorlin R: The coronary circulation, myocardial ischemia, and angina pectoris. I and II. Mod Concepts Cardiovasc Dis 35:111, 1975
3. Hall RJ, Gibson RV: Anterior T-wave changes in the ECG of an athlete. Br Med J 27:38, 1978
4. Hanne-Paparo N: T-wave abnormalities in the electrocardiograms of top-ranking athletes without demonstrable organic heart disease. Am Heart J 81:743, 1971

5. Cohen DH, Kauffman LA: Magnetic determination of the relationship between the ST segment shift and the injury current produced by coronary artery occlusion. Circ Res 36:414, 1975
6. Samson WE, Scher AM: Mechanism of ST segment alteration during acute myocardial injury. Circ Res 8:780, 1960
7. Vicent GM, Abildskov JA, Burgess MJ: Mechanisms of ischemic ST segment displacement. Evaluation by direct current recordings. Circulation 56:559, 1977
8. Elharrar V, Zipes DP: Cardiac electrophysiologic alteration during myocardial ischemia. Am J Physiol Heart Circ Physiol 2:329, 1977
9. Case RB, Nasser MG, Crampton RS: Biochemical aspects of early myocardial ischemia. Am J Cardiol 24:766, 1969
10. De Mello WC: The healing-over process in cardiac and other muscle fibers. P. 323. In Demello WC (ed): Electrical Phenomena in the Heart. Academic Press, Orlando, Florida, 1972
11. Hurst JW: The Heart. McGraw-Hill, New York, 1982
12. Bayley RH, LaDue JS: Differentiation of the electrocardiographic changes produced in the dog by prolonged temporary occlusion of a coronary artery from those produced by postoperative pericarditis. Am Heart J 28:233, 1944
13. Horan LG, Flowers NC, Johnson JC: Significance of the diagnostic Q wave of myocardial infarction. Circulation. 43:428, 1971
14. Horan LG, Flowers NC, Tollesan WJ, Thomas JR: The significance of diagnostic Q waves in the presence of bundle branch block. Chest 58:214, 1970
15. Marriot HJ: Practical Electrocardiography. Williams & Wilkins, Baltimore, 1984
16. Roberts WC, Gardin JM: Location of myocardial infarcts: A confusion of terms and definitions. Am J Cardiol 42:872, 1978
17. Holland RP, Brooks H: The QRS complex during myocardial ischemia. An experimental analysis in the porcine heart. J Clin Invest 57:541, 1976
18. Van Dam RT, Durrer D: Experimental study on the intramural distribution of the excitability cycle and on the form of the epicardial T-wave in the dog heart in situ. Am Heart J 61:537, 1961
19. Kennamen R, Prinzmetal M: Myocardial infarction complicated by left bundle branch block. Am Heart J 51:78, 1956
20. Stern W, Tzironi D, Stern E: Diagnostic accuracy of ambulatory ECG monitoring in ischemic heart disease. Circulation 52:1045, 1975
21. Crawford MH, Medosa CA, O'Rourke RA, et al: Limitations of continuous ambulatory electrocardiogram monitoring for detecting coronary artery disease. Ann Intern Med 89:1, 1978
22. Stern S, Tzironi D: Early detection of silent ischemic heart disease by 24 hour electrocardiographic monitoring of active subjects. Br Heart J 36:481, 1974
23. Wolf E, Tzironi D, Stern S: Comparison of exercise test and 24 hour ambulatory electrocardiographic monitoring in detection of ST-T changes. Br Heart J 36:481, 1974
24. Allen RD, Gettes LS, Phalan C, Arrington D: Painless ST-segment depression in patients with angina pectoris. Chest 69:467, 1976
25. Schang SJ, Pepire CJ: Transient asymptomatic ST-segment depression during daily activity. Am J Cardiol 39:397, 1977
26. Bala Subramanian V, Lahiri A, Green HL, et al: Ambulatory ST-segment monitoring. Br Heart J 46:419, 1980
27. Mazeri A, Sereri S, deNes M, L'Abbatle A: "Variant" angina. One aspect of a continuous spectrum of vasospastic myocardial ischemia. Am J Cardiol 42:1019, 1978
28. Figueras J, Singh BN, Banz W, et al: Mechanism of rest and nocturnal angina: observation during continuous hemodynamic and electrocardiographic monitoring. Circulation 59:955, 1979
29. Kunkes SH, Richard AP, Smith H, et al: Silent ST segment deviations and extent of coronary artery disease. Am Heart J 100:813, 1980
30. Nademanee K, Singh BN, Guerrero J, et al: Accurate rapid compact analog method for the quantification of frequency and duration of myocardial ischemia by semiautomated analysis of 24-Hour Holter ECG recordings. Am Heart J 103:802, 1982
31. Goldhammer S, Scherf D: Electrokardiographische Untersuchunger be: Kranker Mit Angina Pectoris ("ambulatorischer Typus"). Z Schr Khin Med 122:134, 1933
32. Rochmis P, Blackburn H: Exercise tests: A survey of procedures safety, and litigation experience in approximately 170,000 tests. JAMA 217:1061, 1971
33. Robb GP and Marks HH: Latent coronary artery

disease: Determination of its presence and severity by the exercise electrocardiogram. Am J Cardiol 13:603, 1964
34. Cumming GR, Durfresne C, Kich L, Samm J: Exercise electrocardiogram patterns in normal women. Br Heart J 35:10551, 1973
35. Wolthius RA, Froelicher VF Jr, Fischer J, Triebwasser JH: The response of healthy men to treadmill exercise. Circulation 55:153, 1977
36. Sheffield LT, Roitman D: Systolic blood pressure, heart rate, and treadmill work at anginal threshold. Chest 63:327, 1973

7

Basic Cellular Electrophysiology of the Heart

Jacek A. Wojtczak, M.D., Ph.D.

The ECG registered from the human thorax or the surface of the heart is the cumulative response of many thousands of cardiac cells that generate action potentials. Because of the orderly propagation of the action potentials through the heart, the optimal sequence of excitation permits coordinated cardiac mechanical function. The use of intracellular microelectrodes enables the action potential to be directly recorded; regional differences in the shape and size of these potentials in the various regions of the heart then become apparent. An understanding and correct interpretation of the ECG tracings throughout the rest of the book require knowledge of some basic facts about the cellular activity of the heart. Therefore, this chapter outlines the physiology of normal cardiac cellular activity, reviews electrophysiologic abnormalities produced by some pathologic conditions (e.g., ischemia, hypoxia, acid–base changes), and summarizes the mechanisms of cardiac dysrhythmias and the actions of antiarrhythmic drugs.

THE RESTING POTENTIAL OF CARDIAC CELLS

The use of intracellular microelectrodes has permitted direct measurement of the resting potential of cardiac cells. A microelectrode is an electrolyte-filled glass needle (usually less than 1 μm in diameter at the tip) that is inserted into the cell by means of a micromanipulator. At the instant the microelectrode tip passes from the outside to the inside of the cell membrane, it records a negative potential called the resting potential. If the cell is quiescent, this negative potential remains at −80 to −90 mV. Some cells in the sinus node and atrioventricular (AV) node possess less negative resting potentials (around −60 mV). The resting membrane potential (RMP) is determined by (1) the concentration gradient for potassium ions (K^+) across the cell membrane, and (2) electrogenic sodium ion (Na^+) extrusion. Figure 7–1 shows the concentrations of ions inside and outside a cardiac cell. The high intracellular concentration of K^+ and low concentration of Na^+ is maintained by a Na^+/K^+ enzyme pump (Na^+/K^+-ATPase) located within the cell membrane.

The enzyme, Mg-dependent ATPase (adenosine triphosphatase), uses energy stored in the form of ATP to pump Na^+ out of the cell and K^+ into the cell. The ratio is 3 Na^+ pumped out for 2 K^+ pumped in. Thus, the Na^+/K^+ pump generates a net outward movement of positive charges across the membrane (electrogenic sodium extrusion), contributing to the electronegativity of the cell interior. However, the RMP is predominantly determined by the K^+ gradient

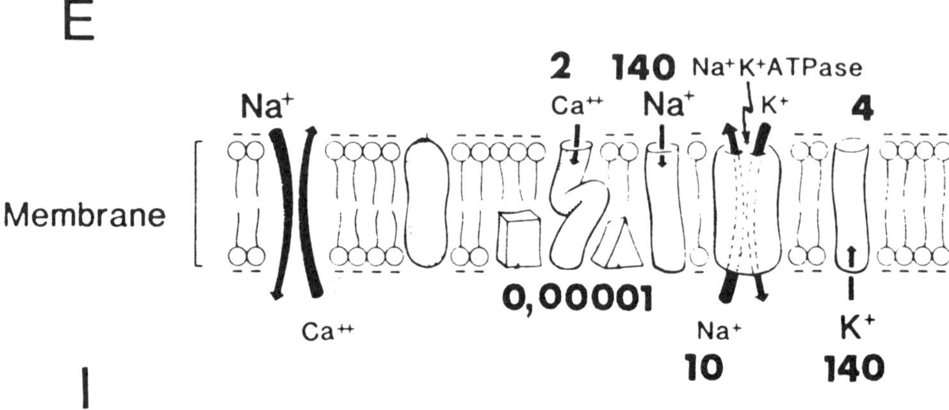

Fig. 7–1 Schematic representation of the cardiac cellular membrane with principal passive (Na^+, Ca^{++}, K^+) and active transporting systems (Na^+/K^+ pump and Na^+/Ca^{++} exchanger). Also shown are concentrations of different ions (in mM) in the extracellular space (E) (Na^+ 140, K^+ 4, Ca^{++} 2) and the intracellular space (I) (Na^+ 10, K^+ 140, Ca^{++} 0,0001).

since, at rest, the cardiac cell membrane is permeable to K^+ but relatively impermeable to other ions such as Na^+, Ca^{++}, or Cl^-. Potassium ions tend to diffuse out of the cell, down their concentration gradient. Impermeable cellular anions which are associated with cell proteins cannot follow, and, therefore, a net negative charge is built up at the cell interior. Thus, the RMP is generally close to, but always less negative than, the equilibrium (reversal) potential (E_k) for K^+.

The equilibrium (reversal) potential for any ion can be defined as the potential at which the electrochemical driving force on that ion is zero and can be calculated by using the Nernst equation. If the intracellular concentration (Ci) of K^+ is 140 mM and the extracellular concentration (C_e) is 4 mM, the value of E_k would be as follows:

$$E_k = (RT/nF) - \log_n Ce/Ci = -92 \text{ mV}$$

where R is the gas constant, T is absolute temperature, F is Faraday's constant, and n is the valency of the ion.

Any loss of intracellular K^+ or increase in extracellular K^+ (i.e., hyperkalemia) will reduce (make less negative) the RMP of cardiac cells. Inhibition of the Na^+/K^+ pump as induced by toxic doses of digitalis will also drastically depolarize cardiac cells by reducing the K^+ gradient across the membrane (less K^+ is pumped back into the cell) and by inhibiting electrogenic Na^+ extrusion. Ischemia and hypoxia will also inhibit the Na^+/K^+ pump by lowering the ATP levels necessary for normal function of the enzyme, leading to a loss of intracellular K^+. Moreover, due to inadequate perfusion during the ischemic event, K^+ released from the cells accumulates in the extracellular space producing pronounced depolarization of the cardiac cells.

ACTION POTENTIALS IN CARDIAC CELLS

When the cardiac cell membrane is depolarized close to its threshold potential (−65 mV), it suddenly becomes highly permeable to Na^+, which enters the cell and produces depolarization. This sudden influx of Na^+ is due to massive opening of membrane sodium channels.[1] In addition, K^+ permeability, which is high at rest, is transiently decreased at the moment of sudden depolarization. Thus, the cells are easily depolarized to above zero potential (up to +30 mV), producing the cardiac action potential (Fig. 7–2).

Depolarization induced by influx of Na^+ is

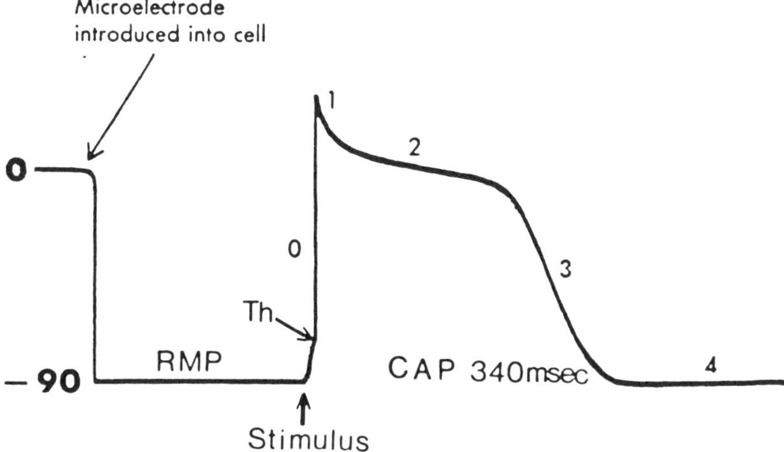

Fig. 7–2 Resting membrane potential (RMP) and cardiac action potential (CAP) of a ventricular muscle cell. A glass microelectrode in the extracellular space records zero potential. When it passes through the membrane there is an abrupt jump of the potential in a negative direction down to −90 mV at the RMP, which is maintained until the cell is stimulated by an electrical impulse from the stimulator. When the impulse is strong enough to bring the cell to the threshold (Th) potential (around −65 mV), the cell produces an action potential during which the potential inside the cell remains far above the level of the resting potential for 340 msec. The cardiac action potential has four characteristic phases numbered 0 to 3. Phase 0: rapid depolarization; phase 1: initial repolarization; phase 2: plateau; and phase 3: terminal repolarization. The diastolic phase between action potentials is called phase 4. In the cell shown from ventricular muscle, intracellular RMP remains constant during phase 4, but in pacemaker cells the RMP gradually becomes less negative (slow phase 4 diastolic depolarization).

responsible for the first phase (upstroke) of the cardiac action potential, called phase 0. These action potentials are very long (200 to 400 msec) in comparison with action potentials in other excitable membranes, such as skeletal muscle (10 msec) or neurons (1 to 3 msec). Sodium channels are quickly inactivated (within a few milliseconds), so that sodium current cannot be the only inward current responsible for the prolonged depolarization seen in phase 2 of the cardiac action potential. The second inward current is carried predominantly by calcium ions.[2] Because of differences in dynamics, Na^+ current is often described as the fast inward current, whereas Ca^{++} current is a slow inward current. Figure 7–3 shows the recording of these currents obtained during a voltage-clamp experiment, in which the membrane potential is stabilized at an elected level and current flowing through the membrane at this potential is registered. The relationship of the currents to the action potential is shown and it is evident that the Ca^{++} current is responsible for the prolonged depolarization during phase 2 (plateau). In the next phase of the action potential (phase 3 terminal repolarization), membrane current reverses direction from inward to outward. This is due to the decay of the slow, inward Ca^{++} current and the emergence of the outwardly flowing K^+ current (Fig. 7–3). Thus, the terminal repolarization and the duration of the action potential depend on both phenomena.

Calcium and potassium currents flow through different sets of calcium and potassium channels, respectively. All the channels seem to have similar gating mechanisms, but their kinetics are different. The function of Ca^{++} channels, but not Na^+ or K^+ channels, depends on the level of membrane (protein) phosphorylation. Phosphorylation increases the number of open Ca^{++} channels, which can be induced by stimulation of β-receptors. β Stimulation activates

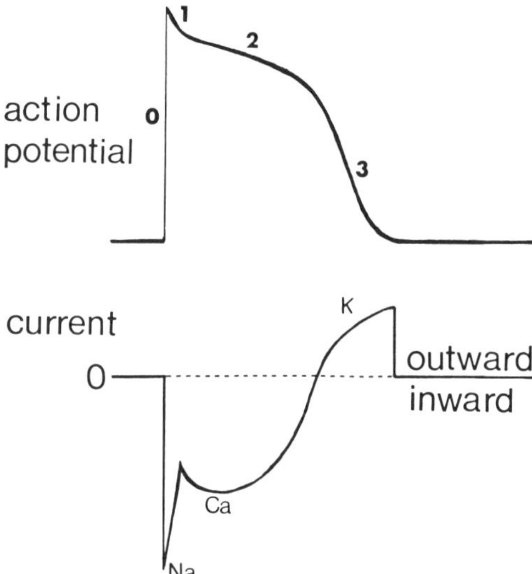

Fig. 7–3 Recording of currents flowing during the action potential. Such a recording can be obtained when the membrane potential is stabilized at an elected level using a voltage clamp. Depolarizing inward currents are carried by sodium (Na) and calcium (Ca) ions, while the repolarizing current is carried by potassium (K) ions.

adenylate cyclase and thus increases production of cyclic adenosine monophosphate (cyclic AMP). Cyclic AMP activates cyclic AMP-dependent protein kinases, which phosphorylate the Ca^{++} channels. By increasing phosphorylation and the number of open Ca^{++} channels, catecholamines increase the magnitude of inward Ca^{++} current flowing during the plateau of the action potential. Since contractile activation is closely related to the amount of Ca^{++} flowing into the cell during each action potential, force of contraction will be markedly increased by catecholamines and other hormones that activate β-receptors. By contrast, calcium antagonists bind directly to the Ca^{++} channels, changing their conformation to a closed state; thus they reduce the magnitude of the inward Ca^{++} current.

Potassium channels carrying outward K^+ current are varied in their properties. Depending on the kinetics of the channels through which they flow, these currents are called K_1, X_1, or X_2. Further information on these complex channels can be found in Noble (ref. 3).

In addition to the three types of currents flowing through the passive membrane channels that open and close, two other currents generated by membrane ion-exchange mechanisms are of importance in the generation of cardiac action potentials. The first is the outward current generated by electrogenic Na^+ extrusion (electrogenic Na^+/K^+ pump). The second is the inward current generated by the Na^+/Ca^{++} exchanger. The importance of the electrogenic Na^+/K^+ pump in the generation of the resting potential was discussed above. During the upstroke of the action potential, Na^+ flows into the cell and automatically stimulates the Na^+/K^+ pump (stimulated by Na^+ inside and K^+ outside). Since the Na^+/K^+ pump is electrogenic (pumps more Na^+ out than K^+ in), it generates a net outward current of positive charges. This accelerates repolarization (shortens the action potential), acting synergistically with K^+ currents. Inhibition of the electrogenic Na^+/K^+ pump by cardiac glycosides produces membrane depolarization (less negative resting potential) and a marked prolongation of the action potential duration (less outward repolarizing current is present). The Na^+/Ca^{++} exchanger cannot be classified as a pump since it does not directly utilize high energy substrates. It is located in the cell membrane and protects the cell against Ca^{++} overloading. It uses the gradient of Na^+ across the cell membrane to remove Ca^{++} from the cell. If the gradient is increased, more Ca^{++} is removed; if the gradient is decreased, less Ca^{++} is removed and its intracellular concentration rises. The positive inotropic action of the cardiac glycosides can be explained by a gradual inhibition of the Na^+/K^+ pump which decreases the Na^+ gradient across the membrane (less Na^+ is pumped out and its intracellular concentration increases); less Ca^{++} is pumped out (its intracellular concentration increases); therefore, less Ca^{++} is exchanged for Na^+, and Ca^{++} remains in the cell. This exchange mechanism is of prime importance for the regulation of contractile force, and was recently proposed to

Table 7–1. Principal Currents Participating in the Generation of Cardiac Action Potentials

Inward currents
Sodium current
Calcium current
Electrogenic Na^+/Ca^{++} exchange
Outward currents
Potassium currents (K_1, X_1, X_2)
Electrogenic Na^+/K^+ exchange

also have a role in the electrogenesis of the cardiac action potential.[4]

Table 7–1 lists the currents participating in the generation of the cardiac action potential. A chloride ion current has been omitted, since it plays only a small role as a repolarizing current in Purkinje fibers.

AUTOMATICITY AND THE CONDUCTION SYSTEM OF THE HEART

Automaticity is the ability of a cell to depolarize spontaneously, reach threshold potential, and initiate an action potential. After termination of an action potential, cardiac cells enter the diastolic phase (phase 4) with its duration depending on the heart rate. In ventricular and atrial muscle, the resting membrane potential remains at the same level throughout the diastolic phase. However, some cells in the right atrium, clustered together near the inlet of the superior vena cava, possess a unique property of spontaneous depolarization during phase 4. This depolarization is much slower than that occurring during the upstroke (phase 0) of the action potential, and is often called slow phase 4 diastolic depolarization. The group of cells possessing this property is classified as sinoatrial (SA) node cells. Figure 7–4 shows slow diastolic depolarization and the type of action potentials generated by these pacemaker cells. When depolarization reaches threshold (−40 mV), an action potential is discharged. As these action potentials are generated at a rate around 70/min, the SA node overdrives other pacemaker regions in the heart where slow diastolic depolarization occurs at lower rates (e.g., Purkinje fibers).

The resting membrane potential in SA cells is low (−60 mV), precluding the existence of the Na^+ current as the charge carrier. Indeed, both SA node action potentials and phase 4 depolarizations are strongly dependent on Ca^{++} concentration and do not depend on Na^+ gradients. Phase 4 depolarization, which is responsible for the automatic spontaneous activity of SA pacemaker cells, is due to a decay of one of the K^+ currents (X_1 current) and to a steady, background influx of Ca^{++} "leakage" current. Catecholamines increase background Ca^{++} current and decay of the K^+ current and thus increase phase 4 depolarization in SA node cells. Acetylcholine reduces background Ca^{++} current and decay of K^+ current, thereby decreasing phase 4 depolarization. Increasing slow diastolic depolarization brings the cell closer to threshold, and more action potentials are fired by the SA node at a given time. The opposite is true when slow diastolic depolarization is decreased. Therefore, adrenergic stimulation (released nor-

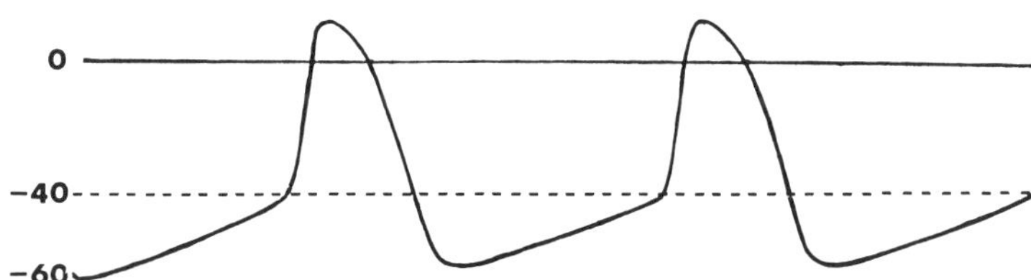

Fig. 7–4 Action potentials generated by sinoatrial (SA) pacemaker cells. Note the low maximal resting potential (−60 mV) steadily decreasing during diastole (slow diastolic depolarization). The upstroke velocity and amplitude of sinus node action potentials is much smaller than that of action potentials from other areas of the heart.

epinephrine around SA cells) leads to sinus tachycardia, while parasympathetic stimulation (release of acetylcholine) leads to sinus bradycardia. Calcium antagonists that block regular Ca^{++} currents during the plateau of the action potential are also able to reduce background Ca^{++} current during phase 4. Since they slow the rate of diastolic depolarization, these drugs exert a marked negative chronotropic effect.

The electrical potential generated spontaneously in SA nodal cells is transmitted to both ventricles through the conduction system of the heart. Figure 7–5 shows a diagramatic representation of this system and gives examples of action potentials generated at the different levels of the heart that vary considerably in their amplitude, duration and shape. These variations are due to different properties of their cell membranes, with some sets of channels being absent or latent. Atrial cells have action potentials with high amplitude but are relatively short (150 to 200 msec) in duration. The cells in the AV node are physiologically depolarized around −60 mV, similar to SA nodal cells. However, the property of slow diastolic depolarization is not as well developed in AV nodal cells. Their action potentials are characterized by low amplitude and a slow upstroke (phase 0) velocity, which is dependent on the slow Ca^{++} current, and their response to sympathetic and parasympathetic stimulation is similar to that of SA nodal cells. Sympathetic stimulation increases the amplitude and upstroke velocity of the action potentials and thus increases conduction velocity in the AV node. Parasympathetic stimulation decreases the amplitude of these potentials and slows down AV nodal conduction.

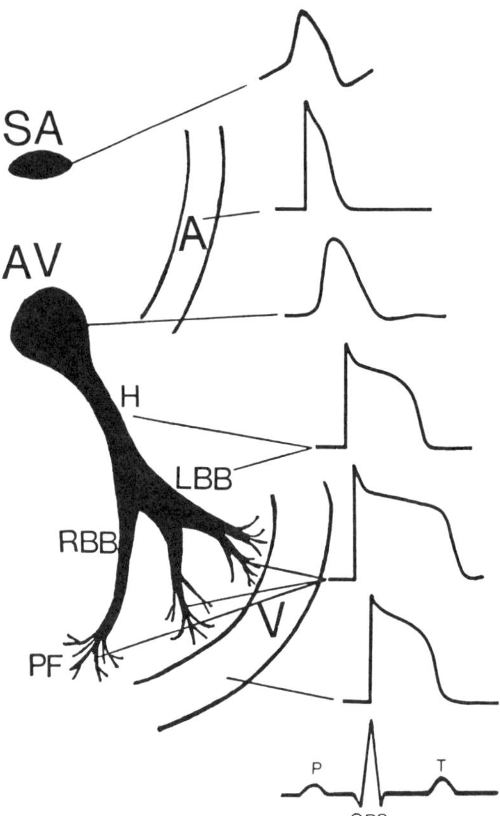

Fig. 7–5 Diagrammatic picture of the conduction system of the heart. Cellular action potentials from various regions differ in duration, shape, and voltage range. SA, sinoatrial node; A, atrium; AV, atrioventricular node; H, bundle of His; LBB, left bundle branch; RBB, right bundle branch; PF, Purkinje fibers; V, ventricle. The corresponding ECG tracing is shown at the bottom.

Digitalis, apart from its direct effects on cardiac cells, can induce central parasympathetic excitation, which indirectly decreases the amplitude of the AV node potential and slows AV nodal conduction. This action is widely used in the treatment of supraventricular dysrhythmias. Calcium antagonists produce the same effect by directly inhibiting AV nodal calcium potentials. Overdose with any of these drugs may lead to advanced heart block at the AV node.

Electrical impulses leaving the AV node enter the bundle of His, the right and left bundle branches, and ultimately the net of terminal Purkinje fibers in the ventricular conduction system. Action potentials generated in Purkinje cells have the highest amplitude and the longest duration (Fig. 7–5).

Surprisingly, the distal Purkinje cells also possess the property of slow phase 4 diastolic depolarization, but the rate of this depolarization is much slower than in SA node cells. Long before the potentials inside the Purkinje cells reach threshold, they are already depolarized by the electrical impulse initiated in the SA node. Phase 4 depolarization in Purkinje cells results from a decay of one of the K^+ currents and a steady background influx of the Na^+ leakage current, whereas in SA node cells the leakage current is carried by Ca^{++}. Fortunately, this type of automaticity found in Purkinje cells is easily suppressed by local anesthetics that inhibit Na^+ fluxes, which are therefore very useful for suppressing ventricular premature beats due to increased automaticity.

The duration of the action potential in the ventricular conduction system increases progressively from the AV node to the distal Purkinje fibers 1 to 2 mm prior to their junction with ventricular muscle. The cells in the ventricular muscle generate action potentials, which have a much shorter duration than do Purkinje cells. The system of cells generating long action potentials in terminal Purkinje fibers protects the left and right ventricles against dangerous, early premature beats descending along the bundle branches. This system below the AV node is often called a peripheral gate, which should not be confused with gates in the ionic channels.

REFRACTORINESS IN CARDIAC MUSCLE

The system of peripheral gates can protect the ventricles against early premature beats due to the long-lasting nature of the cardiac action potential, and the fact that cardiac cells do not become excitable again until the action potential is terminated. This period of inexcitability is called the refractory period. In skeletal muscle it lasts several milliseconds, which corresponds to the duration of the skeletal muscle action potential, whereas in cardiac muscle it lasts several hundred milliseconds. This long refractory period prevents cardiac muscle from being reexcited until the previous contraction is largely completed. This is a very important property in cardiac muscle which acts as a pump.

The refractory period can be divided into the absolute refractory period, defined as the time during which there is no membrane response to a second stimulus, and the relative refractory period, which is the time during which a second stimulus can only induce an action potential with a decreased amplitude, upstroke velocity, and conduction velocity. Slowly propagating action potentials of this kind may underlie conduction abnormalities such as a conduction delay, decremental conduction with block, or even reentrant excitation.

The phenomenon of refractoriness is due to the properties of Na^+ channels. During the action potential, Na^+ channels are first rapidly opened, then inactivated. They remain inactivated throughout the action potential plateau until the repolarization process increases the membrane potential beyond −60 mV. During this time, the membrane is completely inexcitable: the absolute refractory period. Inactivation is then gradually removed as repolarization continues, but it is not removed completely until the membrane potential reaches −90 mV. Often the term effective refractory period is used. This can be defined as a period during which a conducted action potential cannot be evoked, even though the stimulus may produce an active response at the cellular level.

CONDUCTION OF THE CARDIAC IMPULSE

The propagation of electrical impulses depends on the flow of excitatory currents along the muscle fiber from active to resting regions. The larger the excitatory currents generated, the greater the conduction velocity of an impulse travelling along the fiber. The magnitude of excitatory currents and thus the conduction velocity is directly related to the amplitude and the upstroke (phase 0) velocity of the action potential. If the amplitude and the upstroke velocity—rate or rise of the action potential (dV/dt)—is low, the conduction velocity is decreased. The amplitude and dV/dt of action potentials depend on the level of resting membrane potential, since many Na^+ channels are already inactivated if the resting potential is low (e.g., −70 mV). Thus, Na^+ current is much smaller and the amplitude and dV/dt of the action potential, which are dependent on this current, are lower (depressed fast response). When the cells are further depolarized (−60 to −50 mV), all Na^+ channels are inactivated, the cells become unexcitable, and the conduction along the fiber is blocked. However, in the presence of catecholamines, the conducted action potentials can be restored, although their amplitude and upstroke velocity are very low. This occurs via the so-called slow response or calcium potential, since the upstroke is due entirely to the influx of Ca^{++} ions.[5] The conduction velocity of these slow action potentials is very small.

The conduction velocity in cardiac muscle also depends on the diameter of the fiber (the larger the fiber, the faster the conduction) and on the electrical coupling between cardiac cells. Intracellular electrical coupling occurs across low resistance junctions, called gap junctions. Their resistance may increase during pathologic conditions (i.e., ischemia, hypoxia, digitalis intoxication, acidosis, or overdosage of halothane), and conduction velocity may be drastically decreased, leading to a complete conduction block.[6]

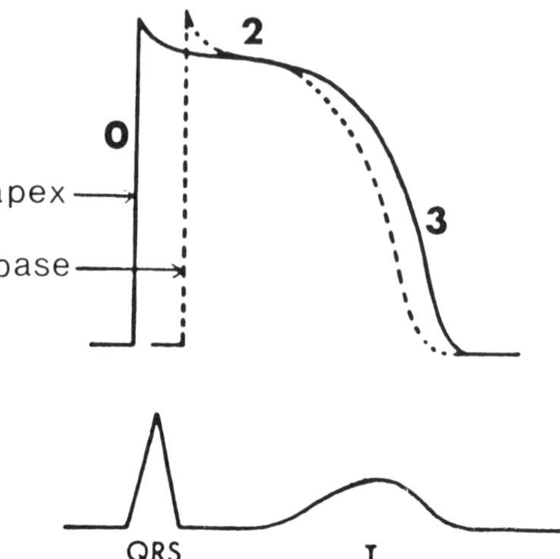

Fig. 7–6 Relationship of the cardiac action potential to the ECG. See explanation in the text.

RELATIONSHIP OF THE CARDIAC ACTION POTENTIAL TO THE ECG

Figure 7–6 shows that the QRS complex of the ECG is related to phase 0, the ST segment to phase 2, and the T wave to terminal repolarization (phase 3) of the action potential. Ventricular depolarization starts at the apex (first cells) and ends in the posterior basal part of the left ventricle (last cells). The QRS complex is due to the current flow between these two regions. If the conduction velocity between different regions of the heart is decreased (the time between the first and last cell to depolarize is longer), this is reflected in the prolongation of the QRS complex and a decrease in its amplitude (decreased amplitude of action potentials). During phase 2 of the action potential, cardiac cells are more or less at the same potential, so no current flows and the ECG signal is isoelectric (ST segment). During terminal repolarization (phase 3), there is again a potential difference because of slightly different durations of the action potentials in different cells that generate current flow reflected by the occurrence of the T wave. If the repolarization process is disturbed by disease, which produces changes in plateau height and duration of action potentials, current may flow between diseased and normal cells during phase 2, producing elevation or lowering of the ST segment (depending on the direction of current flow) and marked changes in the shape and polarity of the T wave.

EFFECTS OF DISEASE ON THE ELECTROPHYSIOLOGIC CHARACTERISTICS OF CARDIAC CELLS

The electrical membrane events in cardiac cells are directly linked to cellular metabolic processes. Any change in the rate of energy production or use will affect ionic gradients and fluxes. The most dramatic changes in the electrical activity of the heart are induced by myocardial ischemia. After sudden coronary occlusion, cardiac cells are progressively depolarized and the amplitude and upstroke velocity of action potentials are decreased[7]; intercellular coupling is diminished[6]; and conduction velocity is slowed, leading to conduction blocks. The duration of action potentials is decreased during the early stages of acute ischemia; however, during prolonged ischemia (more than 12 hours), action potentials of the surviving, subendocardial Purkinje cells become unusually prolonged.[8] Shortening or prolongation of the repolarization phase creates inhomogeneities in the duration of refractoriness, producing dysrhythmias.

These changes are due to progressive inhibition of phosphorylative oxidation and a decreased level of high-energy phosphates, which slows down the ionic pumps in the cell membranes, mitochondria, and sarcoplasmic reticulum during ischemia. Intracellular Na^+ concentration is progressively increased, while intracellular K^+ is progressively lost. Since tissue perfusion is impeded, K^+ remains in the extracellular space, while metabolites accumulate in the cells. Accumulation of carbon dioxide and lactic acid (due to transiently enhanced anaerobic glycolysis) leads to progressive acidification of the cell interior. The cell can produce some ATP through anaerobic glycolysis, but, as the acidosis becomes more pronounced, anaerobic glycolysis is finally blocked. By contrast, during cell hypoxia with normal perfusion, anaerobic glycolysis can provide some basal level of high-energy phosphates. Thus, the cell is only slightly depolarized during hypoxia, and the amplitude, upstroke velocity, and duration are less affected than during ischemia (Fig. 7–7).

An overdose of cardiac glycosides depolarizes cardiac cells (inhibition of Na^+/K^+ pump, loss of intracellular K^+) and produces changes in phase 0 similar to those of any depolarizing agent (diminished amplitude, upstroke velocity, and conduction velocity). The action potential duration is at first prolonged but in advanced intoxication is markedly shortened. Toxic doses of cardiac glycosides can also induce abnormal automaticity in Purkinje fibers and produce marked intracellular electrical uncoupling.[6]

Marked and prolonged metabolic acidosis

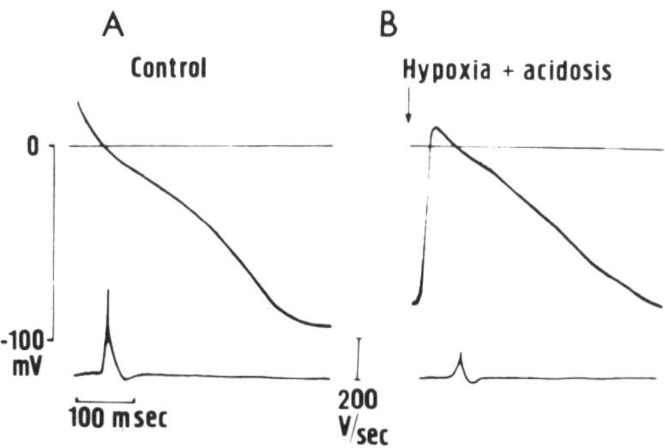

Fig. 7–7 **(A)** Control. **(B)** Effects of prolonged (45 min) hypoxia PO_2 = 15 mmHg) and metabolic acidosis (pH = 6.5) on the action potential in a Purkinje fiber. Differential of the phase 0 (dV/dt) is shown below the action potential. Its amplitude (calibrated in V/sec) reflects the maximal velocity of depolarization (upstroke) which is markedly decreased by hypoxia and acidosis. Purkinje fibers are generally resistant to hypoxia due to the lack of contractile activity and large stores of glycogen substrate for anaerobic glycolysis. (JA Wojtczak, unpublished results.)

produces cell depolarization, which decreases the amplitude and upstroke velocity of action potentials, leading to slow responses. However, transient mild respiratory acidosis may exert slight antiarrhythmic effects, improving the amplitude and upstroke velocity of action potentials. By contrast, any degree of alkalosis may be potentially arrhythmogenic.[9]

Ischemia, hypoxia, digitalis intoxication, alkalosis, stretch, and overdoses of epinephrine can induce abnormal pathologic automaticity in cardiac cells. Often low amplitude, oscillatory action potentials occur after the regular action potential. Potentials that interrupt repolarization of the regular action potential and occur before the membrane potential has returned to baseline or diastole are called early afterdepolarizations[5] (Fig. 7–8). Those that occur after repolarization is complete are called delayed afterdepolarizations.[5,8] Their amplitude usually increases when the rate of stimulation is increased. When they reach the threshold potential they induce "triggered action potentials" (Fig. 7–9) and a burst of tachycardia, so-called triggered dysrhythmia.[9]

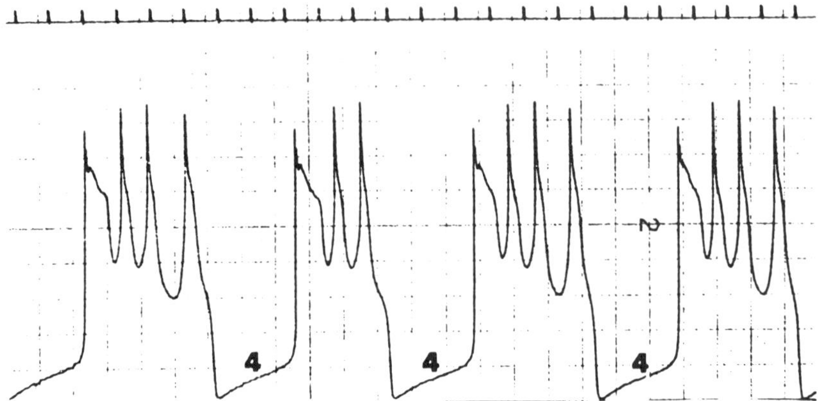

Fig. 7–8 Abnormal automaticity (early afterdepolarization) in Purkinje fiber induced by stretch. Time marks (at the top) occur at 1-second intervals. If the oscillatory action potentials that interrupt repolarization are conducted to the periphery they will cause a burst of extrasystoles with relatively fixed coupling to the preceding beat. In vivo, Purkinje fibers can be stretched during ventricular dilatation associated with decompensated congestive heart failure. (JA Wojtczak, unpublished results.)

MECHANISMS OF CARDIAC DYSRHYTHMIAS

Abnormal Impulse Conduction

Intensive investigations of dysrhythmias both in vitro (glass microelectrodes, extracellular recordings) and in vivo (mapping of excitation sequences in the intact heart) have confirmed previous hypotheses that most serious cardiac dysrhythmias are due to disturbances of conduction with the occurrence of a circus movement (reentry) of excitation.[8] In a heart driven by the sinus node, each impulse dies out after activating the atria and ventricles. The phenomenon of reentry occurs when the propagating impulse does not die out after complete activation of the heart but persists to reexcite the heart after the end of the refractory period. The concept of circus movement of excitation resulting in reentry was first proposed by Mayer in 1908. The prerequisite for the establishment of a reentrant circuit is the occurrence of a unidirectional block of conduction in which excitations cannot be conducted along the fiber in one direction, but can cross the area of block when arriving from the opposite end (Fig. 7–10). The other important conditions that increase the probabil-

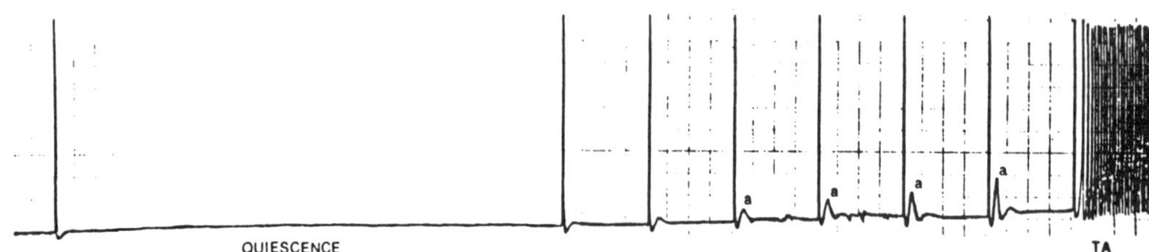

Fig. 7–9 Abnormal automaticity (delayed afterdepolarization) induced by an overdose of norepinephrine in the atrial coronary sinus cell. During quiescence this cell has no ability to generate automatic activity, but stimulation induces afterdepolarizations (a), which at the seventh beat reach the threshold and induce a burst of triggered dysrrhythmias (TA). Delayed afterdepolarizations have been shown to occur in ischemic cells (JA Wojtczak, unpublished results.)

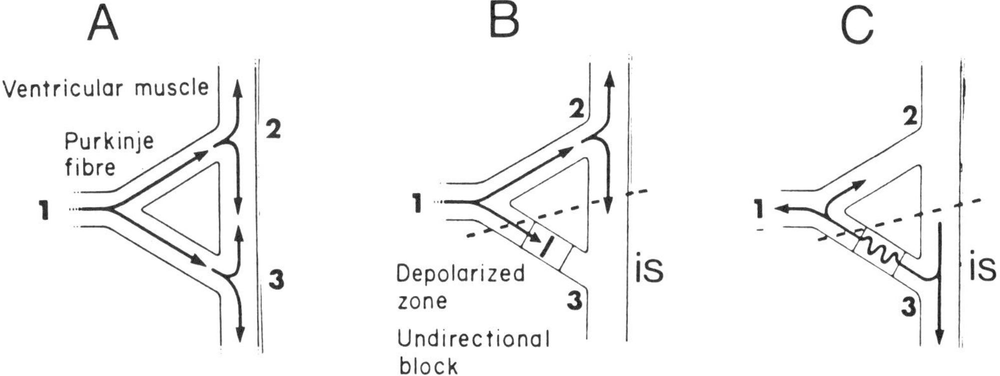

Fig. 7–10 Schematic model of unidirectional block and reentrant dysrhythmias at the junction between peripheral Purkinje fibers (PF) and ventricular muscle (VM). **(A)** Normal activation of VM through branched PF. **(B)** The electrical impulse cannot activate VM through branch 3, which is damaged by ischemia (is), but activates it through branch 2. Conduction in VM, which is damaged by ischemia, is also slow. **(C)** A slowly propagating impulse reaches the depolarized zone in branch 3. As the geometric conditions favor the conduction from VM to PF (large number of VM cells activating few PF cells), the impulse can be conducted in retrograde fashion (from branch 3 to 1 and 2) along the conduction system (if the absolute refractory period is terminated) and result in an ectopic beat.

ity of reentry are (1) slow conduction around the block, (2) shortened refractory period of cells before the block, and (3) a long pathway of activation.

Reentry may also be induced by a single premature excitation that is blocked in regions in which absolute refractory periods or action potentials are prolonged.[8] If this excitation is conducted through some other regions in which refractory periods are of normal duration or are shortened, it may reactivate the area of block from the opposite direction and reenter the fully repolarized cells, generating extrasystoles. The region in which the cells have prolonged refractory periods can be described as a region of functional unidirectional block.

Reentry has been demonstrated to be an important cause of dysrhythmias that occur soon after a coronary artery occlusion. Janse et al.[10] simultaneously recorded 60 unipolar epicardial or intramural electrodes that were placed in the left ventricle of the porcine heart rendered ischemic by acute coronary artery occlusion. These workers found patterns of activation during subsequent episodes of ventricular tachycardia, suggesting a reentry mechanism. The fragmentation of the excitation wave also led to ventricular fibrillation with small reentrant circuits.

Circus movement with excitation resulting in reentry has also been shown to cause serious atrial dysrhythmias, including tachycardia and flutter.[8] Because of its physiologically slow conduction, the AV node is often a site of reentry with resultant nodal tachycardia.[5,8]

Abnormal Impulse Initiation (Automaticity)

The second group of dysrhythmias are due to abnormal impulse initiation. These may result from an increased or decreased rate of depolarization of existing physiologic pacemakers (e.g., sinus bradycardia or tachycardia). In addition, cells that are normally devoid of pacemaker properties (in atrial or ventricular muscle) may develop them due to pathologic conditions, producing abnormal pathologic automaticity. This situation may be induced by the depolarization of cells during ischemia.

A special type of abnormal automaticity that

develops only in cells that are electrically active, but not in those which are quiescent, is shown in Figures 7–8 and 7–9. This type of automaticity requires one or more triggering impulses in order to occur and is called triggered automaticity. The discovery of this type of automaticity changed previously recognized rules of differentiation between reentrant and automatic rhythms.[8] It was previously believed that dysrhythmias due to automaticity, if overdriven by an extrinsic pacemaker, would be suppressed for a period of time after cessation of the overdrive and then eventually return to their prior rate. By contrast, reentrant rhythms were thought to be initiated and totally suppressed by a single or a few appropriately timed premature stimuli. However, it has been clearly shown that triggered automaticity, like reentrant dysrhythmias, can be initiated and also terminated by a single or a few premature excitations.[8]

Disturbances of conduction and automaticity very often coexist. The classic examples are the dysrhythmias that develop during intoxication with cardiac glycosides. Figure 7–11 shows how an increase in automatic activity developing in the Purkinje cells due to adrenergic stimulation, stretch, prolonged ischemia, or digitalis intoxication can alter the pattern and velocity of conduction. Because of the same relationship between automaticity and conduction, conduction velocity in the ventricular conduction system will be faster during tachycardia (overdrive suppression of automaticity more marked) and slower during bradycardia (overdrive suppression of automaticity less marked).

MECHANISMS OF ACTION OF ANTIARRHYTHMIC DRUGS

Since cardiac dysrhythmias are due either to abnormal conduction (reentry) or abnormal initiation of the electrical impulses, antiarrhythmic drugs should correct or modify these abnormalities. Indeed, some antiarrhythmic agents can improve conduction (Fig. 7–12) in specific regions of the heart (Purkinje fibers and their junctions with ventricular muscle), but paradoxically most antiarrhythmic drugs further decrease already disturbed conduction, changing unidirectional block to bidirectional block. Therefore, the circus movement of excitation which results in reentry is no longer possible.[11] This mechanism is seen in ischemic tissue where sensitivity

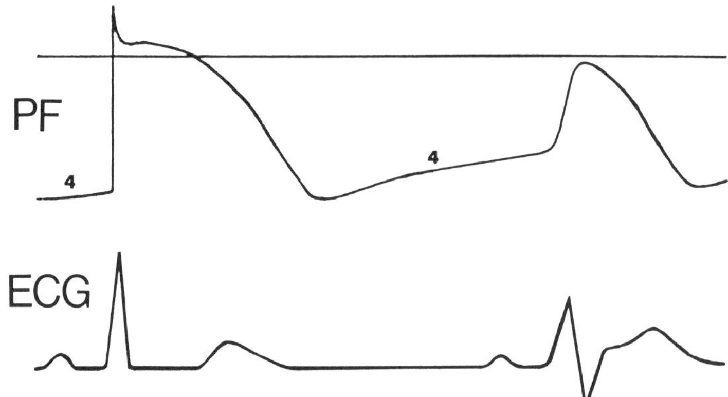

Fig. 7–11 Automaticity and conduction. Action potentials in Purkinje fibers (PF) and the corresponding ECG are shown. Automaticity (phase 4 depolarization) in PF is enhanced considerably after the first beat (e.g., due to local norepinephrine release). The second sinus impulse descending along the conduction system will reach this fiber when it is already considerably depolarized. Thus, the resulting action potential will have a low amplitude and upstroke velocity and will be conducted very slowly. The corresponding ECG shows characteristic prolongation of the QRS complex (due to prolonged conduction) and a change in its shape (due to aberrant conduction).

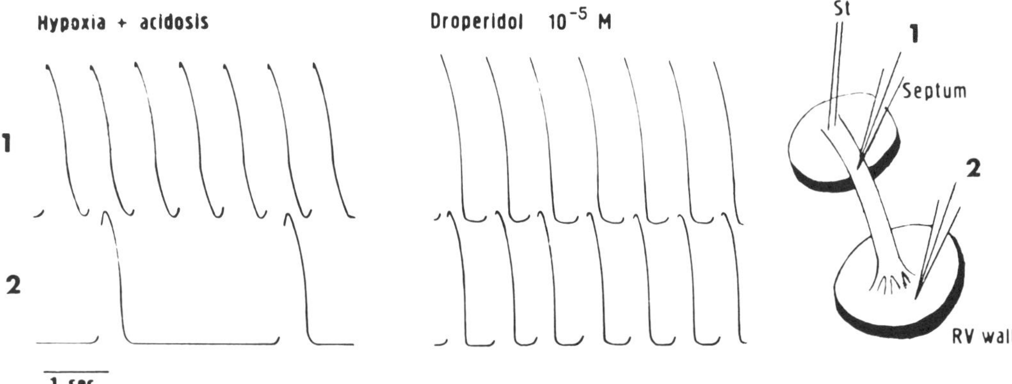

Fig. 7–12 Effects of droperidol on the conduction between terminal Purkinje fibers and ventricular muscle. Conduction block (4:1) induced by hypoxia and acidosis was reversed by droperidol. Similar effects are exerted by lidocaine and diphenylhydantoin. RV, right ventricle. (Wojtczak, unpublished results.)

of the ischemic cells to antiarrhythmic drugs (local anesthetics) is pronounced as a result of intracellular acidosis which increases the amount of the cationic form of the local anesthetic in the myoplasm. The local anesthetics exert their antiarrhythmic effects by inactivating Na^+ channels and thus reducing Na^+ current flow during phase 0, leading to the increased block.

Improvement of conduction is combined with an antiautomatic activity possessed by some antiarrhythmic drugs. Phase 4 automaticity in Purkinje fibers is decreased or suppressed by the majority of antiarrhythmic drugs. Figure 7–13 shows the antiautomatic effects of the neuroleptic drug, droperidol, which exerts similar local anesthetic actions to lidocaine or diphenylhydantoin.[12] It follows from the relationship between automaticity and conduction shown in Figure 7–11 that suppression of automaticity will improve conduction. Some antiarrhythmic drugs are also able to suppress pathologic automaticity (i.e., afterdepolarizations). However, this property is less pronounced among local anesthetics and more common with the calcium antagonists.

Classic antiarrhythmic drugs can either prolong (e.g., quinidine, procainamide) or shorten (e.g., lidocaine, diphenylhydantoin, droperidol) the duration of the action potential. The direction of this change is not as important as the fact that they extend the effective refractory period far beyond repolarization. Even more important is their ability to reduce large inhomogeneities in the duration of repolarization and refractory periods in the neighboring cells. This ability

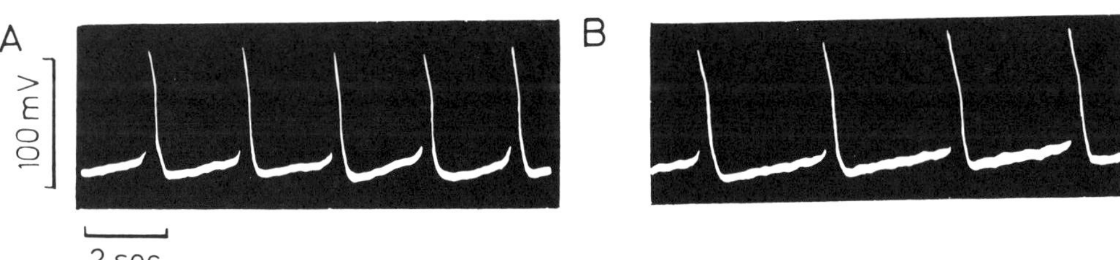

Fig. 7–13 Effects of droperidol on spontaneously beating Purkinje fibers. (A) Control. (B) Droperidol 5 $\times$ 10^{-6} M. Vertical or horizontal bars represent voltage and time calibrations, respectively. (Wojtczak J, Beresewicz A: Electrophysiological effects of the neuroleptanalgesic drugs on the canine cardiac tissue. Naunyn Schmiedebergs Arch Pharmacol 286:211, 1974.)

common to all antiarrhythmic drugs is demonstrated in Figure 7–14 and is due to alterations produced in the peripheral gate mechanism in the ventricles.

ISCHEMIA, ECG, AND ACTION POTENTIALS

It is important to detect myocardial ischemia as early as possible in the operating room. Changes in the ST segment are usually monitored, and the cellular events underlying these ECG changes are shown in Figure 7–15. Cellular depolarization at rest leads to the development of deviation of the TQ (diastolic) segment during ischemia. Since the ECG is usually obtained using AC amplifiers, not DC amplifiers as shown in Figure 7–15, the absolute zero cannot be determined. Therefore, what is usually called ST segment deviation is really the potential difference between the TQ segment and the ST segment. Other complicating factors in using the surface ECG to diagnose ischemia include the fact that the ST segment changes are due to the flow of current between normal and abnormal (ischemic) muscle with the current flowing intracellularly from a region of more positivity to more negativity. If continued progression of ischemia disrupts intracellular electrical connections (gap junctions) and abolishes current flow between regions, the ST-segment changes will decrease, although the injury is more pronounced. In addition, since epicardial and endocardial injury produce changes in the ST segment in opposite directions (Fig. 7–15), and the potential recorded by any ECG lead is determined by the sum of all the currents, extension

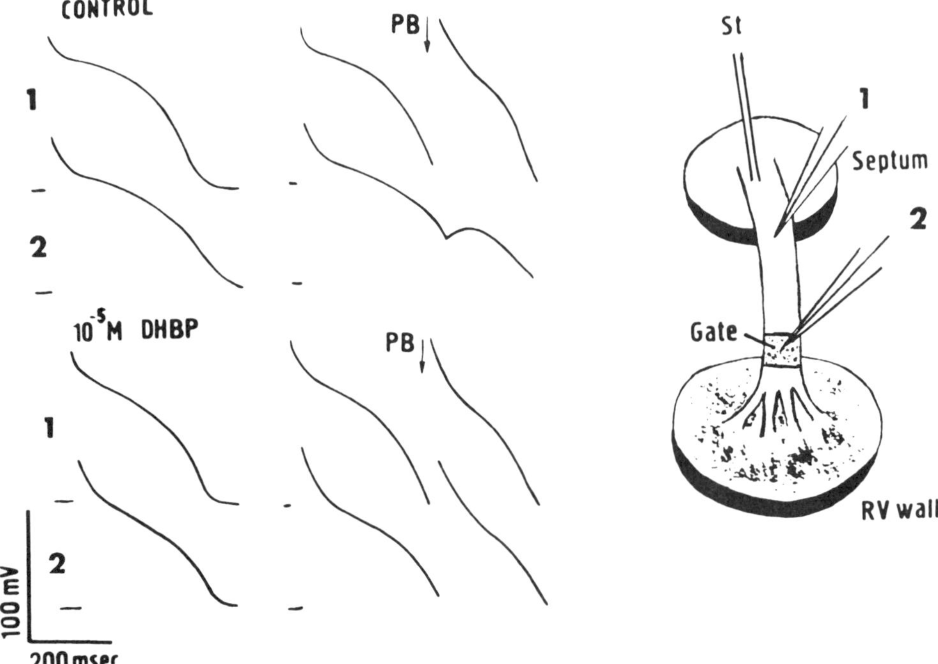

Fig. 7–14 Effects of droperidol (DHBP) on prolonged action potentials in the gate. A premature beat (PB) applied during control conditions **(A)** is blocked and induces a slow response. **(B)** Droperidol, acting as lidocaine and diphenylhydantoin, shortens the long action potential (marked 2) much more than the shorter one (marked 1) permitting unimpaired conduction of the premature beat. (JA Wojtczak, unpublished results.)

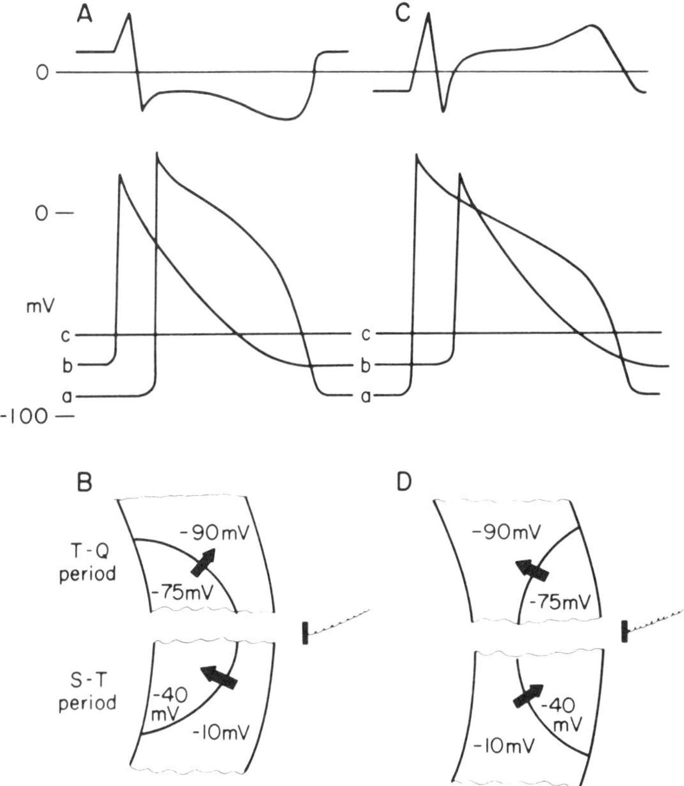

Fig. 7–15 Abnormal repolarization occurring in ischemia. **(A)** ECG showing elevation of the TQ segment and depression of the ST segment relative to zero voltage: the pattern of endocardial injury. Beneath the ECG are three intracellular recordings: *a* is an epicardial cell that has a normal resting membrane potential and is of normal duration, *b* is an endocardial cell that is depolarized in the resting state and has an abbreviated action potential as the result of ischemia, and *c* is an endocardial cell that is depolarized sufficient to render it inexcitable. **(B)** Vector representations of the voltage gradients during rest (TQ period) and activity (ST period). The arrows represent the direction in which positive charges move. Positive charges moving toward the epicardium (during the TQ period) cause positivity in a unipolar epicardial electrode. The converse exists during the ST period. −40 mV is used as an arbitrary example of an average potential in the ischemic area produced because of either early repolarization (b) or failure to depolarize (c). **(C,D)** Comparable patterns for epicardial injury. (Fozzard MA, Das Gupta DS: ST-segment potentials and mapping. Theory and experiments. Circulation 54:533, 1976. By permission of the American Heart Association, Inc.)

of the ischemic process in the opposite region may normalize the ST segment, that is, cancel it out.

Since monitoring ST segments alone may sometimes lead to erroneous interpretations, other methods for reliably detecting myocardial ischemia are needed. Ischemia produces dramatic changes in the shape of the cellular monophasic action potential (MAP) and intracavitary recordings of these potentials using suction electrodes on the subendocardial, ischemic zone of the left or right ventricle were performed by Donaldson et al.[14] in patients with reversible myocardial ischemia. An example of such a recording is shown in Figure 7–16. Monophasic action potentials recorded by the suction electrode accurately reflect both the duration and shape of underlying transmembrane action po-

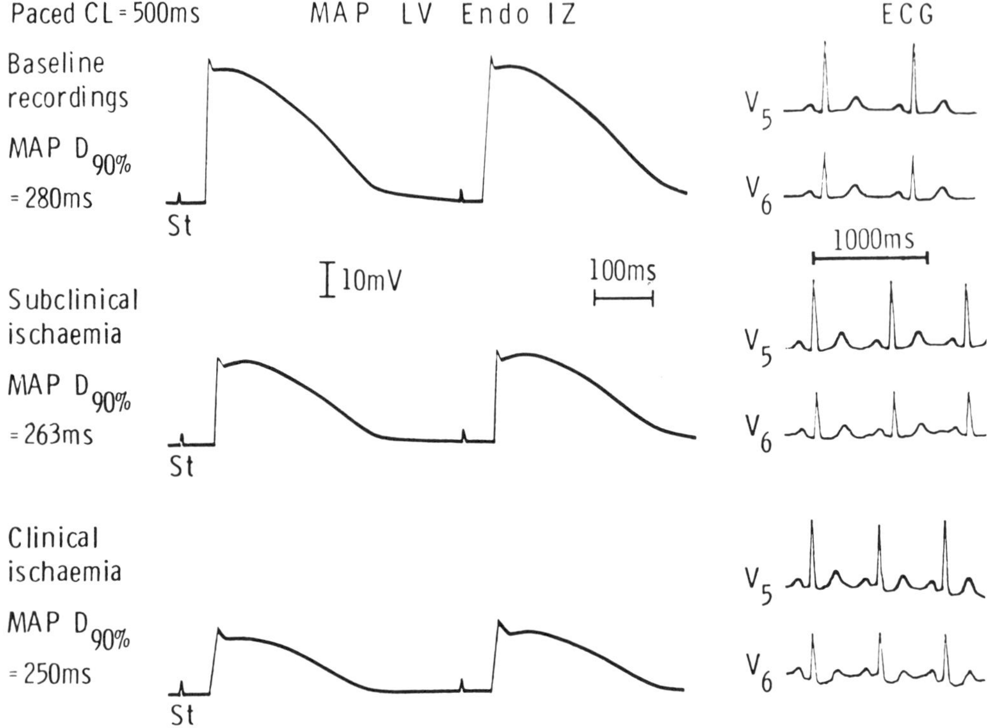

Fig. 7–16 Continuous recordings of the left ventricular endocardial monophasic action potential from the ischaemic zone (Endo IZ) during pacing at the threshold rate for angina until the onset of clinical ischaemia. The baseline tracings correspond to the start of the pacing run. The second tracing was recorded 3 minutes later, before the onset of angina and ECG abnormalities, and shows the characteristic decreases in monophasic action potential amplitude and repolarization time (D 90 percent) of subendocardial ischemia. These changes are more pronounced in the third tracing when both clinical and electrocardiographic evidence of ischaemia was evident. The top unpaced ECGs (leads V5 and V6) were obtained before the pacing run; the other ECGs were recorded within seconds of the corresponding monophasic action potential recordings. (Donaldson RM, Taggart P, Swanton M, et al: Effect of nitroglycerin on the electrical changes of early or subendocardial ischaemia evaluated by monophasic action potential recordings. Cardiovasc Res 18:7, 1984. Reproduced by permission of the Authors and Editors of Cardiovascular Research.)

tentials. Recently, in another series of patients, Donaldson et al.[15] evaluated the therapeutic effects of nitroglycerin on early, subendocardial ischemia with the MAP technique. Both studies showed that intracavitary recordings of MAP provide sensitive indices of regional ischemia in man, with changes in MAP preceding angina and ECG changes by up to 5 minutes, and the effects of drugs being measured on a beat-to-beat basis. Potentially, this method of monitoring would make possible very early detection of intraoperative ischemia and enable on-line evaluation of the effects of drugs. Thus, the theory and physiology of the cardiac action potential described in this chapter could someday be of practical value in the perioperative setting.

REFERENCES

1. Hodgkin AL, Huxley AF: A quantitative description of membrane current and its application to conduction and excitation in nerve. J Physiol (Lond) 117:500, 1952
2. Reuter M: The dependence of slow inward current in Purkinje fibers on the extracellular calcium concentration. J Physiol (Lond) 192:479, 1967

3. Noble D: The Initiation of the Heartbeat. Clarendon Press, Oxford, 1979
4. Mullins LJ: Ion Transport in Heart. Raven Press, New York, 1981
5. Cranefield PF: The conduction of the cardiac impulse. Futura, Mt. Kisco, New York, 1975
6. Wojtczak J: Intracellular coupling between cardiac cells and its disturbances, p. 283. In Bouman L, Jongsma M (eds): Cardiac Rate and Rhythm. Martinus Nijhoff, The Hague, 1982
7. Downar EM, Janse MJ, Durrer D: The effect of acute coronary artery occlusion on subepicardial transmembrane potentials in the intact porcine heart. Circulation 56:217, 1977
8. Hoffman BF, Rosen MR: Cellular mechanisms for cardiac arrhythmias. Circ Res 49:1, 1981
9. Wojtczak J: Effects of transient acid-base changes on afterdepolarizations and triggered arrhythmias in the dog heart. Anesthesiology 61:A33, 1984
10. Janse MJ, van Capelle FJL, Morsink H, et al: Flow of "injury" current and patterns of excitation during early ventricular arrhythmias in acute regional myocardial ischemia in isolated porcine and canine hearts; evidence for two different arrhythmogenic mechanisms. Circ Res 47:151, 1980
11. Hoffman BF, Rosen MR, Wit AL: Electrophysiology and pharmacology of cardiac arrhythmias. III. The causes and treatment of cardiac arrhythmias. Part A. Am Heart J 89:115, 1975
12. Wojtczak J, Beresewicz A: Electrophysiological effects of the neuroleptanalgesic drugs on the canine cardiac tissue. Naunyn Schmiedebergs Arch Pharmacol 286:211, 1974
13. Fozzard MA, Das Gupta DS: ST-segment potentials and mapping. Theory and experiments. Circulation 54:533, 1976
14. Donaldson RM, Taggart P, Swanton M, et al: Intracardiac electrode detection of early ischaemia in man. Br Heart J 50:213, 1983
15. Donaldson RM, Taggart P, Swanton M, et al: Effect of nitroglycerin on the electrical changes of early or subendocardial ischaemia evaluated by monophasic action potential recordings. Cardiovasc Res 18:7, 1984

8

Electrophysiologic Effects of Anesthetic Agents

Margaret Pratila, M.D.
Vasilios Pratilas, M.D.

In recent years, anesthesiologists have discovered that cardiac electrophysiology can be as informative to them as it has been to cardiac electrophysiologists and cardiologists over the past 30 years. Basic cardiac electrophysiology is reviewed in Chapter 7; this chapter summarizes the effects of some of the anesthetic drugs on cardiac electrophysiology. In addition, underlying pathologic conditions (e.g., coronary artery disease, electrolyte imbalance) or concurrent cardiac medications (e.g., digitalis, β-blockers) that may alter or potentiate the effects of anesthetic drugs are discussed.

GENERAL ANESTHETIC AGENTS

The Halogenated Anesthetics

THE SINOATRIAL NODE

Halothane, enflurane, isoflurane, and methoxyflurane are known to depress sinoatrial (SA) nodal activity (Fig. 8–1).[1–3] A dose-dependent reduction in phase 4 depolarization is the main cause for the slowing of the rate of spontaneous discharge. Reduction in the slope of phase 0, overshoot, and amplitude also occur. These effects can be partially reversed by calcium and potentiated by the calcium channel blocker, verapamil, but are not influenced by atropine or propranolol.[2,3] A significant decrease of the maximum diastolic membrane potential occurs only with 2 MAC halothane, while threshold is unaffected and action potential duration is increased.[3] Clinically, this would be evident as a slowing of the rate on ECG, sinus bradycardia, or, in severe cases, sinus arrest.

The level of the resting membrane potential or, in pacemaker cells, the maximum diastolic membrane potential, influences the action potential that follows excitation of the cell. When the transmembrane potential is near its resting level, the action potential has a rapid rate of rise of phase 0 (Vmax), is of large amplitude, and is more efficient in exciting neighboring tissues and initiating a conducted impulse.[4,5] When the resting membrane potential is reduced (i.e., less negative) toward the threshold level, the action potential has a lower Vmax, a lower amplitude, and is a less effective stimulus to bordering cells.

Patients with arteriosclerosis may have SA nodal cells in a partly depolarized state. The disordered impulse generation within their sinus nodes or impaired conduction of impulses from

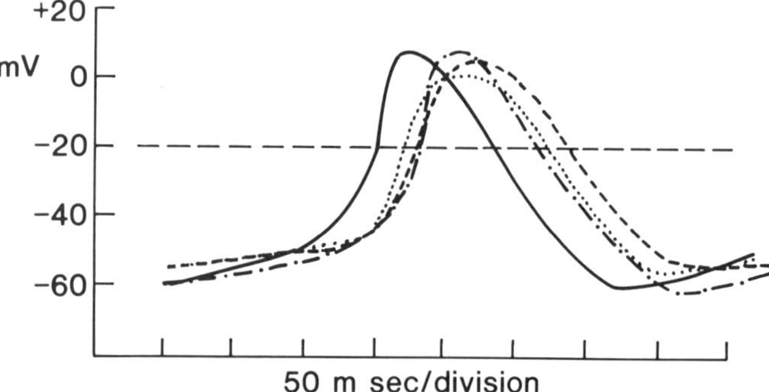

Fig. 8–1 Schematic presentation of the effects of halothane, enflurane, and methoxyflurane on the sinoatrial (SA) node.[2,3] MAC values permit comparison between agents. The control situation is shown as the solid line. See text for explanation.

their sinus node into the atrium (exit block) may not be manifested until halogenated anesthetic agents produce further depolarization. Sick sinus syndrome, a term used for a group of diseases affecting the SA node, may first be evident during anesthesia.[6]

THE ATRIA

Atrial fibers are not very sensitive to the halogenated anesthetics. Dose-dependent decreases of overshoot and slightly prolonged repolarization occur with halothane,[7] methoxyflurane,[8] and enflurane,[9] but no marked changes in resting potential or amplitude occur (Fig. 8–2). Therefore, no effect on the P wave would be expected.

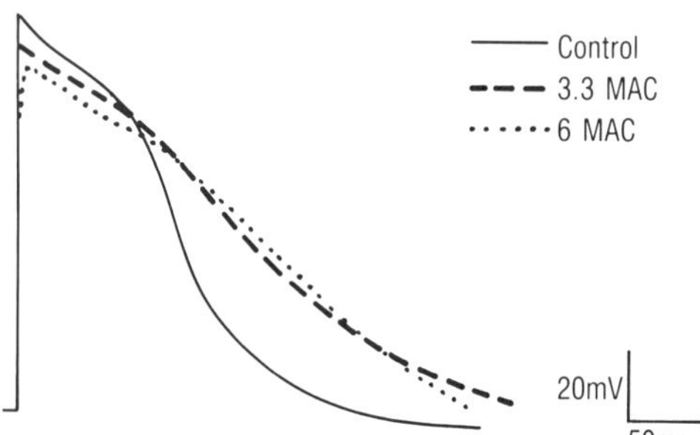

Fig. 8–2 Effects of enflurane on rabbit atrium are minimal. Slightly prolonged repolarization of the action potential is shown.

THE ATRIOVENTRICULAR

It is clinically obvious that currently used volatile anesthetic agents have marked effects on the conduction of electrical activity across the atrioventricular (AV) node. Not uncommonly, P waves unrelated to QRS complexes are seen with ECG monitoring during anesthesia; with termination of the anesthetic agent, the ECG becomes normal.

Unfortunately, there have been few microelectrode studies on AV nodal tissue. The study of Reynolds et al.[10] with methoxyflurane is interesting, showing that AV node activity remained normal even after complete arrest of the SA nodal fibers. This finding correlates well with the frequent development of nodal rhythms during methoxyflurane anesthesia.[11]

The effects of the anesthetic agents on atrioventricular conduction have been studied mainly using His stimulation and recording techniques. Initial studies showed a concentration-dependent depression of AV conduction by halothane, most marked proximal to the His bundle (AH recording).[12] Later studies in chronically instrumented dogs (allowing a true change from an awake to an anesthetized state) indicated that halothane-induced prolongation of AV nodal conduction appears greater at light levels of anesthesia (1 to 1.5 percent) and is a function of changes in autonomic tone rather than increased concentration.[13] If sympathetic activity is eliminated, AH intervals are prolonged at fast rates, but not at slow rates, upon exposure to halothane.[14]

His-bundle studies during 1 to 2 MAC enflurane demonstrated prolonged AV nodal, but not His–Purkinje or ventricular, conduction times.[15] The atrial and AV nodal functional refractory periods, as well as the AV nodal conductivity, were all prolonged by enflurane in a rate-dependent manner. Since halothane does not prolong the atrial effective refractory period, this may explain the decreased incidence of supraventricular dysrhythmias during enflurane anesthesia when compared to halothane.[15] In further support of these experimental findings, it has been shown clinically that 0.75 MAC enflurane has no influence on ventricular pacing when used as a treatment for third-degree heart block produced by cardioplegic solutions during cardiopulmonary bypass.[16]

Isoflurane at 1.25, 2, and 2.5 MAC administered during atrial pacing to dogs produced no changes in the AH interval.[17] The stability of cardiac rhythm seen clinically with isoflurane may be related to this lack of effect on the AV node.

PURKINJE FIBERS

The effect of halothane on Purkinje fibers is both dose and species related.[2,7] At and above 2 percent, depolarization is slowed due to an increase in threshold potential and a decreased rate of rise in phase 4 depolarization. Loss of the plateau occurs due to a steep increase in the slope of phase 2, and the action potential duration may be shortened (with loss of the refractory period) or unchanged when a decrease in phase 3 repolarization occurs. There is a loss of maximum diastolic potential, overshoot, and the amplitude of the action potential. Pruett et al.[18] also showed that enhanced membrane responsiveness occurs. The effects of enflurane are similar to those of halothane, but in spontaneously beating fibers the rate of phase 4 depolarization is enhanced and the maximum diastolic potential is significantly reduced (Fig. 8–3). As with halothane, membrane responsiveness is enhanced.[18] Since membrane responsiveness reflects the fast inward Na^+ current, this effect may be due to alterations in voltage- and/or time-dependent changes in sodium conductance similar to that reported by Chen et al.[19] for lidocaine.

Both enflurane[3] and methoxyflurane[2] produce primary (SA nodal) pacemaker suppression and secondary (Purkinje fibers) pacemaker stimulation.[20] Vassale and Carpentier [21] showed that Purkinje fibers driven at a rate faster than their own rate (overdrive) temporarily suppress spontaneous activity (overdrive suppression). Overdrive causes an initial depolarization (due to interstitial K^+ accumulation) and a delayed

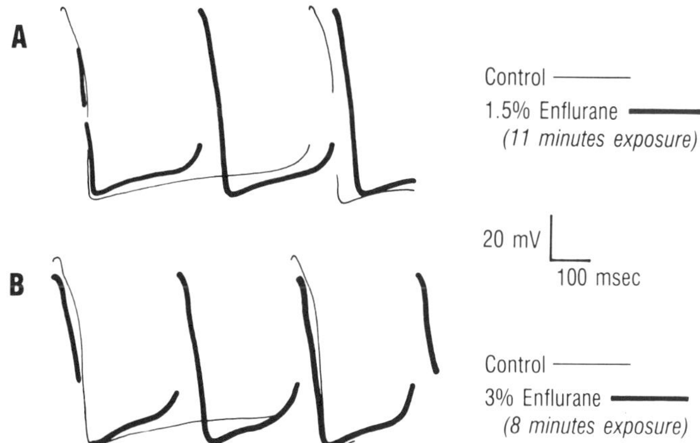

Fig. 8–3 Effects of enflurane on spontaneously firing canine Purkinje fibers at 1.5 percent (0.73 MAC) and 3 percent (1.5 MAC).

hyperpolarization (due to stimulation of the electrogenic Na^+/K^+ pump); and enflurane and methoxyflurane inhibit this postdrive hyperpolarization in a dose-dependent manner (Fig. 8–4),[20] with methoxyflurane being more potent than enflurane. The mechanism of this inhibition could be (1) direct inhibition of the Na^+/K^+ pump, in a manner similar to that of the cardiac glycosides[21]; (2) an indirect effect due to anesthetic-induced structural alterations in the lipid bilayer in which the pump is embedded; or (3) reduction in the Na^+ influx, and thus of sodium loading, during each action potential. Both methoxyflurane and enflurane reduce the slope of phase 0 and the amplitude and duration of phase 2 of the action potential, suggesting inhibition of both the fast Na^+ and slow Ca^{++} current. This has been demonstrated more directly in ventricular muscle.[22]

VENTRICULAR MUSCLE

Halothane depresses intraventricular conduction, but to a lesser extent than conduction through the AV node.[23] Ventricular automaticity is somewhat depressed at 2 percent halothane, while the resting membrane potential is unchanged.[2,24,25] Overshoot, Vmax, and the action potential are decreased, and there is a shortened effective refractory period.[7]

Enflurane has little effect on the resting membrane potential of normal guinea pig action potentials.[22] Amplitude and Vmax were virtually unaffected by even 6 percent enflurane. However, loss of the plateau and decreased action potential duration occurred at higher concentrations. Since the slow inward current is responsible for maintaining the plateau of the action potential, the decrease in duration may

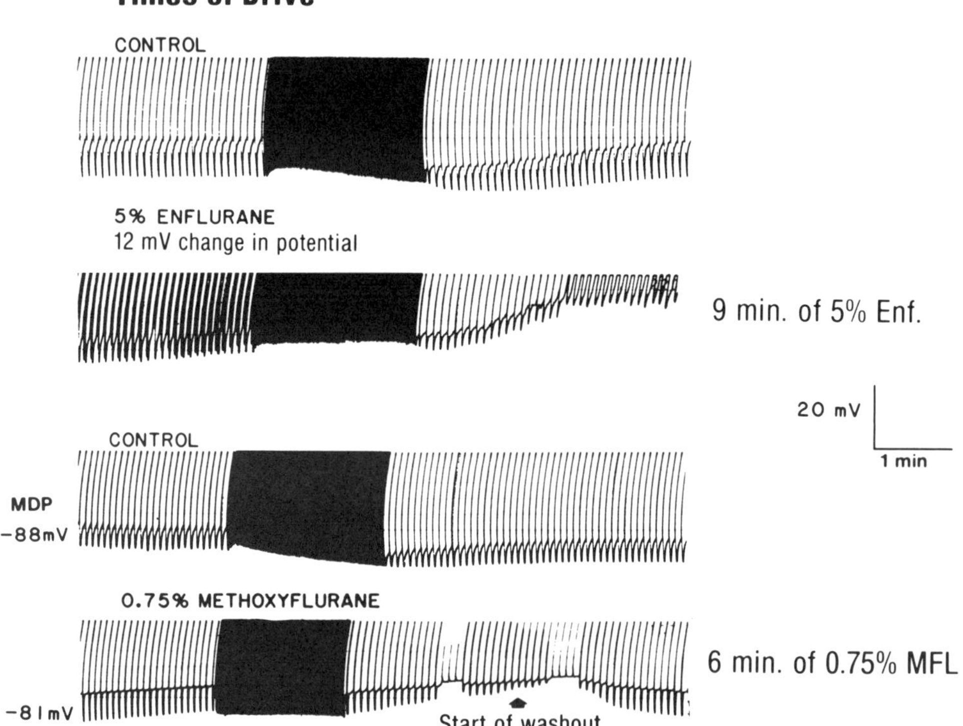

Fig. 8–4 Effects of enflurane and methoxyflurane on postdrive hyperpolarization. MDP, Maximum diastolic potential.

be attributed to depression of the slow inward currents produced by the volatile anesthetic agents.

During phase 2 of the action potential (the plateau), there is inward movement of calcium ions through the kinetically slow ion-transport system.[26] If this system is blocked by verapamil, a marked negative inotropism occurs in the presence of virtually normal action potentials,[27] since the calcium entering via the slow channels contributes to the contractile process.[28] Early researchers showed that halothane produced similar negative inotropism with little effect on cardiac action potentials.[7,29] Slow-channel studies with halothane, enflurane, and methoxyflurane have shown depression of the inward calcium current, with halothane being slightly more depressant than enflurane. Electromechanical dissociation is not uncommon with these drugs and can be seen as hypotension with a virtually normal ECG.

CLINICAL IMPLICATIONS

Halothane produces depression of phase 4 depolarization, thus behaving as an antiarrhythmic drug. It moderates the cardiotoxic effects of digitalis and has therapeutic value in ouabain-induced ventricular tachycardia.[30–32] The site of ectopic pacemaker activity in digitalis-induced ventricular tachycardia is in the left bundle branch or lower, with retrograde activation of the bundle of His, and halothane has been shown to suppress the enhancement of this site produced by digitalis.[33,34] Halothane antagonizes the increased rate of phase 4 depolarization and prevents the increased automaticity in ectopic pacemaker cells.[35,36] Enhanced membrane responsiveness reported with halothane may also help prevent the reentry type of dysrhythmias that occur during digitalis toxicity or ischemia.[37] The competitive action of halothane with calcium on the slow-channel ionic fluxes may also be a factor in its antiarrhythmic properties.[3]

Diethyl ether, methoxyflurane, enflurane, and isoflurane also increase tolerance to digitalis toxicity when given prior to ouabain infusion and restore sinus rhythm when given after ventricular tachycardia has been induced by ouabain.[38] Enflurane also increases membrane responsiveness, which may in part explain its action in moderating digitalis-induced dysrhythmias.[18]

While the effects of the inhalational anesthetic agents on AV nodal conduction remain unclear, it is certain that they do not antagonize the AV nodal depression of digitalis. Effective refractory periods of the ventricles are shortened by the anesthetic agents, as is the case with digitalis. Sympathetic nervous system involvement is a factor in the genesis of digitalis-induced dysrhythmias,[39] and halothane,[40] enflurane,[41] and isoflurane[42] are all reported to decrease sympathetic nervous system activity and to confer increased tolerance to digitalis.

The way in which the volatile anesthetic agents may act as antiarrhythmic agents has been reviewed, but in clinical practice dysrhythmias occur quite frequently. This is particularly true in the presence of catecholamines from either endogenous or exogenous sources. Early papers discussed the underlying mechanism for the dysrhythmias (i.e., increased automaticity or reentry), but all recent evidence is in favor of reentry.[43–45] There are critical threshold levels for both blood pressure and atrial rate associated with these dysrhythmias. A rise in intraventricular systolic pressure causes stretch of Purkinje fibers, which slows conduction velocity and increases the rate of diastolic depolarization, both of which favor reentry.[46] The typical bigeminal beat is believed to be a fusion beat of a reentrant impulse the origin of which is in the upper part of the intraventricular septum with the next normal beat conducted through the AV node.[47]

In comparing presently used volatile anesthetic agents, Joas and Stevens[48] found in dogs that four times the dose of epinephrine was necessary during isoflurane anesthesia as compared with halothane anesthesia to produce premature ventricular contractions. During epinephrine injection in humans, the stability of cardiac rhythm is greatest with isoflurane, second with enflurane, and least with halothane.[49,50] Both Johnston et al. with halothane and Horrigan et al.

with enflurane demonstrated the need for larger doses of epinephrine when the vehicle of injection was lidocaine.[49,50]

Nonhalogenated Agents

The electrophysiologic effects of cyclopropane and ether were studied in the 1960s. Although they are not used in anesthesia today, their effects are interesting because they are unlike those of the halogenated anesthetics. Cyclopropane has little effect on the sinus node, but it increases the rate of rise of phase 4 depolarization in Purkinje fibers and potentiates the increased slope and magnitude of diastolic depolarization produced by epinephrine.[51,52] There is an increased rate of phase 2 repolarization, resulting in loss of the plateau, and dysrhythmias are frequent. Di-ethyl ether is thought to have a direct positive chronotropic effect on atrial muscle, with catecholamine release not being a factor, since pretreatment with reserpine has no influence.[53] Beta-adrenergic stimulation is excluded by use of propranolol, and cholinergic blockade is also excluded since atropine has no influence on atrial rate. This direct stimulant effect of ether on the atrial pacemaker could suppress some dysrhythmias in a manner similar to atrial pacing. This protective effect of ether was used during cyclopropane anesthesia to override ventricular dysrhythmias.

Intravenous Drugs

There has been very little study of intravenous anesthetic drugs from an electrophysiologic point of view. Droperidol has been shown to depress conduction in sheep cardiac Purkinje fibers and papillary muscle.[54–56] It increases the effective refractory period and decreases the rate of phase 0 depolarization, while resting membrane potential and action potential amplitude are unchanged. Bertolo et al.[55] demonstrated its antiarrhythmic properties, showing it effective in preventing ventricular tachycardia produced by halothane/epinephrine exposure and ventricular fibrillation secondary to coronary occlusion. Recently, it has been shown that droperidol also increases the antegrade and retrograde refractory periods of accessory pathways in the Wolff–Parkinson–White syndrome and that it may prevent rapid ventricular responses due to antegrade conduction over the accessory pathway or reciprocal supraventricular tachycardia due to retrograde conduction over the accessory pathway.[57]

Sodium pentobarbital injected directly into the sinus node artery produces a slowing of cardiac rate with SA exit block and nodal rhythm at higher doses.[58] The bradycardia cannot be blocked by atropine and is only partially reversed by norepinepherine. Studies in rabbit cardiac ventricular fibers have shown that barbiturates cause a rapid fall in early phase 3 repolarization (phase of decreased sodium conductance) and a slowing of late repolarization (phase of increased potassium conductance).[59] In addition, Rouse[60] reported a prolongation of AV nodal conduction time in dogs.

Although Morrow[61] reported that barbiturates do not alter the dose of digoxin necessary to produce ventricular automaticity, Atlee and Malkinson[62] showed that thiopentone potentiates halothane–epinephrine-induced dysrhythmias in dogs. This effect of thiopentone was previously demonstrated for cyclopropane–epinephrine-induced dysrhythmias,[63] is localized to the AV node and His bundle, and correlates with Rouse's study.[60]

Ketamine causes a marked increase in heart rate due to central sympathetic stimulation and parasympathetic inhibition.[64] In isolated heart preparations, ketamine produces a negative inotropic effect and a prolonged refractory period, which may explain its reversing both halothane–epinephrine-induced ventricular tachycardia and digitalis-induced dysrhythmias.[65,66] Figure 8–5 shows the increase in action potential duration mainly due to prolongation of the plateau, which correlates well with the prolonged refractory period produced by ketamine.

The effects of meperidine in cat, guinea pig, and rhesus monkey papillary muscle have been studied.[67] In lower concentrations, the main ef-

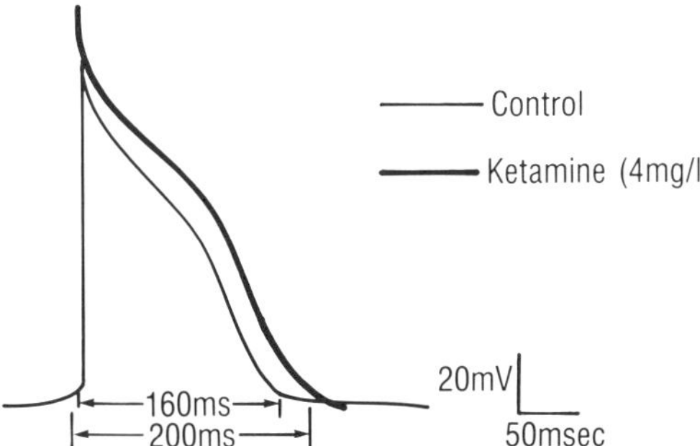

Fig. 8–5 Effect of ketamine 4 mg/L on a guinea pig ventricular cardiac action potential. See text for explanation.

fect is a dose-dependent decrease in the rate of phase 0 depolarization, decreased rate of conduction, and decreased excitability. Resting membrane potential and overshoot are virtually unaffected. In higher concentrations, there are decreases in resting membrane potential and the height of the action potential, with a marked reduction in upshoot velocity. The other narcotics have not been studied in this manner.

The Muscle Relaxants

Only a few electrophysiologic studies have been conducted with this group of drugs. Succinylcholine is known to have profound effects on cardiac rate. A single intravenous dose in children may cause a decrease in cardiac rate, and a second dose may do so in adults.[68,69] Galindo et al.[70] showed that a small dose of succinylcholine (20 mg) can convert a nodal rhythm into a sinus rhythm. These effects can be explained by small doses of succinylcholine stimulating the activity of the SA node, while larger doses depress it. Yasuda et al.[71] studied the effects of succinylcholine and succinylmonocholine on the SA node by direct injection into the sinus node artery. Succinylcholine produced a dose-related positive chronotropic effect through an indirect catecholamine-induced effect. Succinylmonocholine caused a decrease in heart rate due to either cholinergic receptor stimulation or a direct effect. Junctional rhythms may also occur with succinylcholine, since it lowers the cardiac excitability threshold.[72]

Studies with d-tubocurarine have been of a very indirect nature. Dowdy et al.[73] studied the effects of d-tubocurarine in isolated perfused rabbit hearts and observed a quinidine-like action with decreases in the rate of rise of phase 4 depolarization, dV/dt max, threshold of excitability, and conduction velocity. The effective refractory period was increased, and there was slight prolongation of the action potential. Geha et al.[74] studied the effects of pancuronium using His-bundle electrocardiography. AV conduction was shown to be increased, atrial–His bundle conduction time decreased, and His bundle–ventricle time unchanged. This may be of clinical importance.

LOCAL ANESTHETICS

Recently, numerous clinical reports have documented that resuscitation following circulatory collapse from bupivacaine or etidocaine is more difficult than with lidocaine or procaine.[75] Therefore, these drugs, particularly bupivacaine, are discussed in detail. DeJong et al.[76] compared the effects of lidocaine, bupivacaine, and etidocaine at equiconvulsant doses in cats and found increased QRS complex amplitude and aberrant intraventricular conduction with bupivacaine and etidocaine. Nodal and ventricular dysrhythmias occurred with bupivacaine (100 percent) and etidocaine (80 percent), while dysrhythmias were rare with lidocaine (37 percent). These investigators were unable to explain the severe dysrhythmias. By contrast, bupivacaine and etidocaine had previously been reported to protect the heart against epinephrine-induced dysrhythmias, and bupivacaine was shown to have equivalent antiarrhythmic effects to lidocaine in equipotent doses.[77–79]

The direct effects of local anesthetic agents have been studied using isolated rabbit heart preparations.[80] The electrophysiologic effects of lidocaine (class IB antiarrhythmic) are summarized in Figure 8–6 and compared with the class IA drugs. All agents produce dose-related de-

	CLASS I	
	A	**B**
Automaticity (rate of phase 4 depolarization)	↓	↓
Maximum Rate of Depolarization dV/dt max	↓	↓
Threshold of Excitability	↑	0
Conduction Velocity	↓	↑
Effective Refractory Period	↑	↓
Resting Membrane Potential	0	+ Neg
Action Potential Duration	SL ↑	SL ↓
Sympatholytic Effect	0	0
Slow Response	0	0
Drugs --------	**Quinidine** **Procainamide** **Disopyramide**	**Lidocaine** **DPH**

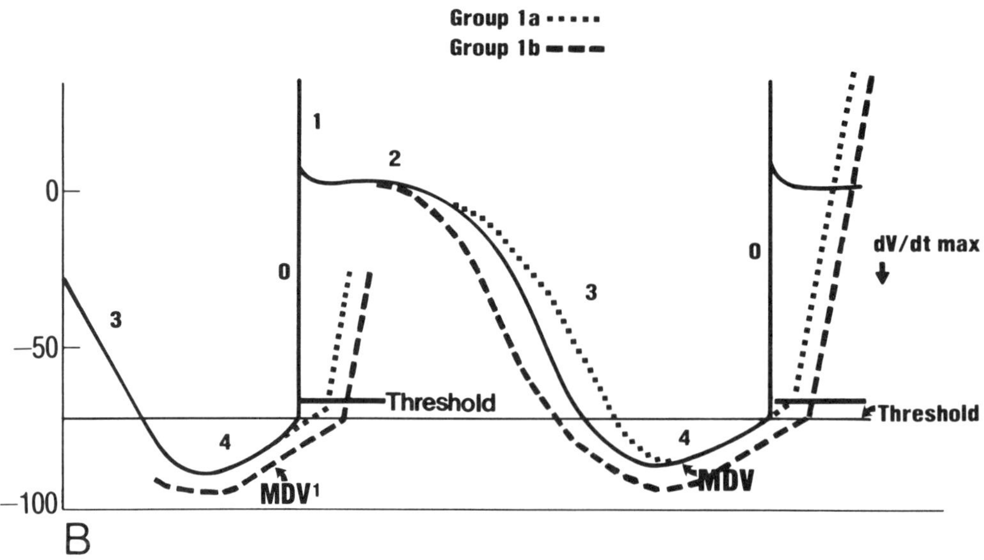

Fig. 8–6 (A,B) Effects of class I A and B antiarrhythmic drugs on the action potential. Lidocaine, an amide-type local anesthetic, is the standard class IB drug.

pression of intraatrial, AV nodal, and intraventricular conduction, and myocardial contractility. The more potent local anesthetic agents depress conduction and contractility at significantly lower concentrations than the less potent drugs. AV nodal conduction was less influenced than intraatrial and intraventricular conduction pathways. In isolated canine Purkinje fibers, slow diastolic depolarization was decreased when exposed to perfusates containing bupivacaine in concentrations of 1 to 10 mg/L.[81] The duration of the action potential decreased, while upshoot velocity and amplitude decreased in a dose-dependent manner, with a resulting decrease in conduction velocity. Conduction block and total inexcitability occurred in more than 50 percent of fibers exposed to the highest bupivacaine concentrations; if fibers were depolarized by hyperkalemia or stretch, these effects were evident at lower bupivacaine concentrations. Bupivacaine also suppressed pathologic oscillations at low levels of membrane potential. Ventricular dysrhythmias due to bupivacaine may therefore be due to slowing of conduction velocity with unidirectional block and reentry. They are obviously not due to increased automaticity or oscillations in membrane potential, which are suppressed by bupivacaine. Bupivacaine had been found to have more marked effects in partially depolarized fibers, suggesting that patients with ischemic heart disease may be more sensitive to the effects of the drug.[82]

Wojtczak et al.[83] also studied the effects of high-dose bupivacaine in guinea pig right atria and canine ventricular Purkinje fibers. Bupivacaine slowed the spontaneous rate of right atrial cells to less than 40 percent of control, and both catecholamines in increasing concentration and alkalosis reversed the bradycardia. The catecholamines restored excitability and conduction in 40 percent of fibers, although conduction remained slow, while alkalosis produced only a transient improvement in conduction velocity. The beneficial effects of catecholamines and alkalosis may be explained by their action on the background calcium current primarily responsible for automaticity in the SA node. Bupivacaine suppresses the fast inward Na^+ current in Purkinje fibers, leading to slowed conduction and inexcitability; high doses of catecholamines partially reverse this effect by leading to hyperpolarization of the resting membrane potential.

REFERENCES

1. Hauswirth O, Schaer H: Effects of halothane on the sino-atrial node. J Pharmacol Exp Ther 158:36, 1967
2. Reynolds AK, Chiz JF, Pasquet AF: Halothane and methoxyflurane. A comparison of their effects on cardiac pacemaker fibers. Anesthesiology 33:602, 1970
3. Bosnjak ZJ, Kampine JP: Effects of halothane, enflurane, and isoflurane on the SA node. Anesthesiology 58:314, 1983
4. Weidmann S: Effects of calcium ions and local anesthetics on electrical properties of Purkinje fibers. J Physiol (Lond) 129:568, 1955
5. Kao CY, Hoffman BF: Graded and decremental responses in heart-muscle fibers. Am J Physiol 194:187, 1958
6. Pratila MG, Pratilas V: Sick-sinus syndrome manifested during anesthesia. Anesthesiology 44:433, 1978
7. Hauswirth O: Effects of halothane on single atrial, ventricular and Purkinje fibers. Circ Res 24:745, 1969
8. Reynolds AK, Chiz JF, Pasquet AF: Pacemaker migration and sinus node arrest with methoxyflurane and halothane. Can Anaesth Soc J 18:137, 1971
9. Pratila MG, Vogel S, Sperelakis N: Effects of enflurane on rabbit atrium. p. 619. In Sperelakis N (ed): Physiology and Pathophysiology of the Heart. Martinus Nijhoff, Boston, 1984
10. Reynolds AK, Chiz JF, Pasquet AF: Pacemaker migration and sinus node arrest with methoxyflurane and halothane. Can Anaesth Soc J 18:137, 1971
11. Jacques A, Hudon F: Effect of epinephrine on the human heart during methoxyflurane anesthesia. Can Anaesth Soc J 10:53, 1963
12. Atlee JL, Rusy BF: Halothane depression of AV conduction studied by electrograms of the bundle of His in dogs. Anesthesiology 36:112, 1972
13. Atlee JL, Houge JC, Malkin CE: Halothane and AV conduction. Awake vs. anesthesia. Anesthesiology 55:A53, 1981

14. Hantler CB, Kroll DA, Tait AR, Knight PR: Cardiac effects of halothane with spinal anesthesia. Anesthesiology 55:A4, 1981
15. Atlee JL, Rusy BF, Kreul JF: Supraventricular excitability in dogs during anesthesia with halothane and enflurane. Anesthesiology 49:407, 1978
16. Zaidan JR, Curling PE, Kaplan JA: Effect of enflurane on pacing threshold. Anesthesiology 55:A59, 1981
17. Blitt CD, Raessler KL, Wightman MA, et al: Atrioventricular conduction in dogs during anesthesia with isoflurane. Anesthesiology 50:210, 1979
18. Pruett JK, Note PS, Grover TE, Augeri JM: Enflurane and halothane effects on cardiac Purkinje fibers. Anesthesiology 55:A65, 1981
19. Chen C, Gettes LS, Katzung BG: Effect of lidocaine and quinidine on steady-state characteristics and recovery kinetics of dv/dt max in guinea pig ventricular myocardium. Circ Res 37:20, 1975
20. Pratila MG, Vogel S, Sperelakis N: Inhibition by enflurane and methoxyflurane of post-drive hyperpolarization in canine Purkinje fibers. J Pharm Exp Ther 229:603, 1984
21. Vassale M, Carpentier R: Overdrive excitation: Onset of activity following fast drive in cardiac Purkinje fibers exposed to norepinephrine. Pflugers Arch 332:198, 1972
22. Lynch C, Vogel S, Pratila MG, Sperelakis N: Enflurane depression of myocardial slow action potentials. J Pharm Exp Ther 222:383, 1982
23. Atlee JL, Homer LD, Tober RE: Diphenylhydantoin and lidocaine modification of AV conduction in halothane anesthetized dogs. Anesthesiology 43:49, 1975
24. Hashimoto K, Endoh M, Kimura T: Effects of halothane on automaticity and contractile force of isolated blood-perfused canine ventricular tissue. Anesthesiology 42:15, 1975
25. Logic JR, Morrow DH: The effect of halothane on ventricular automaticity. Anesthesiology 36:107, 1972
26. Weidmann S: Heart: Electrophysiology. Annu Rev Physiol 36:155, 1974
27. Shigenobu K, Schneider JA, Sperelakis N: Blockade of slow Na^+ and Ca^{++} currents in myocardial cells by verapamil. J Pharm Exp Ther 190:280, 1974
28. Fabiato A, Fabiato F: Calcium and cardiac excitation–contraction coupling. Annu Rev Physiol 41:473, 1978
29. Awalt CH, Frederickson EL: The contractile and cell membrane effects of halothane. Anesthesiology 25:90, 1964
30. Morrow DH, Townley NT: Anesthesia and digitalis toxicity: An experimental study. Anesth Analg 43:510, 1964
31. Reynolds AK, Horne ML: Studies on the cardiotoxicity of ouabain. Can J Physiol Pharmacol 47:165, 1969
32. Morrow DH, Knapp DE, Logic JR: Anesthesia and digitalis toxicity V: Effect of the vagus on ouabain-induced ventricular automaticity during halothane. Anesth Analg 49:23, 1970
33. Damato AN, Lau SH, Bobb GA: Digitalis-induced bundle-branch ventricular tachycardia studied by electrode catheter recordings of the specialized conducting tissue of the dog. Circ Res 28:16, 1971
34. Logic JR, Morrow DH: The effect of halothane on ventricular automaticity. Anesthesiology 36:107, 1972
35. Matsui H, Schwartz A: Mechanism of cardiac glycoside inhibition of the (Na^+-K^+) dependent ATP-ase from cardiac tissue. Biochim Biophys Acta 151:655, 1968
36. Baker PF, Blaustein MP, Hodgkin AL, Steinhardt RA: The influence of calcium on sodium efflux in squid axons. J Physiol (Lond) 200:431, 1969
37. Pruett JK, Gramling ZW: Halothane enhanced membrane responsiveness in canine Purkinje fibers. Fed Proc 38:589, 1979
38. Ivankovich AD, Miletich DJ, Grossman RK, et al: The effect of enflurane, isoflurane, fluroxene, methoxyflurane, and diethyl ether anesthesia on ouabain tolerance in the dog. Anesth Analg 55:360, 1976
39. Pearle DL, Gillis RA: Effect of digitalis on response of the ventricular pacemaker to sympathetic neural stimulation and to isoproterenol. Am J Cardiol 34:704, 1974
40. Skovsted P, Price ML, Price HL: The effects of carbon dioxide on preganglionic sympathetic activity during halothane, methoxyflurane, and cyclopropane anesthesia. Anesthesiology 37:70, 1972
41. Brown FF, Owens WD, Felts JA, et al: Plasma epinephrine and norepinephrine levels during anesthesia. Enflurane -N_2O-O_2 compared with fentanyl–N_2O-O_2. Anesth Analg 61:366, 1982
42. Skovsted P, Sapthavichaikul S: The effects of isoflurane on arterial pressure, pulse rate, auto-

nomic nervous activity and barostatic reflexes. Can Anaesth Soc J 24:304, 1977

43. Hashimoto K, Hashimoto K: The mechanism of sensitization of the ventricle to epinephrine by halothane. Am Heart J 83:652, 1972
44. Hashimoto K, Endoh M, Kimura T: Effects of halothane on automaticity and contractile force of isolated blood-perfused canine ventricular tissue. Anesthesiology 42:15, 1975
45. Zink J, Sasyniuk BI, Dresel PE: Halothane–epinephrine induced cardiac arrhythmias and the role of heart rate. Anesthesiology 43:548, 1975
46. Singer DH, Lazzara R, Hoffman BF: Electrophysiological effects of canine peripheral AV conducting system. Circ Res 26:361, 1970
47. Reynolds AK, Chiz JF: Epinephrine-potentiated slowing of conduction in Purkinje fibers. Res Commun Chem Pathol Pharmacol 9:633, 1974
48. Joas TA, Stevens WC: Comparison of the arrhythmic doses of epinephrine during Forane, halothane, and fluroxene anesthesia in dogs. Anesthesiology 35:48, 1971
49. Johnston RR, Eger EI, Wilson C: A comparative interaction of epinepherine with enflurane, isoflurane and halothane in man. Anesth Analg 55:709, 1976
50. Horrigan RW, Eger EI, Wilson C: Epinephrine-induced arrhythmias during enflurane anesthesia in man: A non-linear dose–response relationship and dose-dependent protection from lidocaine. Anesth Analg 57:547, 1970
51. Davis LO, Temte JV, Helmer PR, et al: Effect of cyclopropane and of hypoxia on transmembrane potentials of atrial ventricular and Purkinje fibers. Circ Res 18:692, 1966
52. Davis LO, Tempte JV, Murphy QR: Epinephrine–cyclopropane effects on Purkinje fibers. Anesthesiology 30:369, 1969
53. Krishna G, Trueblood MS, Paradise RR: The mechanism of the positive chronotropic action of diethyl ether on rat atria. Anesthesiology 42:312, 1975
54. Hauswirth O: Effects of droperidol on sheep Purkinje fibers. Naunyn Schmiedebergs Arch Pharmacol 261:133, 1968
55. Bertolo L, Novakovic L, Penna M: Antiarrhythmic effects of droperidol. Anesthesiology 37:529, 1972
56. Kern R, Einwachter HM, Haas HG: Cardiac membrane currents as affected by neuroleptic agent: Droperidol. Pfluegers Arch 325:262, 1971
57. Gomez-Arnau J, Marquez-Montes J, Avello F: Fentanyl and droperidol effects on the refractoriness of the accessory pathway in the Wolff–-Parkinson–White syndrome. Anesthesiology 58:307, 1983
58. Chiba S, Nakajima T: Effect of sodium pentobarbital on the SA nodal activity of the dog heart in vivo. Tohoku J Exp Med 106(4):381, 1972
59. Daniel EE, Johnston PK, Foulks JG: The mechanism of the effects of sodium pentobarbital and norepineprhine in isolated cardiac muscle. Arch Int Pharmacodyn Ther 138:276, 1962
60. Rouse W: Effects of propranolol and ouabain on the conducting system of the heart in dogs. Am J Cardiol 18:406, 1966
61. Morrow DH: Anesthesia and digitalis toxicity. Effects of barbiturates and halothane in digoxin toxicity. Anesth Analg 49:305, 1970
62. Atlee JL III, Malkinson CE: Potentiation by thiopental of halothane–epinephrine-induced arrhythmias in dogs. Anesthesiology 57:285, 1982
63. MacCannell KL, Dresel PE: Potentiation by thiopental of cyclopropane–adrenaline cardiac arrhythmias. Can J Physiol Pharmacol 42:627, 1964
64. Traber DL, Wilson RO, Priano LL: The effect of beta-adrenergic blockade on the cardiopulmonary response to ketamine. Anesth Analg 49:604, 1970
65. Dowdy EG, Kaya K: Studies of the mechanism of cardiovascular responses to CI-581. Anesthesiology 29:931, 1968
66. Ivankovich AD, El-Etr AA, Janeczko GH: The effects of ketamine and of Innovar anesthesia on digitalis tolerance in dogs. Anesth and Analg 54:106, 1975
67. Grundy HF, Tritthart H: Effects of pethidine and nalorphine on the mechanical and electrical activities of mammalian isolated ventricular muscle. Br J Pharmacol 46:13, 1971
68. Leigh MD, McCoy DC, Belton MK, et al: Bradycardia following intravenous administration of succinylcholine chloride to infants and children. Anesthesiology 18:698, 1957
69. Lupprian KG, Churchill-Davidson HD: Effect of suxamethonium on cardiac rhythm. Br Med J 2:1774, 1960
70. Galindo A, Wyte SR, Witherhold JW: Junctional rhythm induced by halothane anesthesia. Anesthesiology 37:261, 1972
71. Yasuda L, Hirano T, Amahak, et al: Chronotropic effects of succinylcholine and succinylmonocholine on the sino-atrial node. Anesthesiology 57:289, 1982

72. Galindo A, Davis T: Succinylcholine and cardiac excitability. Anesthesiology 23:32, 1962
73. Dowdy EG, Dugger PN, Fabian LW: Effects of neuromuscular blocking agents on isolated digitalized mammalian hearts. Anesth Analg 44:608, 1965
74. Geha DG, Rozelle BC, Raessler KL: Pancuronium bromide enhances atrio-ventricular conduction in halothane anesthetized dogs. Anesthesiology 46:342, 1977
75. Albright GA: Cardiac arrest following regional anesthesia with etidocaine or bupivacaine. Anesthesiology 51:285, 1979
76. DeJong RH, Ronfeld RA, DeRosa RA: Cardiovascular effects of convulsant and supraconvulsant doses of amide local anesthetics. Anesth Analg 61:3, 1982
77. Chapin JC, Kushings LG, Munson ES, Schick LM: Lidocaine, bupivacaine, etidocaine, and epinephrine induced arrhythmias during halothane anesthesia in dogs. Anesthesiology 52:23, 1980
78. Boettner RB, Dunbar RW, Haley JV, Morrow DH: A comparison of the anti-arrhythmic effects of bupivacaine and lidocaine. South Med J 65:1328, 1972
79. Dunbar RW, Boettner RB, Gatz RN, Pennington RE: The effect of mepivacaine, bupivacaine, and lidocaine on digitalis induced ventricular arrhythmias. Anesth Analg 29:761, 1970
80. Block AB, Covino BG: Effect of local anesthetic agents on cardiac conduction and contractility. Reg Anesth 6:55, 1981
81. Wojtczak JA, Pratila V, Griffin RM, Kaplan JA: Cellular mechanisms of cardiac arrhythmias induced by bupivacaine. Anesthesiology 61:A37, 1984
82. Pratila MG, Pratilas V: Dysrhythmia occurring during epidural anesthesia with bupivacaine. The Mount Sinai J of Med 49:130, 1982
83. Wojtczak JA, Griffin RM, Pratilas V, Kaplan JA: Is it possible to resuscitate a bupivacaine-intoxicated heart? Anesthesiology 61:A207, 1984

9

Intraoperative Myocardial Ischemia

Richard M. Griffin, M.D.
Joel A. Kaplan, M.D.

Coronary artery disease (CAD) is prevalent in modern society and a leading cause of death among middle-aged men. Inevitably, these patients require anesthesia for myocardial revascularization or noncardiac surgery. Some will have well-documented anginal symptoms with the extent and severity of their CAD evaluated by careful history, physical examination, and laboratory investigation; and they will be treated with nitrates, β-blockers, or calcium channel blockers. However, other patients with silent or undiagnosed CAD will also be at increased risk for the development of ischemia during anesthesia. Patients undergoing major noncardiac surgical procedures do not have the benefit of receiving myocardial revascularization, while still being exposed to the multitude of risk factors predisposing to myocardial ischemia that occur during the perioperative period. Moreover, the anesthetic and monitoring techniques used may not be ideal due to the varying nature and short duration of some noncardiac surgical procedures.

INCIDENCE OF PERIOPERATIVE MYOCARDIAL ISCHEMIA AND INFARCTION

Many studies have investigated the incidence of postsurgical myocardial infarction or reinfarction. In the normal surgical population, the incidence of postoperative myocardial infarction is on the order of 0.13 to 0.66 percent.[1–4]

Preoperative myocardial infarction significantly increases the risk for the development of subsequent postoperative reinfarction. Topkins and Artusio[4] found that 43 (6.5 percent) of 658 patients reinfarcted, while Knapp et al.[3] reported that 26 (6 percent) of 427 patients developed an infarction postoperatively. In a series of 240 patients with severe CAD, Arkins et al.[5] found that 54 (22.6 percent) subsequently died in the 2 months following surgery. Tarhan et al.[2] collected data on 422 patients with previous myocardial infarctions and found that 28 (6.6 percent) experienced another infarction during the first postoperative week.[2] Six years later

Steen et al.,[6] reviewing data from the same institution, still found that 6.1 percent of patients developed a reinfarction within 1 week of surgery. The time interval between the first infarction and surgery markedly influenced the subsequent risk of reinfarction.[2,4,6] If the first infarction occurred within 3 months prior to surgery, the incidence of reinfarction was 27 to 37 percent. Between 3 and 6 months, this fell to 11 to 16 percent and thereafter stabilized at 4 to 5 percent. Recently, these results have been markedly improved by Rao et al.,[1] who used aggressive invasive hemodynamic monitoring and prompt treatment of hemodynamic aberrations to produce reinfarction rates of 5.8 percent and 2.3 percent, respectively, for previous infarctions less than 3 months and 4 to 6 months old. Thereafter, the reinfarction rate dropped to 1 to 1.7 percent. In this study, the mortality after reinfarction was 36 percent, which is also significantly lower than that reported in previous studies (over 50 percent).

Other studies have attempted to define the incidence of ECG changes occurring in the perioperative period in selected groups of patients who may be at an increased risk for the development of myocardial ischemia. Chamberlain and Edmons-Seal[7] performed preoperative and postoperative 12-lead ECGs in 217 patients with ischemic heart disease or hypertension. Twenty-two percent developed significant ECG deterioration (2.3 percent sustained frank myocardial infarction), and 33 percent had minor ECG changes, of which 68 percent became worse with a subsequent ECG on the fourth postoperative day. These workers postulated that persistence of ECG changes indicated that severe myocardial muscle injury may have occurred. Driscoll et al.[8] studied 145 patients with documented arteriosclerosis with pre- and postoperative ECGs and found that 23 percent developed fresh ischemic changes. The problem with these early studies from the 1960s using serial ECGs to detect ischemic changes is that monitoring was not continuous; therefore, the onset of ischemia was unknown and transient episodes of ischemia were probably missed.

To overcome this problem, 24-hour continuous recordings of the ECG on magnetic tape were developed.[9] Using this technique, Coleman and Jordan[10] found that 8 out of 36 healthy patients developed ST-segment changes during induction and anesthesia and, in a high-risk group of 20 patients with CAD, 36 episodes of ST-segment depression were recorded.[11] Slogoff and Keats[12] recently evaluated the incidence of ischemia in patients undergoing myocardial revascularization, utilizing an almost continuous (every 2 minutes) recording of leads II and V_5 of the ECG. They found that 36.9 percent of the patients had ST-segment changes and almost half of these occurred prior to the induction of anesthesia. Patients who had ischemic changes on arrival in the operating room had a 6 percent infarction rate, compared with 7.4 percent in patients with intraoperative ST-segment changes, and 2.5 percent in patients without any signs of ischemia. An alternative to the retrospective method of Holter monitoring is the intraoperative use of an exercise ECG monitor to instantaneously display ST-segment changes. Using this approach, Roy et al.[13] monitored 11 patients without and 29 patients with known CAD during a variety of surgical procedures. No patients in the control group developed significant ST-segment depression and 11 of the 29 patients with CAD demonstrated significant ST-segment depression, for an incidence of 38 percent. Griffin and Kaplan[14] also studied patients with and without known CAD using a Quinton ST-segment analyzer. None of the patients without CAD displayed ST-segment changes, while 20 percent of patients with CAD had significant changes. Despite the small numbers of patients in these studies, it does appear that ST-segment changes are frequently found during anesthesia if the ECG is subject to closer-than-normal scrutiny. Moreover, the incidence of ischemia detected intraoperatively may be affected by the lead system employed. Roy et al., using multiple lead systems, showed that 9 out of 11 episodes of ischemia were missed on the standard operating room monitor which displayed only lead II.[13]

FACTORS PREDISPOSING TO THE DEVELOPMENT OF ISCHEMIA

It is important to identify those factors that may cause perioperative ischemia and myocardial infarction in order to define appropriate measures for their prevention and treatment. The presence of preexisting CAD is a major risk factor for the subsequent development of perioperative ischemia.[4,5,7,8,12–14] Coriat et al.[11] found that patients with disabling angina (class III and IV) had the highest incidence of myocardial ischemia. Many groups have studied the incidence of perioperative myocardial infarction in patients with CAD with or without previous coronary artery bypass grafting (CABG).[15–19] Patients without prior CABG who developed perioperative infarction usually had three-vessel CAD. The infarction rate in the CABG group has been very low, supporting the protective effect of prior CABG before noncardiac surgery.[15–19]

Anesthesia, especially during induction, periods of surgical stress, and emergence, may produce adverse hemodynamic changes that affect the myocardial oxygen balance. Hypertension and tachycardia during intubation may produce myocardial ischemia in healthy patients[10] and in those with CAD.[12,13] Intraoperative hypotension in patients with ischemic heart disease has been associated with the development of postoperative ECG changes[7] and postoperative infarction in patients with preoperative myocardial infarction.[1,6,16,18] Rao et al.[1] found a higher incidence of reinfarction in patients who developed episodes of intraoperative hypotension or hypertension (with or without tachycardia). Slogoff and Keats[12] found that tachycardia (heart rate over 100 beats/min), but not hypotension or hypertension, correlated best with myocardial ischemia and infarction.

Although the concept is attractive that a particular anesthetic technique may affect the incidence of perioperative myocardial ischemia and infarction, numerous studies have failed to demonstrate any benefits of different anesthetic regimens.[2–4,6,20,21] In the prospective study conducted by Rao et al.[1] patients receiving nitrous oxide, oxygen, a muscle relaxant, and a narcotic had a higher incidence of reinfarction compared with other anesthetic drugs, but for no apparent reason. However, the pitfalls of subjecting such data to multiple retrospective analysis has thrown some doubt on these findings.[22] The retrospective study by Steen et al.[6] included two groups of patients who had transurethral resections of the prostate under either general (50 patients) or spinal (44 patients) anesthesia. The incidence of perioperative myocardial infarction was similar in both groups, and it appears that regional or general anesthesia is equally safe if properly conducted with maintenance of normal hemodynamic parameters.

The effect of the type and duration of surgery on the development of perioperative infarction and ischemia has also been extensively studied. Several studies have demonstrated an increased risk of reinfarction following intrathoracic or abdominal surgery.[1,2,6,21] However, the data on duration of surgery are not clear. Topkins and Artusio[4] found no correlation between the length of surgery and occurrence of perioperative myocardial infarction in patients with or without prior infarctions, while the studies from the Mayo Clinic were positive regarding the incidence of reinfarction and duration of surgery.[2,6] Similarly, in the study of Rao et al.,[1] surgery longer than 4 hours increased the incidence of reinfarction in the retrospective group but had no influence on the prospective group of patients. This finding may reflect the advantages of intensive hemodynamic monitoring with prompt treatment of hemodynamic aberrations during prolonged surgery, which may be associated with major physiologic and hemodynamic changes.

ELECTROCARDIOGRAPHIC LEAD SYSTEMS FOR THE DETECTION OF ISCHEMIA

The ECG was originally used in the operating room to diagnose rhythm disturbances.[23,24] For this purpose, standard limb lead II was used, since its axis parallelled the electrical axis of the heart, thereby producing a large P-wave deflection. However, it has long been known that the precordial leads are superior to the standard leads for the detection of myocardial ischemia.[24,25] With the development of the exercise ECG test for the detection of latent coronary insufficiency, many lead systems were introduced for simplicity and good performance during muscular effort. In a comparative study of different chest lead configurations, Blackburn et al.[26] found that for the detection of ischemia the most sensitive exploring electrode position was at the V_5 position. Furthermore, of all the lead configurations tested, the CM_5 lead was superior for the detection of significant ischemia and least affected by variations in body build, electrical frontal plane position, and noise (see Chapter 2). However, these results were not confirmed in another study of postexercise ECG testing utilizing visual and computerized techniques.[27] ST-segment depression and slope were compared using standard lead V_5 and the bipolar leads CM_5 and CC_5 in two groups of subjects, one with known CAD and one without. Lead CM_5 was found to be less sensitive than V_5 for the detection of ischemia, and lead CC_5 was more comparable to V_5. Both bipolar leads were less affected by noise than standard lead V_5.

Dalton[28] reported use of lead V_5 monitoring during cardiac surgery by attaching the exploring precordial lead to a sterile spinal needle inserted subcutaneously following skin preparation. Kaplan and King[29] first demonstrated the value of monitoring lead V_5 with a modern multilead system during both cardiac and noncardiac surgery. These investigators were able to monitor leads I, II, III, aVR, aVL, aVF, and V_5 using a five-wire system and demonstrated that

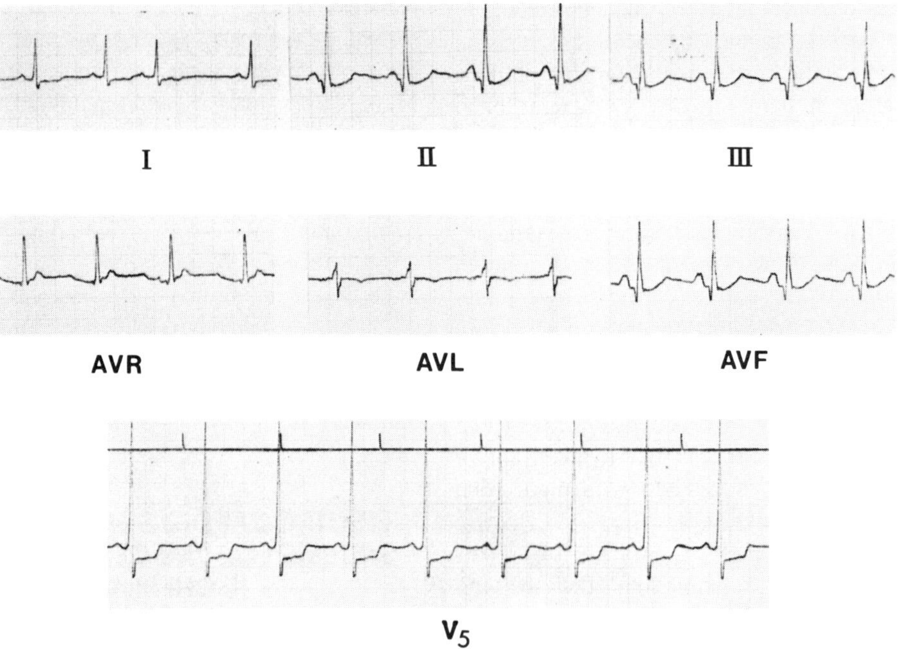

Fig. 9–1 ECG showing 3 mm of horizontal ST-segment depression in V_5 with no changes in other leads. (Kaplan JA, King SB: The precordial electrocardiographic lead (V_5) in patients who have coronary artery disease. Anesthesiology 45:570, 1976.)

significant ST-segment depression in V_5 could occur in the absence of any changes in the standard leads (Fig. 9–1).

In 1979, Kaplan[30] recommended that a five-electrode ECG system be used during all cardiac surgery. Four disposable ECG pads are placed on the extremities, with a fifth placed in the V_5 position covered with Steri-drape. The electrodes are positioned before the induction of the anesthesia, and the V_5 electrode is included in the skin preparation without detrimental effect on the ECG tracing. Standard and augmented limb leads can be displayed in addition to lead V_5 using an ECG monitor with a lead selector switch (Fig. 9–2). Before surgery, all seven leads are displayed and recorded to serve as a baseline reference. During induction of anesthesia and surgery, leads II and V_5 can be displayed simultaneously (Fig. 9–3) in order to monitor anterior and inferior ischemic changes, respectively.

Many operating room ECG monitors are equipped with a three-electrode system, and, therefore, are unable to monitor a true lead V_5. Modified bipolar leads CM_5 or CS_5 can be employed in this case, as described in Chapter 2. Although the comparability of ST-segment changes obtained with various bipolar leads and those recorded with a true V_5 lead during stress testing is disputed,[26,27] any of these leads is satisfactory during anesthesia[14] (Fig. 9–4).

Blackburn and co-workers[26,31] showed that 89 percent of significant ST-segment depression following exercise was found in precordial lead V_5 of a 12-lead ECG. Furthermore, these investigators showed that 100 percent of the ST-segment changes could be detected by recording leads II, aVF, and anterior precordial leads V_3 to V_6. Mason et al.[32] demonstrated the value of multiple-lead ECG recording during and after exercise. Nineteen of 67 patients with angina showed a positive test in only one lead. Overall, 30 patients showed anterior ischemia (leads I and V_3–V_6), and 8 showed inferior ischemia

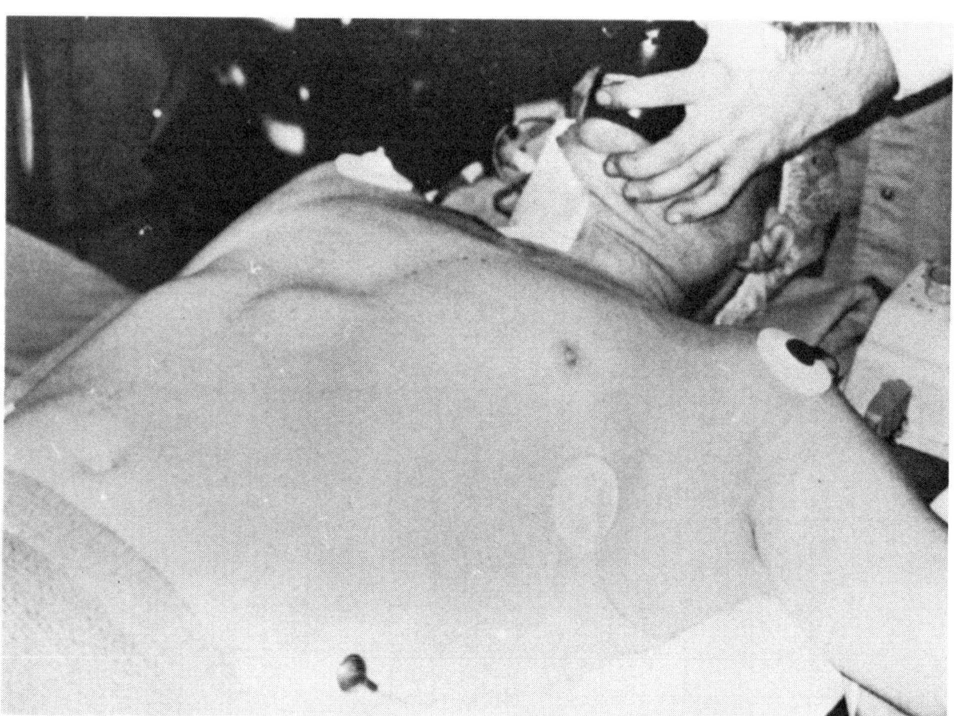

Fig. 9–2 Photograph of lead placement and HP switchable ECG monitor system (upper corner). (Kaplan J: Cardiac Anesthesia. Grune & Stratton, 1979, by permission.)

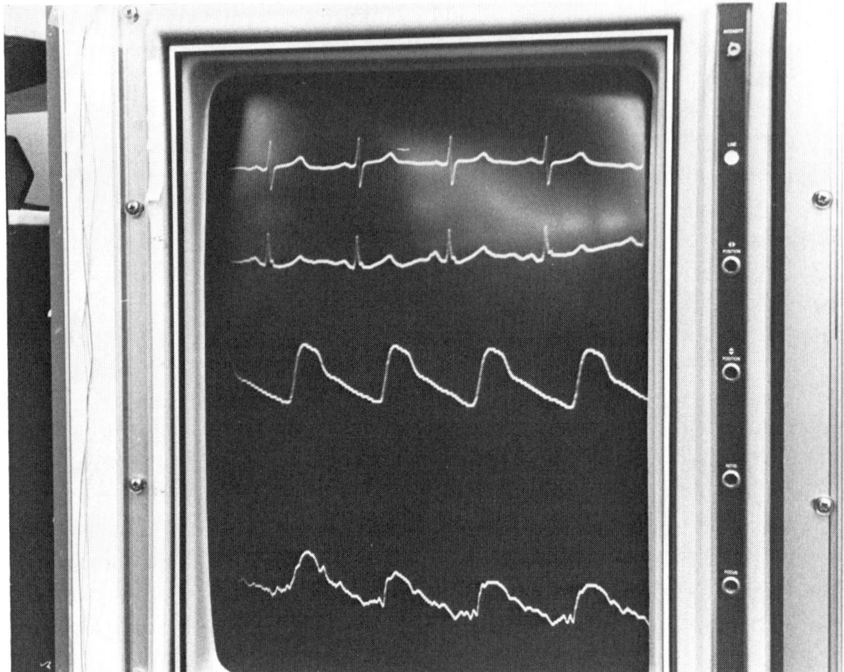

Fig. 9–3 Photograph of simultaneous display of leads V_5 (top) and II (bottom) on monitor.

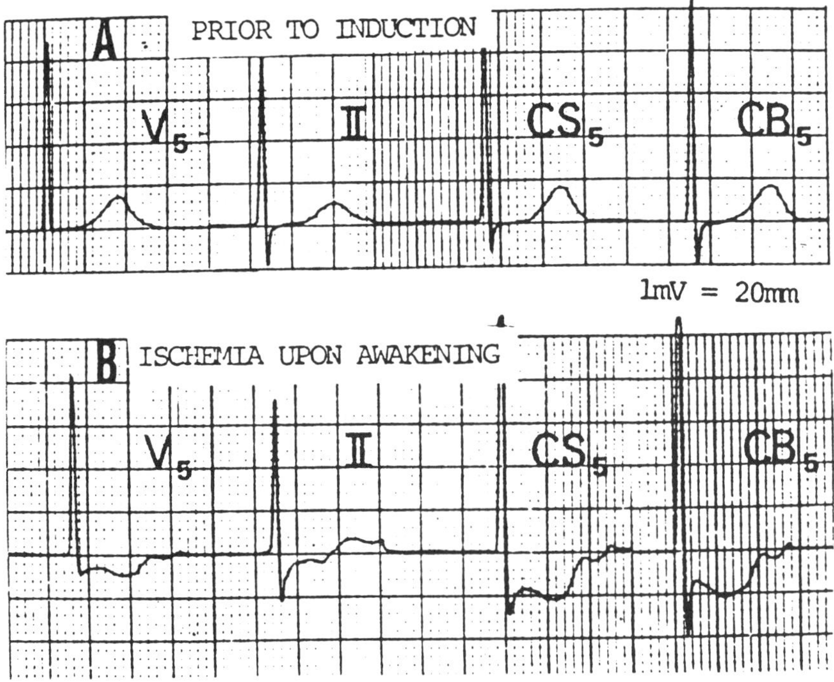

Fig. 9–4 Leads V_5, II, CS_5, and CB_5 during surgery. **(A)** Prior to ischemia. **(B)** During ischemia.

(leads II, III, and aVF). Multiple-lead ECGs are usually not used during anesthesia for routine monitoring since the anesthesiologist may not be able to assimilate the amount of information provided by the continuous simultaneous display of 12 ECG leads. Nonetheless, especially in high-risk cases, the anterior, inferior, and posterior surfaces of the heart should be monitored for the development of ischemia. The inferior surface of the heart overlies the diaphragm, and ischemia is seen in leads II, III, and aVF. Lead II is most often used to detect inferior ischemia, which may remain undetected if only anterior leads are employed,[32,33] since it is also helpful in detecting rhythm problems.

True posterior ischemia may not be detected by leads looking at the inferior or the anterolateral surface of the heart. Anatomically, the posterior wall of the left ventricle lies adjacent to the esophagus. An esophageal ECG inserted 40 to 50 cm into the esophagus will reflect the electrical potential of the posterior surface of the heart and, therefore, may be used for the detection of posterior myocardial ischemia and infarction[34,35] (see Chapter 2). The esophageal ECG lead is suitable for use in the anesthetized patient, and Kates et al.[36] demonstrated its value in patients undergoing CABG. In their study, a patient with posterior ischemia developed significant ST-segment elevation on the esophageal ECG, but not in leads II and V_5 (Fig. 9–5).

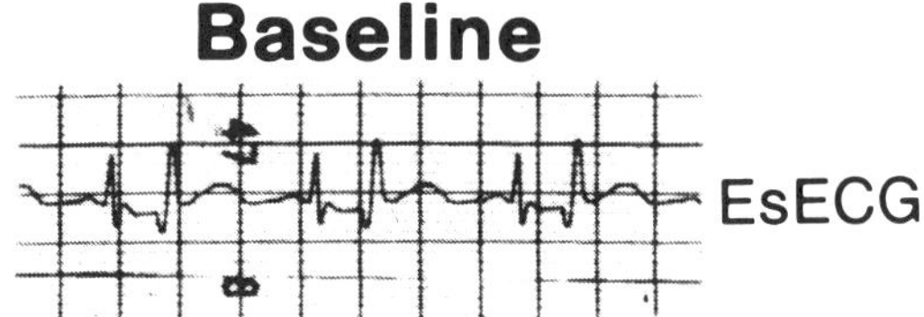

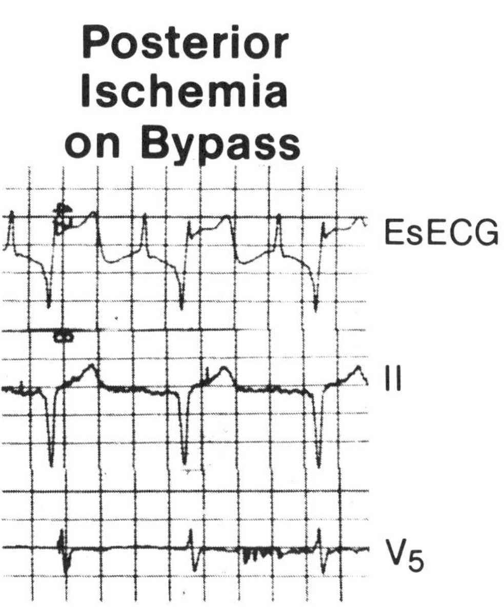

Fig. 9–5 Tracing of EsECG, II, V_5 showing posterior ischemia. (Reprinted with permission from the International Anesthesia Research Society from Kates RA, Zaidan JR, Kaplan JA: Esophageal lead for intraoperative electrocardiographic monitoring. Anesth Analg 61:781, 1982.)

Acute myocardial ischemia and infarction are not confined to the left ventricle. Right ventricular (RV) infarction may occur in isolation or, more frequently, along with inferoposterior infarction of the left ventricle. Cohn et al.[37] described the hemodynamic consequences of right ventricular infarction along with acute left ventricular inferior wall infarction. Six patients developed hypotension, engorged neck veins, and heart block, and hemodynamic measurements disclosed that RV filling pressure equaled or exceeded left ventricular end-diastolic pressure (LVEDP). However, these clincial and hemodynamic findings are variable and their time of onset unpredictable. The diagnosis can be confirmed by techniques to detect RV dilatation, dysfunction, and necrosis. However, these diagnostic criteria are time consuming, and RV infarction may rapidly lead to serious hemodynamic dysfunction. Having previously found a 43 percent incidence of RV infarction in an autopsy study, Erhard and colleagues[38,39] first proposed the use of a right-sided precordial lead for early diagnosis. Subsequently, Klein et al.[40] used lead V_4R in conjunction with clinical and laboratory criteria to diagnose right ventricular infarctions in a series of 110 patients presenting with acute inferior myocardial infarctions. Right ventricular infarctions were detected in 58 patients (52.7 percent), of whom 82.7 percent developed ST-segment elevation. The V_4R lead had a reasonably high sensitivity, specificity, and predictive value for right ventricular infarction and ischemia. Although its use has not been reported during anesthesia, the V_4R lead may prove beneficial for monitoring those patients with previous inferior infarction or with evidence of right-sided occlusive disease on coronary arteriography.

ANALYSIS OF THE ST SEGMENT

The patterns of ST-segment change that fulfill the criteria of myocardial ischemia have been extensively studied in subjects with and without CAD undergoing exercise stress testing in the laboratory. Since anesthesia and surgery may be regarded as a potentially stressful situation, these criteria may be applied to anesthetized patients.

For the accurate diagnosis of ischemia, a knowledge of the normal morphology of the ST segment and the response to exercise is essential. A normal resting ECG complex is shown in Figure 9–6. The J point is the junction between the S wave and the ST segment. Exercise causes a downward displacement of the J point, such that the baseline is depressed below the isoelectric line in the resting tracing (Fig. 9–6). The ST segment normally becomes upsloping and slightly concave and returns to the baseline (PR junction) within 0.04 to 0.06 seconds after the J point. J-point depression with an upsloping ST segment may be the earliest indication of myocardial ischemia. This is differentiated from the normal J-point depression produced with exercise by the upsloping ST segment. Salzman et al.[41] attempted to quantify J-point slope and suggested that a J-point slope of 30 degrees above horizontal was probably not indicative of ischemia. Stuart and Ellestad[42] concluded that an upsloping ST segment was indicative of ischemia if the ST segment was depressed at least 2.0 mm below the baseline of the PR segment at 0.08 seconds from the J point (Fig. 9–7). With ongoing ischemia, the J-point depression evolves into progressive horizontal depression of the ST segment (Fig. 9–8). Significant myocardial ischemia is present when there is greater than 1 mm of ST-segment depression measured 0.06 seconds from the J point.[43] The ST-segment depression may be convex in form or downsloping (Fig. 9–8). The magnitude of ST-segment depression correlates with the amount of myocardium involved and the extent to which it is made ischemic.[43,44] There is also a relationship between the severity of CAD and the ST-segment configuration induced by exercise. Robb and Marks[45] were able to demonstrate an increased mortality and worse prognosis for patients with downsloping ST-segment depression as compared with horizontal depression. Goldshlager et al.[46] compared ST-segment depression with extent of disease as demonstrated by coronary angiography and found a correlation between downsloping ST-segment depression and increasing number of diseased vessels. Downsloping ST-segment de-

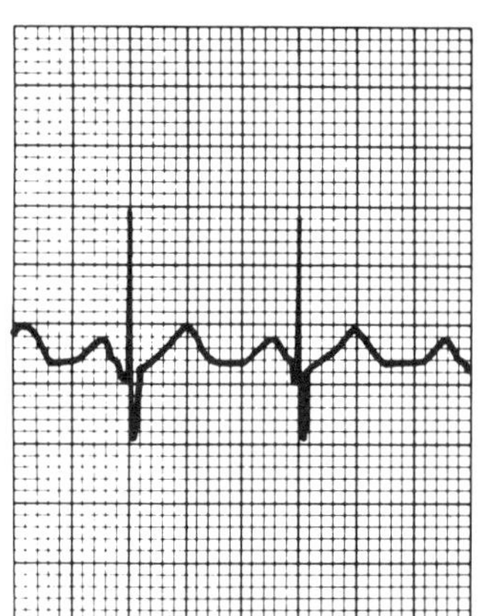

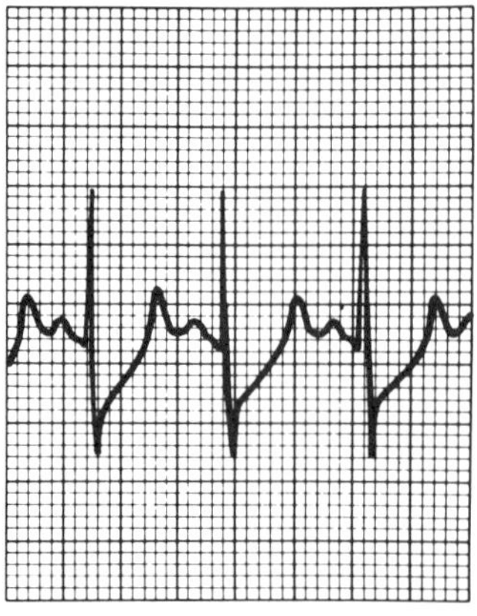

Fig. 9–6 Normal resting ECG complex (left), and an exercise ECG tracing showing depression of the J point and an upsloping ST segment (right). (Ellestad MH: Stress Testing: Principles and Practice. FA Davis, Philadelphia, 1975.)

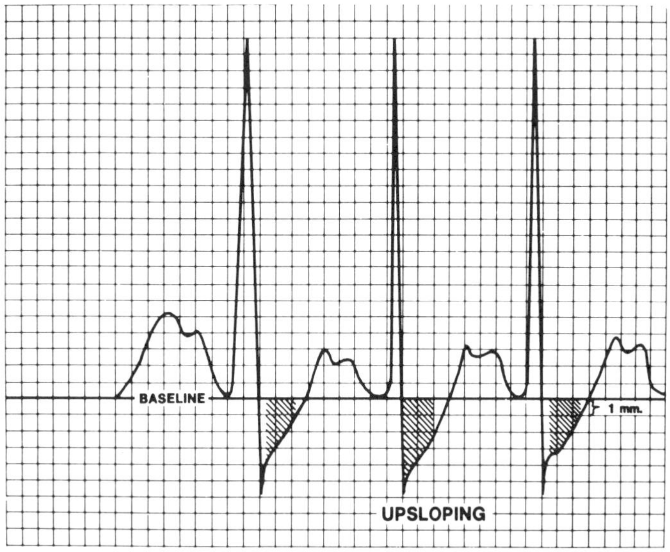

Fig. 9–7 Upsloping ST-segment depression showing early ischemia. (Ellestad MH: Diagnostic and prognostic information derived from exercise testing. p. 33. In Wenger NK (ed): Exercise and the Heart. FA Davis, Philadelphia, 1978.)

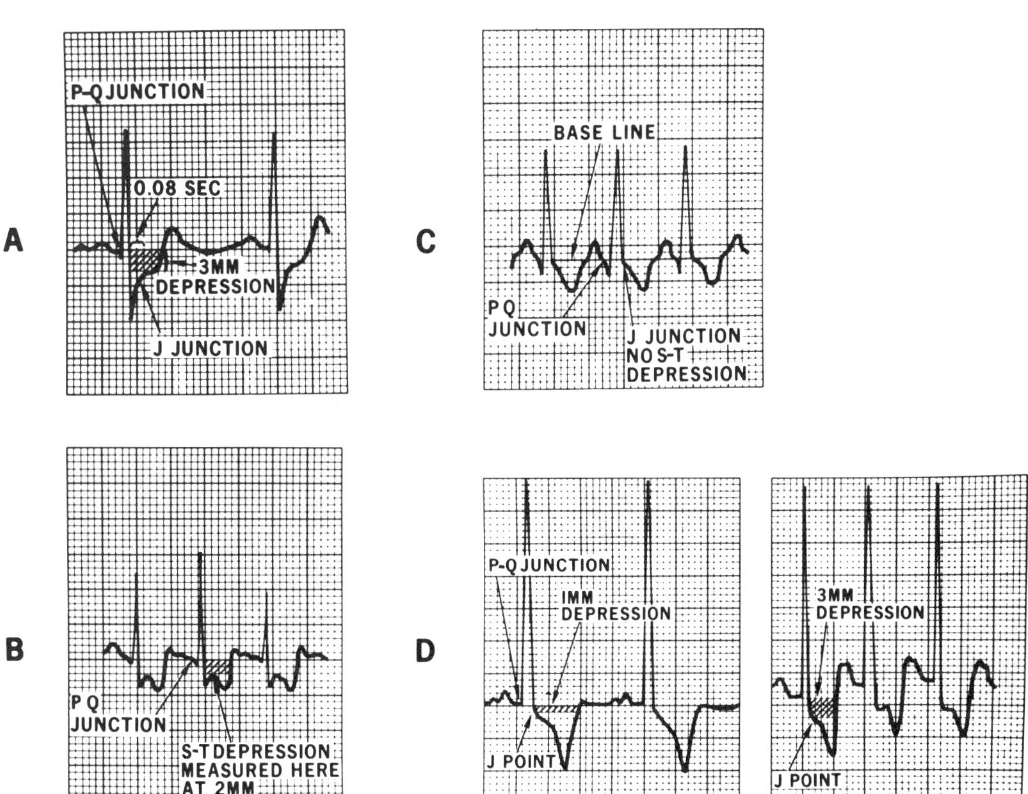

Fig. 9–8 Tracings showing ST-segment depression. **(A)** Horizontal ST-segment depression is measured from a point 0.06 seconds after the J point. **(B)** Convex ST-segment depression is measured from the top of the curve to the PQ junction. **(C,D)** With downsloping ST segments, the depression is measured at the point where the ST segment changes slope. (Ellestad MH: Stress Testing: Principles and Practice. FA Davis, Philadelphia, 1975.)

pression represents profound myocardial ischemia and possibly even transmural ischemia. ST-segment elevation greater than 1 mm is also indicative of severe transmural ischemia.

ST-segment changes have been reported in normal subjects. Using ambulatory ECG monitoring in 50 normal males, Armstrong et al.[47] demonstrated a 30 percent incidence of transient ST-segment depression. Posture and positional changes can also affect the ST segment.[48] Patients with nonspecific T-wave abnormalities in their resting ECG may develop ST-segment depression while standing or with hyperventilation.[49] Intermittent ST-segment depression associated with respiration has been observed during stress testing in apparently normal subjects and may be a preliminary finding to the subsequent development of classical ischemia.[43] Ellestad et al.[43,44] postulated that in a left ventricle with slightly decreased compliance, different rates of filling during inspiration and expiration could produce an increased end-diastolic pressure, hence ST-segment depression for a few beats. Drugs such as digitalis and diuretics, by depletion of potassium or hypokalemia per se, disturbances of conduction such as left bundle branch block (LBBB) or Wolff–Parkinson–White syndrome, and LV hypertrophy with strain can all affect the ST segment.

When ST-segment elevation occurs in the absence of any obvious hemodynamic or rhythm disturbances, coronary artery spasm (Prinzmetal's angina) should be suspected as the cause of the myocardial ischemia. Coronary artery spasm has been reported during anesthesia,[50] where the diagnosis is especially important, since appropriate treatment with verapamil or nitroglycerin is effective.

INTRAOPERATIVE ANALYSIS OF THE ST SEGMENT

For the accurate evaluation of ST-segment changes, it is essential that the ECG monitor be properly calibrated before use so that a signal of 1 mV will produce a vertical deflection of 10 mm. It is also important that the ECG signal displayed on the oscilloscope be an accurate representation of the true signal. This becomes a major consideration when the ST segment is subject to computer analysis. Many of the oscilloscopes currently used in the operating room can distort the ST segment and T wave of the ECG. This is largely the result of electronic filtering circuits used to remove artifacts from the ECG, such as baseline wandering and 60-cycle interference. The lower end of the normal frequency response of the ECG is 0.14 cycles/sec, below which electrical signals are attenuated by low-frequency filters. On some monitors this filter may be selected as the diagnostic mode and should be used to evaluate ST-segment changes. However, in this mode the ECG is very susceptible to baseline wandering caused by respiration, movement, or electrode artifact. The baseline may be stabilized by further filtering of low-frequency signals up to 4 cycles/sec in the monitor mode. Unfortunately, the addition of more filtration may cause spurious shifts in the ST segment due to the absence of the usual low-frequency components.[51,52] An isoelectric ST segment may become elevated or depressed, resembling ischemia (Fig. 9–9). Moreover, elevated or depressed ST segments may be shifted toward the isoelectric line, effectively masking ongoing ischemia.

Changes in the ST segment indicative of ischemia may be evaluated visually or subjected to analysis by computer. Computer analysis was first applied to stress testing as an alternative to close scrutiny of tracings that may inevitably introduce an element of human error.[53] Accurate computer analysis of changes in ST-segment configuration depends on selection of ECG complexes which are unaffected by artifact. Rosner et al.[54] described one of the first digital computer systems for analyzing the exercise ECG in 1967. The subsequent development of computer averaging techniques over several beats with the rejection of ectopic beats has reduced the amount of random noise and enabled studies of the ECG during and after graded exercise.[55] Computer analysis of the ECG has also established precise numerical measurements for the objective ECG diagnosis of ischemia.[56] However, the useful-

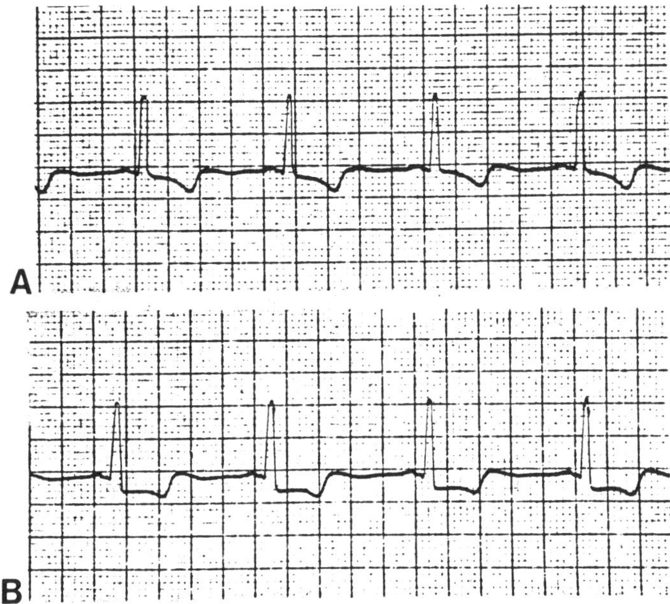

Fig. 9–9 **(A)** Control. **(B)** Tracing demonstrating artifact introduced by low-frequency filtering. (Arbeit SR, Rubin IL, Gross H: Dangers in interpreting the electrocardiogram from the oscilloscope monitor. JAMA 211:453, 1970. Copyright 1970, American Medical Association.)

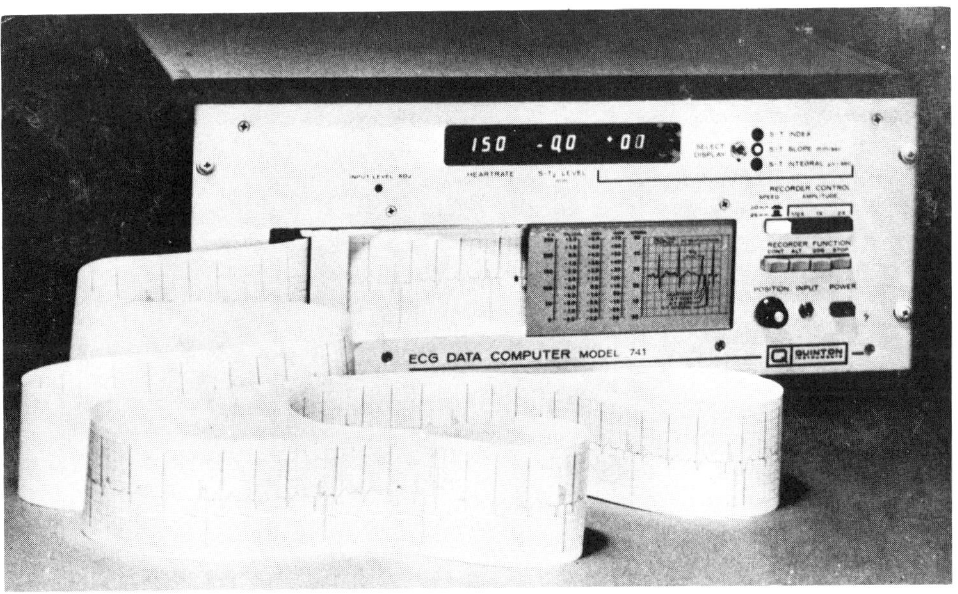

Fig. 9–10 Photograph of the Quinton ST-segment analyzer.

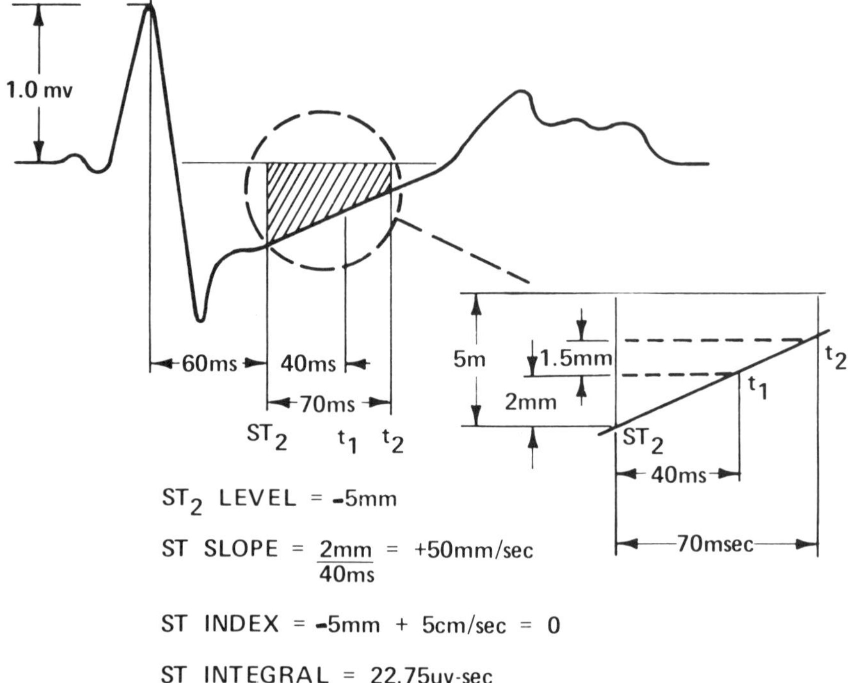

Fig. 9–11 Diagram of ST segment and derived parameters. ST_2 level/ST slope/ST index/ST integral. The ST_2 level is the change in the ST segment (in millimeters). ST slope is measured between ST_2 and T_1 (in millimeters per second). The ST index is the sum of the ST_2 level and ST slope without a unit value. The ST integral is the area of ST depression measured as an integrated voltage between ST_2 and T_2.

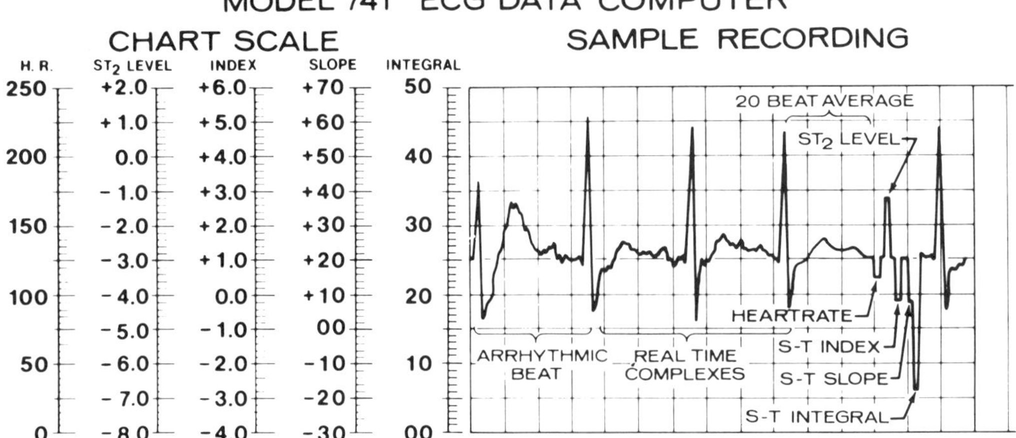

Fig. 9–12 Tracing of ECG and histogram.

ness of derived parameters and the criteria for defining ischemia when computerized techniques are employed are still controversial.[26,27]

The technology of computerized segment monitoring is equally applicable to the conscious and the anesthetized patient. Roy et al.[13] first described the use of a computerized exercise testing system to detect ischemia during anesthesia. During induction, leads V_4, V_5, and V_6 were continuously recorded on paper; for the remainder of the procedure, leads V_5 and II were continuously displayed and leads II, aVF, V_3, V_4, V_5, and V_6 were recorded on paper every 3 minutes. The diagnosis of ischemia was aided by a continuous digital readout of the magnitude of ST-segment depression and an averaged picture of the last 16 QRST complexes in lead V_5. Every 20 minutes a written histogram retrospectively demonstrated the amount of ST-segment displacement over 1-minute intervals. Recently, Griffin and Kaplan[14] evaluated the use of a simple ST-segment computer during anesthesia. The device received a signal from an ECG preamplifier and displayed in digital form the ST_2 level, ST index, ST slope, and ST integral (Figs. 9–10 and 9–11). The computations are performed on an ECG complex produced from the average of the previous 20 beats. The averaged beat is recorded on paper followed by a histogram of all the derived ST-segment information (Fig. 9–12). Although the averaging process of the computer greatly reduces the amount of random noise, interference from electrocautery is a major problem, since the ECG trace is completely lost and a further 20 beats have to elapse before another useful analysis can be obtained. Although the written record was unaffected in the exercise monitor used by Roy et al.,[13] the computer also would not accept any data for processing during electrocautery.

Kotrly et al.[57] reported the use of a modified microcomputer-based ECG that displayed, as a trend line, the summed ST-segment deviations from the isoelectric line in leads V_5, aVF, and $-V_1$. The trend line is continuously displayed for 20 minutes and thereafter may be retained in hard copy form. In addition, the three ECG complexes can be electronically stored every 10 minutes (Figs. 9–13 and 9–14). This ST-segment analyzer has been recently updated and currently analyzes leads I, II, and V_5.

The value of computer monitoring of the ST segment is being evaluated. The visual quantification of ST segment shifts in absolute terms as a digital display or trend line may provide the anesthesiologist with an almost instanta-

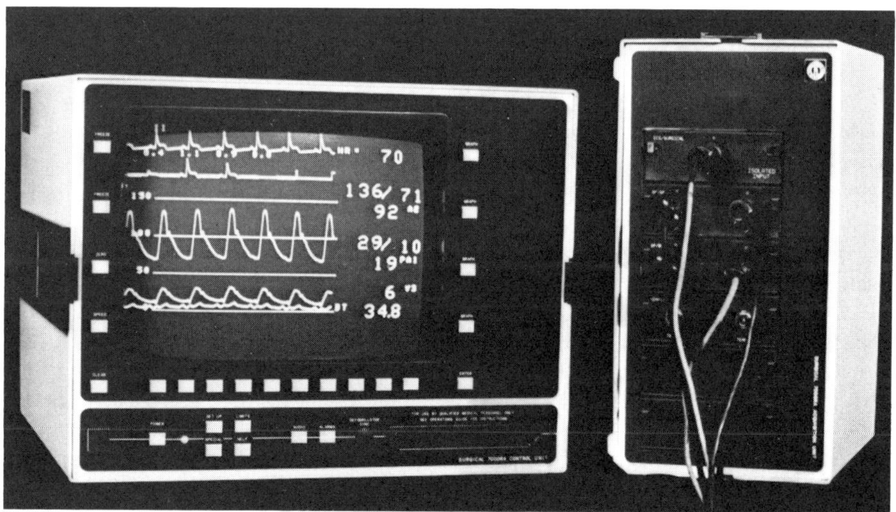

Fig. 9–13 Photograph of the Marquette monitoring system with the ST-segment analyzer.

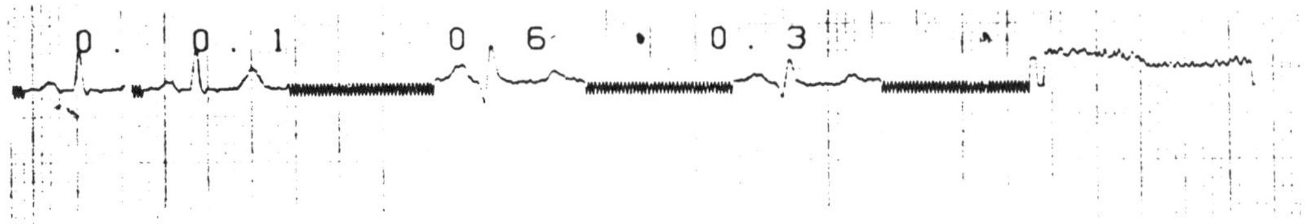

Fig. 9–14 Marquette ST-segment analysis. From left to right are leads I, II, and V_5. The ST-segment trend line (28 minutes) is shown at the far right. It can be seen that the ST-segment trend line has returned back toward the baseline during the past 15 minutes. The change in ST segment from baseline (in millimeters) is shown above each of the leads.

neous and simple means for the early and accurate ECG diagnosis of ischemia.

REFERENCES

1. Rao TLK, Jacobs KH, El-Etr AA: Reinfarction following anesthesia in patients with myocardial infarction. Anesthesiology 59:499, 1983
2. Tarhan S, Moffitt EA, Taylor WF, Giuliani ER: Myocardial infarction after general anesthesia. JAMA 220:1451, 1972
3. Knapp RB, Topkins MJ, Artusio JF: The cerebrovascular accident and coronary occlusion in anesthesia. JAMA 182:332, 1962
4. Topkins MJ, Artusio JF: Myocardial infarction and surgery: A five year study. Anesth Analg 43:716, 1964
5. Arkins R, Smessaert AA, Hicks RG: Mortality and morbidity in surgical patients with coronary artery disease. JAMA 190:485, 1964
6. Steen PA, Tinker JH, Tarhan S: Myocardial reinfarction after anesthesia and surgery. JAMA 239:2566, 1978
7. Chamberlain DA, Edmonds-Seal J: Effects of surgery under general anesthesia on the electrocardiogram in ischemic heart disease and hypertension. Br J Med 2:784, 1964
8. Driscoll AC, Hobika JH, Etsten BE, Proger S: Clinically unrecognised infarction following surgery. N Engl J Med 264:633, 1961
9. Holter NJ: New method for heart studies. Continuous electrocardiography of active subjects over long periods is now practical. Science 134:1214, 1961
10. Coleman AJ, Jordan C: Cardiovascular responses to anaesthesia. Influence of beta-adrenoreceptor blockade with metoprolol. Anaesthesia 35:972, 1980
11. Coriat P, Harari A, Daloz M, Viars P: Clinical predictors of intraoperative myocardial ischemia in patients with coronary artery disease undergoing non-cardiac surgery. Acta Anaesthesiol Scand 26:287, 1982
12. Slogoff S, Keats AS: Does perioperative myocardial ischemia lead to postoperative myocardial infarction? Anesthesiology 62:107, 1985
13. Roy WL, Edelist G, Gilbert B: Myocardial ischemia during noncardiac surgical procedures in patients with coronary artery disease. Anesthesiology 51:393, 1979
14. Griffin RM, Kaplan JA: Comparison of ECG leads V_5, CS_5, CB_5, and II by computerized ST segment analysis. Anesth Analg 65:S65, 1986
15. Mahar LJ, Steen PA, Tinker JH, et al: Perioperative myocardial infarction in patients with coronary artery disease with and without aorta-coronary artery bypass grafts. J Thorac Cardiovasc Surg 76:533, 1978
16. Scher KS, Tice DA: Operative risks in patients with previous coronary artery bypass. Arch Surg 111:807, 1976
17. McCollum CH, Garcia-Rinaldi R, Graham JM, DeBakey ME: Myocardial revascularization prior to subsequent major surgery in patients with coronary artery disease. Surgery 81:302, 1977
18. Bernhard VM, Johnson SD, Peterson JJ: Carotid artery stenosis. Association with surgery for coronary artery disease. Arch Surg 105:837, 1972
19. Crutchley P, Kaplan JA, Hug CC, et al: Noncardiac surgery in patients with prior myocardial revascularization. Can Anaesth Soc J 30:629, 1983.
20. Stein I, Caginalp N: The postoperative electrocardiogram. Angiology 17:323, 1966
21. Eerola M, Eerola R, Kaukinen S, Kaukinen L: Risk factors in surgical patients with verified

preoperative myocardial infarction. Acta Anaesthesiol Scand 24:219, 1980
22. Lowenstein E, Yusef S, Teplick R: Perioperative myocardial reinfarction: A glimmer of hope— A note of caution. Anesthesiology 59:493, 1983
23. Cannard TH, Dripps RD, Helwig J Jr, Zinsser HF: The electrocardiogram during anesthesia and surgery. Anesthesiology 21:194, 1960
24. Russell PH, Coakley CS: Electrocardiographic observation in the operating room. Anesth Analg 48:784, 1969
25. Wood FC, Wolferth CC: Angina pectoris. The clinical and electrocardiographic phenomenon of the attack and their comparison with the effects of experimental temporary occlusion. Arch Intern Med 47:339, 1931
26. Blackburn H, Taylor HL, Okamoto N, et al: Standardization of the exercise electrocardiogram. A systemic comparison of chest lead configurations employed for monitoring during exercise. p. 101. In Karoonen MJ, Barry AJ (eds): Physical Activity and the Heart. Charles C Thomas, Springfield, Illinois, 1967
27. Froelicher VF Jr, Wolthius R, Keiser N, et al: A comparison of two bipolar exercise electrocardiographic leads to lead V_5. Chest 70:611, 1976
28. Dalton B: A precordial ECG lead for chest operations. Anesth Analg 55:740, 1976
29. Kaplan JA, King SB: The precordial electrocardiographic lead (V_5) in patients who have coronary artery disease. Anesthesiology 45:570, 1976
30. Kaplan JA: Electrocardiographic monitoring. p. 117. In Kaplan JA: Cardiac Anesthesia. Grune & Stratton, Orlando, Florida, 1979
31. Blackburn H, Katigbak R: What electrocardiographic leads to take after exercise? Am Heart J 67:184, 1964
32. Mason RE, Likar I, Biern RO, Ross RS: Multiple lead exercise electrocardiography. Experience in 107 normal subjects and 67 patients with angina pectoris and comparison with coronary cinearteriography in 84 patients. Circulation 36:517, 1967
33. Kirstner JR, Miller ED, Epstein RM: More than V_5 needed. Anesthesiology 47:75, 1977
34. Goldman MJ: The Principles of Clinical Electrocardiography. Appleton-Lange, East Norwalk, Connecticut, 1964
35. Scherlis L, Wener J, Grishman A, Sandberg AA: The ventricular complex in esophageal electrocardiography. Am Heart J 41:246, 1951
36. Kates RA, Zaidan JR, Kaplan JA: Esophageal lead for intraoperative electrocardiographic monitoring. Anesth Analg 61:781, 1982
37. Cohn JN, Guiha NH, Broder MI, Limas CJ: Right ventricular infarction: Clinical and hemodynamic features. Am J Cardiol 33:209, 1974
38. Erhardt LR: Clinical and pathological observations in different types of acute myocardial infarction. A study of 84 patients deceased after treatment in a coronary care unit. Acta Med Scand (suppl) 560, 1974
39. Erhardt LR, Sjogren A, Wahlberg I: Single right-sided precordial lead in the diagnosis of right ventricular involvement in inferior myocardial infarction. Am Heart J 91:571, 1976
40. Klein HO, Turdjman T, Nino R, et al: The early recognition of right ventricular infarction: Diagnostic accuracy of the electrocardiographic V_4 lead. Circulation 67:558, 1983
41. Salzman SH, Hellerstein HK, Radke JD, et al: Quantitative effects of physical conditioning on the exercise electrocardiogram of middle aged subjects with arteriosclerotic heart disease. p. 388. In Blackburn H (ed): Measurements in Exercise Electrocardiography. Charles C Thomas, Springfield, Illinois, 1969
42. Stuart RJ, Ellestad MH: Upsloping ST segment in exercise stress testing. Am J Cardiol 37:19, 1976
43. Ellestad MH, Cooke BM Jr, Greenberg PS: Stress Testing: Principles and Practice. FA Davis, Philadelphia, 1980
44. Ellestad MH, Cooke BM Jr, Greenberg PS: Stress testing: Clinical application and predictive capacity. Prog Cardiovasc Dis 21:431, 1979
45. Robb GP, Marks H: Post-exercise electrocardiogram in arteriosclerotic heart disease. JAMA 200:918, 1967
46. Goldshlager N, Selzer A, Cohn K: Treadmill stress tests as indicators of presence and severity of coronary artery disease. Ann Intern Med 85:277, 1976
47. Armstrong WF, Jordon JW, Morris SN, McHenry PL: Prevalence of and magnitude of ST segment and T wave abnormalities in normal men during continuous ambulatory electrocardiography. Am J Cardiol 49:1638, 1981
48. Lachman AB, Semler JH, Gustafson RH: Postural ST-T wave changes in the radioelectrogram simulating myocardial ischemia. Circulation 31:557, 1965
49. Holmgren A, Strom G: Vasoregulatory asthenia in a female athlete and Da Costa's syndrome

in a male athlete successfully treated by physical training. Acta Med Scand 164:113, 1959

50. Briard C, Coriat P, Commin P, et al: Coronary artery spasm during noncardiac surgical procedures. Anesthesia 38:467, 1983
51. Berson AS, Pipberger HV: The low-frequency response of electrocardiographs, a frequent source of recording errors. Am Heart J 71:779, 1966
52. Arbeit SR, Rubin IL, Gross H: Dangers in interpreting the electrocardiogram from the oscilloscope monitor. JAMA 211:453, 1970
53. Acheson RM: Observer error and variation in interpretation of electrocardiograms in epidemiological study of coronary heart disease. Br J Prev Social Med 14:99, 1960
54. Rosner SR, Leinbach RC, Presto AJ, et al: Computer analysis of the exercise electrocardiogram. Am J Cardiol 20:356, 1967
55. Davies CT, Kitchin AH, Knibbs AV: Computer quantitation of ST segment response to graded exercise in untrained and trained normal subjects. Cardiovasc Res 5:201, 1971
56. Sheffield LT, Holt JH, Lester FM, et al: On-line analysis of the exercise electrocardiogram. Circulation 40:935, 1969
57. Kotrly KJ, Kotter GS, Mortara D, Kampine JP: Intraoperative detection of myocardial ischemia with an ST segment trend monitoring system. Anesth Analg 63:343, 1984

10

A Practical Approach to the Detection of Dysrhythmias

John Manos, M.D.
Daniel M. Thys, M.D.

INTRAOPERATIVE DYSRHYTHMIAS

The detection of dysrhythmias has proved one of the most useful and important indications for the use of intraoperative electrocardiography.[1] Interest in the intraoperative detection of cardiac dysrhythmias has grown since 1847, when the first cardiac arrest during surgery was reported.[2] While earlier in this century occasional cases of dysrhythmia in anesthetized patients were described, the first large series of ECG studies during anesthesia, was published by Kurtz et al.[3] in 1936. These workers observed dysrhythmias in 79 percent of 109 patients receiving cyclopropane, ether, procaine, ethylene, nitrous oxide, vinylether, chloroform, or tribromethanol.[4] Other studies documenting the incidence of intraoperative dysrhythmias associated with contemporary agents and techniques were reviewed by Katz et al.[4] and are summarized in Table 10–1.[5–9]

Dysrhythmias are most common at times of endotracheal intubation and extubation. Patients with preexisting cardiac disease have a higher incidence of ventricular dysrhythmias than patients without known heart disease (60 percent versus 37 percent). In a study of patients undergoing cardiac surgery, Angelini et al.[10] reported that 29 of 50 patients (58 percent) having valve surgery and 35 of 78 patients (45 percent) having coronary revascularization developed significant postoperative dysrhythmias. These dysrhythmias tended to correlate with the severity of the heart disease, led to a prolonged hospital stay, and were responsible for up to 80 percent of the surgical mortality in their series.

The following features have been shown to be possible contributors to the etiology of dysrhythmias during the perioperative period:

1. *Anesthetic agents.* Halogenated hydrocarbons such as halothane or enflurane have been shown to produce dysrhythmias, probably by a reentrant mechanism.[11] In addition, these agents, especially halothane, have been shown to sensitize the myocardium to both endogenous and exogenous cathecholamines. Drugs, such as cocaine and ketamine, that block the reuptake of norephinephrine, can facilitate the development of epinephrine-induced dysrhythmias.[12]

2. *Abnormal arterial blood gases or electrolytes.* Edwards et al.[13] showed that hyperventilation to a $PaCO_2$ of 30 or 20 mmHg lowered a

Parts of this chapter are reproduced with modification from Kaplan JA and Thys DM: The electrocardiogram and anesthesia. p. 155. In Miller RD (ed): Anesthesia. 2nd Ed. Churchill Livingstone, New York, 1985.

Table 10–1. Incidence of Intraoperative Dysrhythmias

Study	Year	Total Patients	Dysrhythmias	Patients with Dysrhythmias (%)
Dodd et al.[5]	1962	569	170	29.9
Kuner et al.[6]	1967	154	95	61.7
Vanik and Davis[7]	1968	5,013	901	17.9
Russel and Coakley[8]	1969	3,177	494	15.5
Bertrand et al.[9]	1971	100	84	84
Total		9,013	1,744	19.3

normal serum potassium to 3.64 or 3.12 mEq/L, respectively. If serum and total body potassium start at low levels, it is possible to decrease the serum potassium into the 2-mEq/L range by hyperventilation and thus precipitate severe cardiac dysrhythmias. Alterations of blood gases or electrolytes may lead to dysrhythmias either by producing reentrant mechanisms or by altering phase 4 depolarization of conduction fibers.

3. *Endotracheal intubation.* This may be the most common cause of dysrhythmias during surgery. These dysrhythmias occasionally can be associated with severe hypertension.[14] Several authors have emphasized the hemodynamic alterations which may occur during endotracheal intubation.[15]

4. *Reflexes.* Vagal stimulation may produce sinus bradycardias and allow ventricular escape mechanisms to occur. In addition, specific reflexes such as the occulocardiac reflex can produce severe rhythm disturbances during surgery.[16]

5. *Central nervous system stimulation.*[17] Many ECG abnormalities have been reported with intracranial pathology, especially subarachnoid hemorrhage, including changes in QT intervals, development of Q waves, ST-segment changes, and the occurrence of U waves. The mechanism of these dysrhythmias appears to be due to changes in the autonomic nervous system.

6. *Location of surgery.* Dental surgery is often associated with dysrhythmias, since profound stimulation of both the sympathetic and parasympathetic nervous systems often occurs.[18] Junctional rhythms commonly occur and may be due to stimulation of the autonomic nervous system via the fifth cranial nerve.

7. *Preexisting cardiac disease.* Studies by Angelini et al.[10] have shown that patients with known cardiac disease have a much higher incidence of dysrhythmias during anesthesia than patients without known cardiac disease.

8. *Insertion of catheters or wires in the heart.* This may lead to dysrhythmias. It is seen with the placement of the Swan-Ganz catheter, often leading to premature ventricular contraction.

Dysrhythmias may also be attenuated or eliminated by general anesthesia.[19] This could be due to relief of anxiety and loss of sympathetic stimulation, an antiarrhythmic property of the anesthetic agent itself, or the correction of abnormalities of respiration, blood gases,and electrolytes.

The diagnosis and treatment of important intraoperative dysrhythmias can be simplified by using the following six questions when looking at a rhythm and attempting to decide whether treatment is necessary:[20]

1. What is the heart rate?
2. Is the rhythm regular?
3. Is there one P wave for each QRS complex?
4. Is the QRS complex normal?
5. Is the rhythm dangerous?
6. Does the rhythm require treatment?

The following are common intraoperative dysrhythmias that require diagnosis and treatment and to which the six key questions should be applied.

Sinus Bradycardia

The pacemaker site is in the sinus node, but the rate is slower than normal. Etiologic factors include drug effects, acute inferior myocardial infarction, hypoxia, vagal stimulation, and high sympathetic blockade (Fig. 10–1). Sinus bradycardia accounts for 11 percent of intraoperative dysrhythmias.[6]

1. *Heart rate:* 40 to 60 beats/min. In patients on chronic β-adrenergic blocking therapy, the dysrhythmia is defined as a heart rate of less than 50 beats/min.[21]
2. *Rhythm:* The rhythm is regular except for occasional escape beats from other pacemaker sites.
3. *P : QRS:* There is a 1 : 1 relationship between the P waves and the QRS complexes.
4. *QRS complex:* Normal.
5. *Significance:* Heart rates below 40 beats/min are poorly tolerated even in healthy patients and should be evaluated on the basis of their effect on cardiac output. Treatment is recommended if hypotension, ventricular dysrhythmias or signs of poor peripheral perfusion are observed. A sinus bradycardia may be part of the so-called sick sinus syndrome in which sinus node dysfunction can precipitate bradycardias, heart block, tachydysrhythmias, or alternating bradytachydysrhythmias.[22]
6. *Treatment:* There is usually none, but a progression from atropine (0.3 to 2 mg IV) to ephedrine (5 to 25 mg IV) to isoproterenol (1.4 μg IV) to a temporary transvenous pacemaker insertion may be necessary for severe or refractory sinus bradycardias.

Sinus Tachycardia

The pacemaker site is in the sinoatrial (SA) node, but the rate is faster than normal. Sinus tachycardia is the most commonly occurring dysrhythmia in the perioperative period. It occurs with such frequency that it is not included in most incidence studies. Common causes include pain, inadequate anesthesia, hypovolemia, fever, hypoxia, hypercarbia, heart failure, and drug effects.

1. *Heart rate:* The rate is greater than 100 beats/min and can go up to 170 beats/min, which may be seen with a severe episode of hyperpyrexia (Fig. 10–2).
2. *Rhythm:* Regular.
3. *P : QRS:* 1 : 1
4. *QRS complex:* Normal. There may be associated ST-segment depression with severe increases in heart rate and resulting myocardial ischemia.
5. *Significance:* Prolonged tachycardias in patients with underlying heart disease can precipitate congestive heart failure due to the increased myocardial work required. The tachycardia decreases coronary perfusion time, which can cause secondary ST-T-wave changes and can precipitate angina pectoris in patients with coronary artery disease. A major diagnostic problem is encountered when the heart rate is 150 beats/min since this is a common rate for either a sinus tachycardia, paroxysmal atrial tachycardia (PAT), or atrial flutter with a 2:1 block.[23] These three dysrhythmias can sometimes be separated by the use of carotid sinus massage, intravenous administration of edrophonium, or atrial or esophageal ECG leads

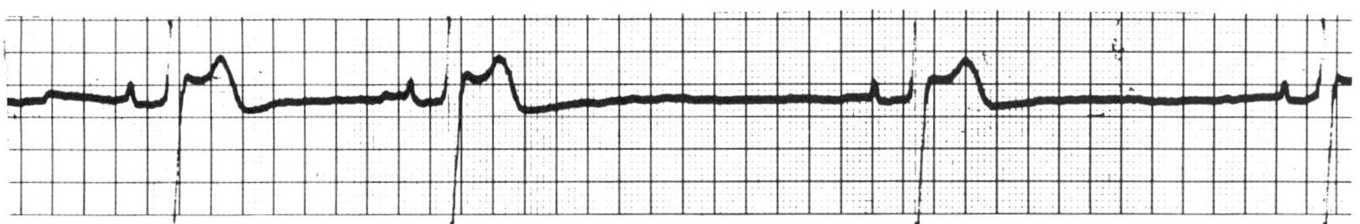

Fig. 10–1 Episode of severe sinus bradycardia in a patient with first-degree AV block.

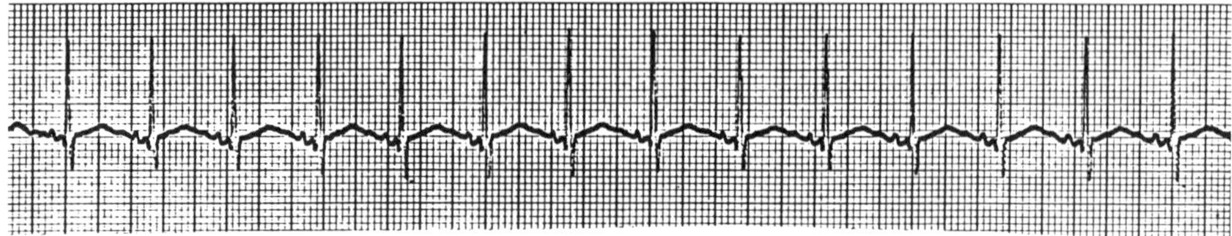

Fig. 10–2 Sinus tachycardia with heart rate of 115 beats/min.

in order to identify the P waves on the ECG more accurately.

6. *Treatment:* The underlying disorder should be treated. If necessary, while determining the cause, propranolol should be used in patients with ischemic heart disease who develop ST segment changes in order to prevent further myocardial ischemia.

Sinus Dysrhythmia

The pacemaker impulse arises from the sinoatrial node, but the dysrhythmia is manifested by alternating periods of slower and more rapid heart rates. The P-R interval is normal as is the QRS complex (Fig. 10–3). Most commonly but not invariably the rate increases with inspiration and decreases with expiration. It occurs more often in children than in adults.

1. *Heart rate:* 60 to 100 beats/min.
2. *Rhythm:* Irregular.
3. *P : QRS:* 1:1.
4. *QRS complex:* Normal.
5. *Significance:* Normal finding.
6. *Treatment:* None.

Premature Atrial Contractions

An ectopic pacemaker site in either the left or right atrium initiates the premature atrial contraction (PAC). The shape of the P wave is abnormal and possibly inverted. The P-R interval may be shorter or longer than normal, depending on the site of the ectopic focus and the refractoriness of the atrioventricular AV nodal pathway. The PAC spreads not only through the AV node and ventricular conduction system, but also in a retrograde fashion reaches the sinoatrial (SA) node, thus resetting the sinus pacemaker. The interval from the PAC to the next sinus beat is therefore a normal sinus cycle (i.e., no compensatory pause). The absence of a compensatory pause is an important distinguishing feature between PACs and premature ventricular contractions (PVCs). Occasionally, PACs may find part of the ventricular conduction system refractory. In that case, they will travel down an aberrant pathway and create an abnormal QRS complex. They are then called PACs with ventricular aberration and can very easily be confused with PVCs. Since the recovery period of the right ventricular (RV) conduction system outlasts that of the left, the most common form

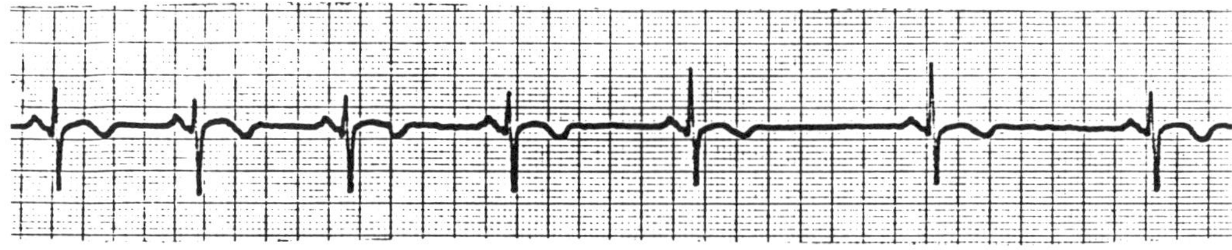

Fig. 10–3 Sinus dysrhythmia. Note the normal PR interval and QRS complex.

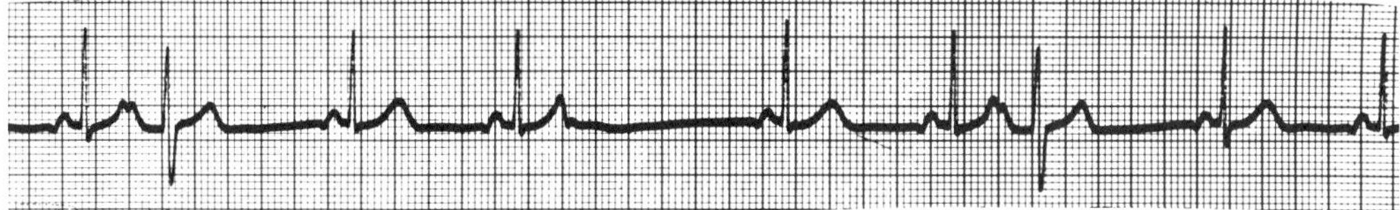

Fig. 10–4 Premature atrial contraction. Note that the RR interval between the first and the third beats is shorter than the RR interval between the third and fifth beats.

of aberration appears as a right bundle branch block (RBBB). Helpful points in separating a PAC with aberration from a PVC are as follows: (1) there is a preceding P wave, usually abnormally shaped; (2) the QRS complex has a RBBB configuration; (3) there is an rSR^1 in V_1; and (4) the initial vector forces are identical with the preceding beat, but are usually the opposite with a PVC. Other characteristics of PACs are as follows:

1. *Heart rate:* Variable, depending on frequency of PACs.
2. *Rhythm:* Irregular.
3. *P : QRS:* Usually 1:1, the P waves have various shapes and may even be lost in the QRS or T waves. Occasionally, the P wave will be so early as to find the ventricle refractory and a nonconducted beat will occur.
4. *QRS complex:* Usually normal unless there is ventricular aberration, as mentioned above (Fig 10–4).
5. *Significance:* PACs represented 10 percent of the total intraoperative dysrhythmias seen in one study.[6] They have little clinical significance, but frequent PACs may portend other more serious supraventricular dysrhythmias or be a sign of digitalis intoxication.
6. *Treatment:* Rarely necessary but digitalis, a β-adrenergic blocking agent, or verapamil may be considered if hemodynamic function is impaired.

Paroxysmal Atrial Tachycardia

A run of rapidly repeated supraventricular premature beats from a site other than the SA node characterizes paroxysmal atrial tachycardia (PAT). The inclusion of tachycardias originating in the AV node allows for the current more clinically useful classification of paroxysmal supraventricular tachycardia (SVT). The rhythm is usually abrupt in both its onset and termination.

1. *Heart rate:* 150 to 250 beats/min.
2. *Rhythm:* Usually regular unless the impulse originates from multiple atrial foci.
3. *P : QRS:* There is a 1:1 relationship, although the P wave is often hidden in the QRS complex or T wave.
4. *QRS Complex:* Generally normal, but ST-T changes indicative of ischemia may be noted (Fig. 10–5). Aberration of ventricular conduction may occur, thus complicating the differential diagnosis with ventricular tachycardia. SVT may also be confused with sinus tachycardia, atrial flutter, and atrial fibrillation. In differentiating these rhythms, carotid sinus massage and edrophonium (5 to 10 mg IV) may be used to slow the rate. Esophageal ECG leads to better define atrial activity may also be helpful.
5. *Significance:* Paroxysmal SVT can be seen in 5 percent of normal young adults and in patients with Wolff–Parkinson–White or other aberrant conduction pathway syndromes. During anesthesia it comprises 2.5 percent of all dysrhythmias,[6] and it has been associated with intrinsic heart disease, systemic illness, thyrotoxicosis, digitalis toxicity, pulmonary embolism, and pregnancy.[24] Under anesthesia it can be precipitated by changes in the autonomic nervous system, drug effects, or volume shifts and can produce severe hemodynamic deterioration.[25] At times, the PAT may be associated with AV block due to the fast atrial rate

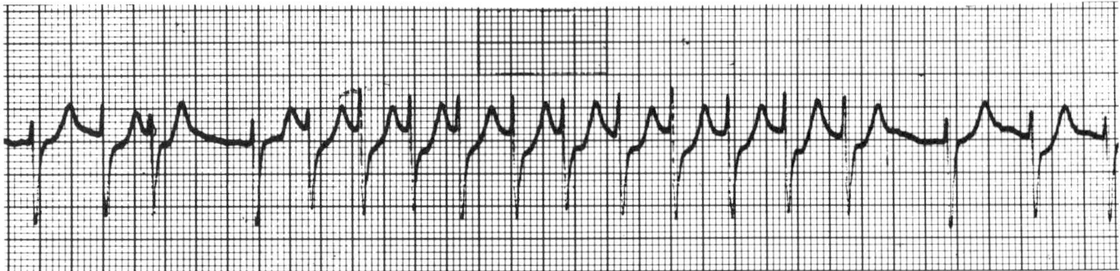

Fig. 10–5 Paroxysmal atrial tachycardia.

and slow AV conduction. PAT with 2 : 1 block represents digitalis intoxication in many patients.

6. *Treatment:* This dysrhythmia often must be treated because of its rapid rate and associated poor hemodynamic function. Several steps can be taken to treat this dysrhythmia:[26]

a. Vagal maneuvers such as carotid sinus massage, which should only be applied to one side
b. Verapamil (5 to 10 mg IV)—terminates AV nodal reentry successfully in about 90 percent of cases and has become the drug of choice[27] (It should be avoided in patients with known WPW, since it may lead to increased conduction through the abnormal pathway.)
c. Propranolol in 0.5-mg IV bolus doses
d. Edrophonium (Tensilon) in 5 to 10-mg IV bolus doses
e. Phenylephrine, if the patient is hypotensive—100-μg IV bolus doses in an effort to increase the blood pressure and achieve a reflex vagal slowing of the heart rate
f. Intravenous digitalization with one of the short-acting digitalis preparations: ouabain 0.25 to 0.5 mg IV or digoxin 0.5 to 1.0 mg IV[28]
g. Rapid overdrive pacing, in an effort to capture the ectopic focus[29]
h. Cardioversion with appropriate synchronization[30]

Atrial Flutter

This represents a faster discharge from an irritable focus in the atria than does a rapid atrial tachycardia. Since it is so fast, it is usually associated with atrioventricular block. Classic sawtooth flutter waves (F waves) are usually present (Fig. 10–6). The characteristics of atrial flutter are as follows:

1. *Heart rate:* The atrial heart rate is 250 to 350 beats/min, with a ventricular rate of about 150 beats/min.

2. *Rhythm:* The atrial rhythm is regular. The ventricular rhythm may be regular if a fixed

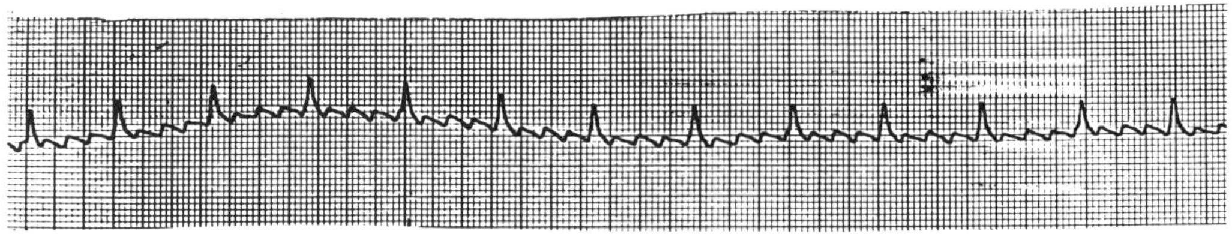

Fig. 10–6 Atrial flutter with classic sawtooth flutter waves (F waves).

AV block is present or irregular if a variable block exists.

3. *P : QRS:* Usually there is a 2:1 block with an atrial rate of 300 beats/min and a ventricular rate of 150 beats/min, but it may vary between 2:1 and 8:1. F waves are best seen in leads V_1, II, or the esophageal lead.

4. *QRS complex:* Normal. T waves are lost in the F waves.

5. *Significance:* It usually indicates the presence of severe heart disease. It has been seen with increased incidence in patients with coronary artery disease, mitral valve disease, pulmonary embolism, hyperthyroidism, trauma to or malignancies of the heart, and myocarditis.

6. *Treatment*
   a. The initial treatment of choice is synchronous DC cardioversion using very low voltage (10 to 40 watt-sec), which is effective in more than 90 percent of cases.[31]
   b. Rapid atrial pacing effectively terminates atrial flutter in many patients and results in a return to sinus rhythm or atrial fibrillation with a slow ventricular rate.[32]
   c. Verapamil, 5 to 10 mg IV, is given.[27]
   d. Digitalis, with or without propranolol, is given.

Atrial Fibrillation

This is an excessively rapid and irregular atrial focus with no P waves appearing on the ECG, but, instead, a fine fibrillatory activity called f waves. This is the most irregular rhythm and is thus called irregularly irregular and may be associated with a pulse deficit (Fig. 10–7). The characteristics are as follows:

1. *Heart rate:* The atrial rate is 350 to 500 beats/min and the ventricular rate between 60 to 170 beats/min.
2. *Rhythm:* Irregularly irregular.
3. *P : QRS:* P wave is absent and replaced by f waves or no obvious atrial activity at all.
4. *QRS complex:* Normal.
5. *Significance:* The etiologic factors of atrial fibrillation are similar to those of atrial flutter. This rhythm is almost invariably associated with significant cardiac disease. The clinical significance and treatment of atrial fibrillation are also similar to that of atrial flutter except for two important considerations. The loss of an atrial kick secondary to inefficienct contraction of the atria will reduce ventricular filling and may significantly compromise cardiac output. In addition, atrial fibrillation may lead to the formation of atrial thrombi with resultant pulmonary and systemic embolization.
6. *Treatment:* Digitalis is most commonly used to slow the ventricular rate. Propranolol or verapamil may be added. If the fibrillation is of recent onset, cardioversion may be used to reestablish sinus rhythm.

Junctional Rhythms

The AV node itself shows no intrinsic phase 4 depolarization. Therefore, cells in the node cannot act as pacemakers. Ectopic activity, however, may be initiated from sites just above and below the node. It would make sense to consider these dysrhythmias as AV junctional

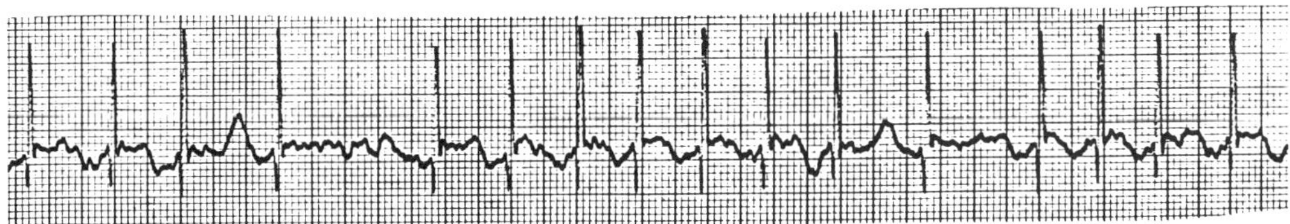

Fig. 10–7 Atrial fibrillation.

in nature. The resultant P wave will be abnormal and, depending on the position of the ectopic pacemaker, may be very close to, buried in, or following the QRS complex. Depending on the rate of fire of the ectopic pacemaker, the resultant rhythm will be nodal premature, nodal quadrigeminy, trigeminy or bigeminy, nodal rhythm, or nodal tachycardia.

1. *Heart rate:* Variable, 40 to 180 beats/min (nodal bradycardia to tachycardia) (Fig. 10–8).
2. *Rhythm:* Regular.
3. *P : QRS:* 1:1 but there are three varieties.[33]
   a. *High-nodal rhythm:* The impulse reaches the atrium before the ventricle; therefore, the P wave precedes the QRS but has a shortened P-R interval (less than 0.1 second).
   b. *Mid-nodal rhythm:* The impulse arrives in the atrium and the ventricle at the same time, and the P wave is lost in the QRS.
   c. *Low-nodal rhythm:* The impulse reaches the ventricle first and then the atrium so that the P wave follows the QRS complex.
4. *QRS complex:* Normal, unless altered by the P wave.
5. *Significance:* Junctional rhythms are common under anesthesia (about 20 percent of the cases), especially with halogenated anesthetic agents. The junctional rhythm frequently decreases blood pressure and cardiac output by about 15 percent, but it can decrease it by up to 30 percent in patients with heart disease.[34]
6. *Treatment:* Usually no treatment is required, and the rhythm reverts spontaneously. If hypotension and poor perfusion are associated with the rhythm, treatment is indicated. Atropine, ephedrine, or isoproterenol can be used in an effort to increase the activity of the SA node so it will take over as the pacemaker. A small dose of succinycholine (10 mg IV) may revert a nodal rhythm to a sinus rhythm during anesthesia with halothane or enflurane.[35] This probably works as a result of the effect of succinylcholine as a sympathetic ganglionic stimulator. In some cases, propranolol may correct the rhythm disturbance if it is due to sympathetic stimulation.

Premature Ventricular Contractions

PVCs are a result of ectopic pacemaker activity arising from below the AV junction. The PVC originates in and spreads through the myocardium or ventricular conducting system resulting in a wide (0.12 seconds) bizarre QRS complex. The ST segment usually slopes in the opposite direction of the main deflection of the QRS complex. There is no P wave associated with a PVC but retrograde depolarization of the atria or blocked sinus beats may obscure the diagnosis (Fig. 10–9).

The most important entity in the differential diagnosis is PACs with aberrant ventricular conduction. The distinction should be made whenever possible. Note that while a PAC will normally reach the SA node and reset the sinus

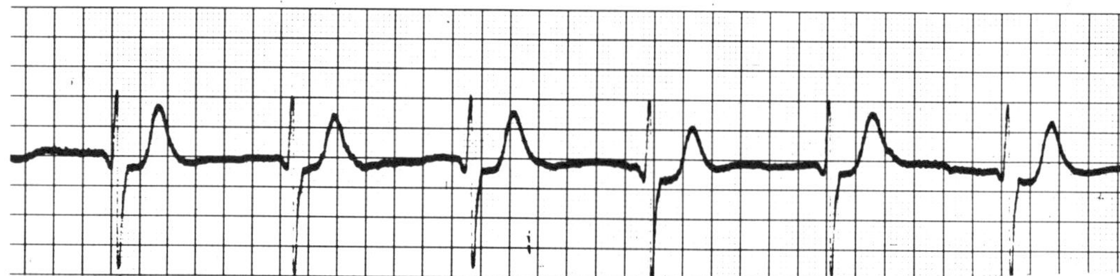

Fig. 10–8 Junctional rhythm. Note that the P waves are buried in the QRS complex.

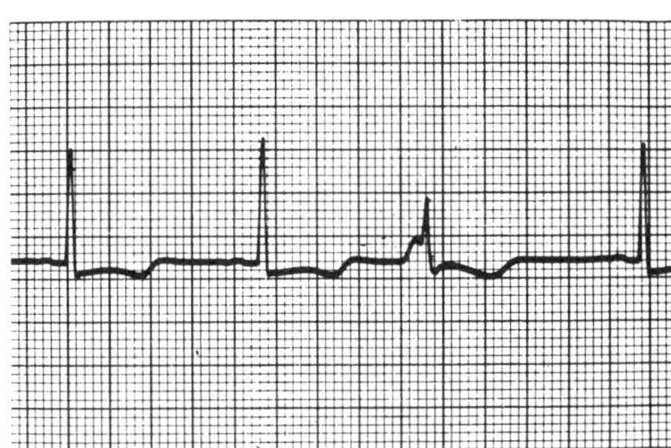

Fig. 10–9 Premature ventricular contraction.

rhythm, such an occurrence is rare when the ectopic pacemaker is in the ventricle. Therefore, a PVC will block the next depolarization from the SA node, but the following sinus beat occurs on time. The result is a compensatory pause consisting of the interval from PVC to the expected normal QRS, which is blocked at the AV node, plus a normal sinus interval. PVCs are common during anesthesia accounting for 15 percent of observed dysrhythmias.[6] They are much more common in anesthetized patients with preexisting cardiac disease. Other than heart disease, known etiologic factors include electrolyte and blood gas abnormalities, drug interactions, brain stem stimulation, and trauma to the heart.

1. *Heart rate:* Depends on the underlying sinus rate and frequency of the PVCs.
2. *Rhythm:* Irregular.
3. *P : QRS:* No P wave with the PVCs.
4. *QRS complex:* Wide and bizarre with a width of more than 0.12 seconds.
5. *Significance:* The new onset of PVCs must be considered life threatening because in certain clinical situations it may progress to ventricular tachycardia or fibrillation. These situations include coronary artery insufficiency, myocardial infarction, digitalis toxicity with hypokalemia, and hypoxemia. PVCs are more likely to lead to fibrillation if they are multiple, multifocal, bigeminal, or occur near the vulnerable period of the preceding ventricular depolarization (the so-called R-on-T phenomenon).[36]
6. *Treatment:* The first step is to correct any underlying abnormalities such as low potassium or arterial oxygen tension. Lidocaine is then usually the treatment of choice with an initial bolus dose of 1.5 mg/kg IV. Recurrent PVCs can be treated wtih a lidocaine infusion of 1 to 4 mg/min; additional therapy can be supplied with propranolol, bretylium, procainamide, quinidine, verapamil, disopyramide, atropine, or overdrive pacing.

Ventricular Tachycardia

These are a run of rapidly repeated ectopic beats arising from the ventricle, which are potentially life threatening. Diagnostic criteria include the presence of fusion beats, capture beats, and AV dissociation (Fig. 10–10).[37] The characteristics of ventricular tachycardia are as follows:

1. *Heart rate:* 100 to 200 beats/min.
2. *Rhythm:* Usually regular but may be irregular if the ventricular tachycardia is paroxysmal.
3. *P : QRS:* No fixed relationship, since ven-

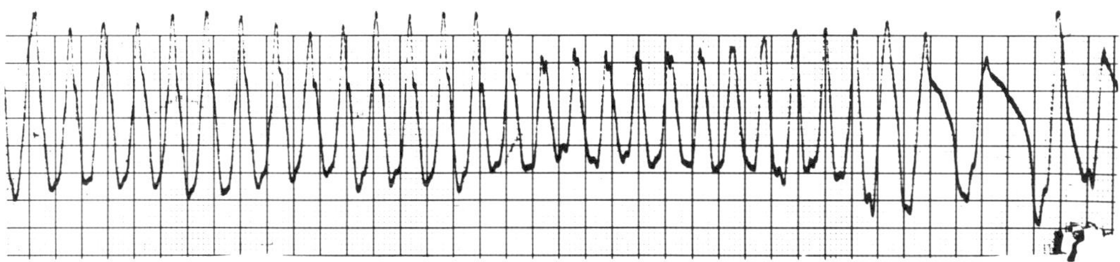

Fig. 10–10 Ventricular tachycardia.

tricular tachycardia is a form of AV dissociation in which the P waves can be seen marching through the QRS complex.

4. *QRS complex:* Wide, more than 0.12 seconds in width.

5. *Significance:* Acute onset is life threatening and requires immediate treatment.

6. *Treatment:* Lidocaine and/or immediate cardioversion is usually required. Recurrent episodes may require therapy with any or all of the drugs listed under the treatment of PVCs.

Ventricular Fibrillation

Ventricular fibrillation is an irregular rhythm resulting from a rapid discharge of impulses from one or more foci in the ventricles. The ventricular contractions are erratic and are represented on the ECG by bizarre patterns of various sizes and configurations. P waves are not seen (Fig. 10–11). Important causes of the dysrhythmia include myocardial ischemia, hypoxia, hypothermia, electric shock, electrolyte imbalance, and drug effects. The characteristics are as follows:

1. *Heart rate:* Rapid and grossly disorganized.
2. *Rhythm:* Totally irregular.
3. *P : QRS:* None seen.
4. *QRS complex:* Not present.
5. *Significance:* There is no effective cardiac output, and life must be sustained by artificial means, such as external cardiac massage.
6. *Treatment:* Cardiopulmonary resuscitation must be initiated immediately and then defibrillation performed as rapidly as possible. External defibrillation should be performed with a DC defibrillator, using 200 to 400 watt-sec.[37] Supportive pharmacologic therapy may include propranolol, bretylium, or lidocaine. In some instances, epinephrine is used to coarsen the fibrillation in an attempt to be able to defibrillate the patient.[36]

Asystole

During asystole, no ventricular activity is present. Asystole is the second most common rhythm disorder (after ventricular fibrillation) during cardiac arrests. The characteristics are as follows:

1. *Heart rate:* None present.
2. *Rhythm:* Straight line on the ECG.
3. *P : QRS:* None present.
4. *QRS complex:* Absent.
5. *Significance:* Difficult to treat and an attempt should be made to convert it to ventricular fibrillation.
6. *Treatment:* Maintain cardiopulmonary resuscitation while administering calcium chloride, isoproterenol, epinephrine, sodium bicarbonate, and, if necessary, inserting a transvenous pacemaker.

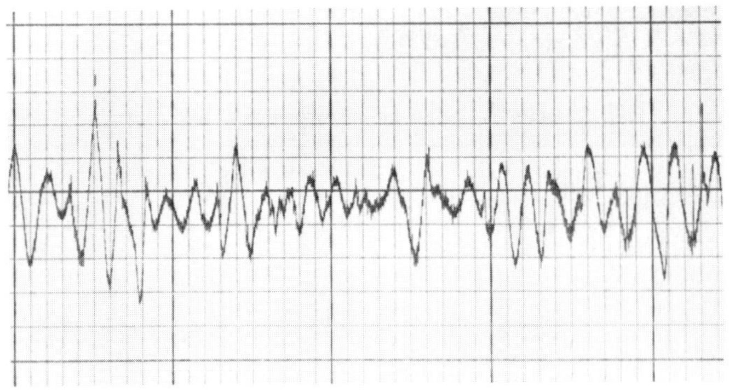

Fig. 10–11 Ventricular fibrillation.

REFERENCES

1. Kaplan JA: Cardiac Anesthesia. Grune & Stratton, Orlando, Florida, 1979
2. Beecher HK: First anesthesia death with some remarks suggested by it on the fields of the laboratory and the clinic in the appraisal of new anesthestic agents. Anesthesiology 2:443, 1941
3. Kurtz CM, Bennett JH, Shapiro H: Electrocardiographic studies during surgical anesthesia. JAMA 106:434, 1936
4. Katz RL, Bigger JT: Cardiac arrhythmias during anesthesia and operation. Anesthesiology 33:193, 1970
5. Dodd RB, Sims WA, Bone DJ: Cardiac arrhythmias observed during anesthesia. Surgery 51:440, 1962
6. Kuner J, Enescu V, Utsu F, et al: Cardiac arrhythmias during anesthesia. Dis Chest 52:580, 1967
7. Vanik PE, Davis HS: Cardiac arrhythmias during halothane anesthesia. Anesth Analg 47:299, 1968
8. Russel PH, Coakley CS: Electrocardiographic observation in the operating room. Anesth Analg 48:784, 1969
9. Bertrand CA, Steiner NV, Jameson AG, Lopez M: Disturbances of cardiac rhythm during anesthesia and surgery. JAMA 216:1615, 1971
10. Angelini L, Feldman MI, Lufschonowski R, et al: Cardiac arrhythmias during and after heart surgery: Diagnosis and management. Prog Cardiovasc Dis 16:469, 1974
11. Atlee JL, Rusy BF: Ventricular conduction times and AV nodal conductivity during enflurane anesthesia in dogs. Anesthesiology 47:498, 1977
12. Koehntop DE, Liao JC, Van Bergen FH: Effects of pharmacologic alterations of adrenergic mechanisms by cocaine, tropolone, aminophylline, and ketamine on epinephrine-induced arrhythmias during halothane-nitrous oxide anesthesia. Anesthesiology 46:83, 1977
13. Edwards R, Winnie AL, Ramamurthy S: Acute hypocapnic hypokalemia: An iatrogenic anesthetic complication. Anesth Analg 56:786, 1977
14. Fox EJ, Sklar GS, Hill CH, et al: Complications related to the pressor response to endotracheal intubation. Anesthesiology 47:524, 1977
15. Stoelting RK: Circulatory changes during direct laryngoscopy and tracheal intubation: Influence of duration of laryngoscopy with and without prior lidocaine. Anesthesiology 47:381, 1977
16. Katz RL, Bigger JT: Cardiac arrhythmias during anesthesia and operation. Anesthesiology 33:193, 1970
17. Smith M, Ray CT: Cardiac arrhythmias, increased intracranial pressure, and the autonomic nervous system. Chest 61:125, 1972
18. Alexander JP: Dysrhythmia and oral surgery. Br J Anaesth 43:773, 1971
19. Borg DE: Paradox of cardiac arrhythmias in anaesthesia. Br J Anaesth 41:709, 1969
20. Kaplan JA: Electrocardiographic monitoring. p. 117. In Kaplan JA (ed): Cardiac Anesthesia. Grune & Stratton, Orlando, Florida, 1979
21. Kaplan JA, Dunbar RW, Bland JW, et al: Propranolol and cardiac surgery: A problem for the anesthesiologist? Anesth Analg 54:571, 1975
22. Slapa WJ: The sick sinus syndrome. Am Heart J 92:648, 1976
23. Moe GK, Mendez C: Physiologic basis of premature beats and sustained tachycardia. N Engl J Med 288:250, 1973
24. Jones RM, Broadbeht MP, Adams AP: Anaesthetic considerations in patients with paroxysmal supraventricular tachycardia. Anaesthesia 39:307, 1984
25. Sprague DH, Mandel SD: Paroxysmal supraventricular tachycardia during anesthesia. Anesthesiology 46:75, 1977
26. Chung EK: Tachyarrhythmias in Wolff–Parkinson–White syndrome: Antiarrhythmia therapy. JAMA 237:376, 1977
27. Rinkenberger RL, Prystowsky EN, Heger JJ: Effects of intravenous and chronic oral verapamil administration in patients with supraventricular tachyarrhythmias. Circulation 62:996, 1980
28. Zipes DP: Specific arrhythmias, diagnosis and treatment. p. 709. In Braunwald E (ed): Heart Disease. WB Saunders, Philadelphia, 1984
29. Escher DJW, Furman S: Emergency treatment of cardiac arrhythmias: Emphasis on use of electrical pacing. JAMA 214:2028, 1970
30. Kleiger RE: Cardioversion of paroxysmal arrhythmias. JAMA 213:107, 1970
31. Glassman E: Direct current cardioversion. Am Heart J 82:128, 1971
32. Camm J, Ward D, Spunell R: Response of atrial flutter to overdrive atrial pacing and intravenous disopyramide phosphate, singly and in combination. Br Heart J 44:240, 1980
33. Scherlag BJ, Lazzara R, Helfant RH: Differentiation of "AV junctional rhythms." Circulation 48:304, 1973

34. Haldemann G, Schoer H: Haemodynamic effects of transient atrioventricular dissociation in general anesthesia. Br J Anaesth 44:159, 1972
35. Galindo A, Wyte SR, Wetherhold JW: Junctional rhythm induced by halothane anesthesia—Treated with succinylcholine. Anesthesiology 37:261, 1972
36. Cranefield PF: Ventricular fibrillation. N Engl J Med 289:732, 1973
37. Geddes LA, Tacker WA, Rosborough J, et al: The electrical dose for ventricular defibrillation with electrodes applied directly to the heart. J Thorac Cardiovasc Surg 68:593, 1974

11

Electrolyte Disturbances and the ECG

James B. Eisenkraft, M.D.

The basic mechanisms of automaticity and rhythmicity of the heart muscle originate in the distribution of ions across cell membranes. Changes in electrolyte concentrations in the body may change the distribution, and hence, flux of ions, thereby producing alterations in the recorded electrocardiograph. Electrolyte abnormalities may cause specific configurational changes in each complex or its components.[1] More severe abnormalities may result in progressive changes that may eventually affect the normal sequential relationship among complexes, causing dysrhythmias. Finally, chronic electrolyte abnormalities may cause degenerative anatomic changes in the myocardium. These may result in nonspecific ECG changes, reflecting the extent of the lesion rather than the specific causative agent. Potassium (K^+), calcium (Ca^{++}), sodium (Na^+), and magnesium (Mg^{++}) are the electrolytes considered in this chapter.

POTASSIUM

Within the ranges of electrolyte concentrations seen in clinical disorders, K^+ is the electrolyte most likely to change the electrophysiologic properties of the heart.[2]

Hyperkalemia

Hyperkalemia is usually iatrogenic.[3] Causes include the following:

Administration of K^+ salts (orally or IV)
K^+-conserving diuretics
Blood transfusions ($[K^+]$ = 30 mEq/L in old stored blood)[4]
K^+-containing drugs (e.g., potassium penicillin)
Massive hemolysis
Crush syndrome
Acute and chronic renal disease
Diabetic acidosis
Malignant hyperthermia
Administration of succinylcholine to patients with burns,[5] trauma,[6] certain neurologic[7] and muscular disorders
Infections (pneumonias)
Hyperkalemic periodic paralysis[8]

EFFECTS ON THE ECG

ECG effects are secondary to effects on the atrial and ventricular action potentials (Fig. 11–1). Increasing $[K^+]$ produces shortening of the action potential and more rapid phase 3 repolarization due to an increased membrane perme-

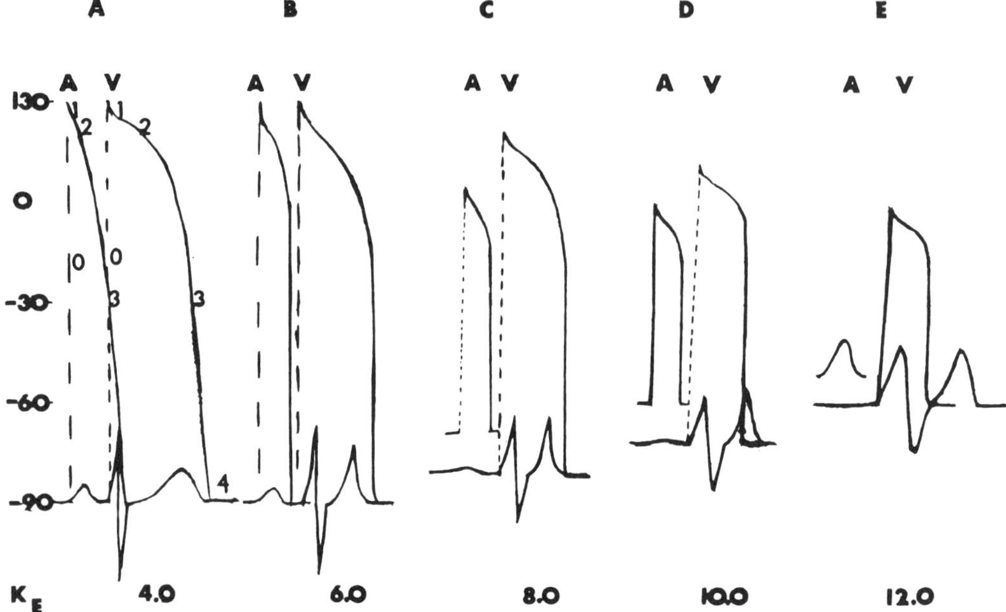

Fig. 11–1 Effect on hyperkalemia on the atrial (A) and ventricular (V) action potential and ECG. The scale on the left shows the transmembrane potential in millivolts. K_E represents the extracellular potassium concentration in milliequivalents per liter. (Surawicz B: Relationship between electrocardiogram and electrolytes. Am Heart J 73:815, 1967.)

ability to K^+ (Fig. 11–1A,B), and a reduction in the resting membrane potential (less negative) due to a decreased transmembrane concentration gradient for K^+ (Fig. 11–1C to E).

RELATIONSHIP TO POTASSIUM CONCENTRATIONS

$[K^+]$ 5.5 to 6.5 mEq/L: The earliest ECG change is peaking of the T wave. Note that the slope of the terminal portion of the T wave tends to parallel the slope of phase 3 repolarization. The QRS complex is normal and the QTc (QT interval corrected for heart rate) interval is normal or slightly decreased (Fig. 11–1B).

$[K^+]$ 6.5 to 7.0 mEq/L: The QRS becomes widened (intraventricular block). As $[K^+]$ increases, there is a rough correlation between QRS duration and K^+ concentration.

$[K^+] > 7.0$ mEq/L: P-wave amplitude decreases and P wave widens due to slower atrial conduction. The PR interval is increased due to slower atrioventricular (AV) transmission (AV nodal block). The ventricular rate may be irregular, regular, slow, or rapid (Fig. 11–1C).

$[K^+]$ 8.0 mEq/L: P wave frequently disappears (intraatrial block) or may wander in and out of the QRS complex. The disappearance of the P wave at a time when the ventricular complex is still well defined indicates that atrial excitability is lost at a lower K^+ concentration than that at which ventricular excitability is lost. The resting membrane potential and the action potential amplitude of the atrial fibers are decreased more than those of the ventricular fibers.

Disappearance of the P wave does not indicate cessation of sinoatrial (SA) node activity—only paralysis of the atria. The P wave is absent because the impulse from the SA node produces no propagated response, only a small local atrial depolarization. The impulse that originates in the SA node may be propagated to the ventricles through specialized atrial fibers without ever deplorizing the atrial muscle. This may result in a sinoventricular conduction in the presence of a SA block.

When the P waves are absent, an erroneous diagnosis of atrial fibrillation may be made, especially when the ventricular rhythm is irregular.

$[K^+]$ *10 mEq/L:* Wide aberrant QRS complexes appear (Fig. 11–1D,E).
$[K^+]$ *11 mEq/L:* Biphasic deflections due to fusion of QRS complexes with ST segment and T waves, appear. The ST segment may deviate significantly from baseline, simulating the picture of acute myocardial injury.
$[K^+]$ *12 to 14 mEq/L:* Ventricular asystole or fibrillation occurs.

Fibrillation may or may not be preceded by an increase in the ventricular rate. Ventricular fibrillation most likely results from reentry facilitated by slow intraventricular conduction and a short duration ventricular action potential.

Marked hyperkalemia may be associated with patterns simulating myocardial infarction, such as ST elevations, inverted T waves, and even transient Q waves. These pseudoinfarct patterns should revert to normal when the serum $[K^+]$ is lowered.

DYSRHYTHMIAS

Hyperkalemia has a biphasic effect on automaticity. It first decreases the resting membrane potential, enhancing automaticity. It also decreases the rate of rise of phase 4 depolarization, which reduces automaticity. The overall effect on automaticity is therefore variable.[1,9]

Dysrhythmias that may be associated with hyperkalemia include the following.

Sinus bradycardia
First-degree heart block
Junctional rhythm
Idioventricular rhythm
Ventricular tachycardia
Ventricular arrest
Ventricular fibrillation

The ECG patterns and dysrhythmias of hyperkalemia can be corrected by increasing concentrations of Ca^{++} and Na^+; they can be made more abnormal by decreasing the concentration of Ca^{++} and possibly of Na^+ as well. Hypermagnesemia may also render the heart insensitive to hyperkalemia, while Mg^{++} ions attenuate the electrophysiologic response to elevated $[K^+]$.

Hypokalemia

Hypokalemia usually results from excessive losses of K^+ from the gut or kidney.[10] Causes include the following:

Vomiting and/or nasogastric suction
Diarrhea, laxatives
Malabsorption, sprue
Alkalosis
Diuretic therapy
Renal dialysis
Hyperadrenalism, steroid therapy
Diabetes mellitus
Hyperinsulinism
Malignant disease
Hepatic cirrhosis
Familial hypokalemic periodic paralysis

EFFECTS ON THE ECG

Hypokalemia causes an increase in the resting membrane potential and prolongs the duration of the action potential. Figure 11–2 shows the relationship among the action potential, ECG, and potassium level. As $[K^+]$ decreases, the slope of phase 2 becomes progressively steeper, while that of phase 3 becomes less steep (Fig. 11–2B–D). The repolarization slope (phase 3) becomes slower and changes from convex to

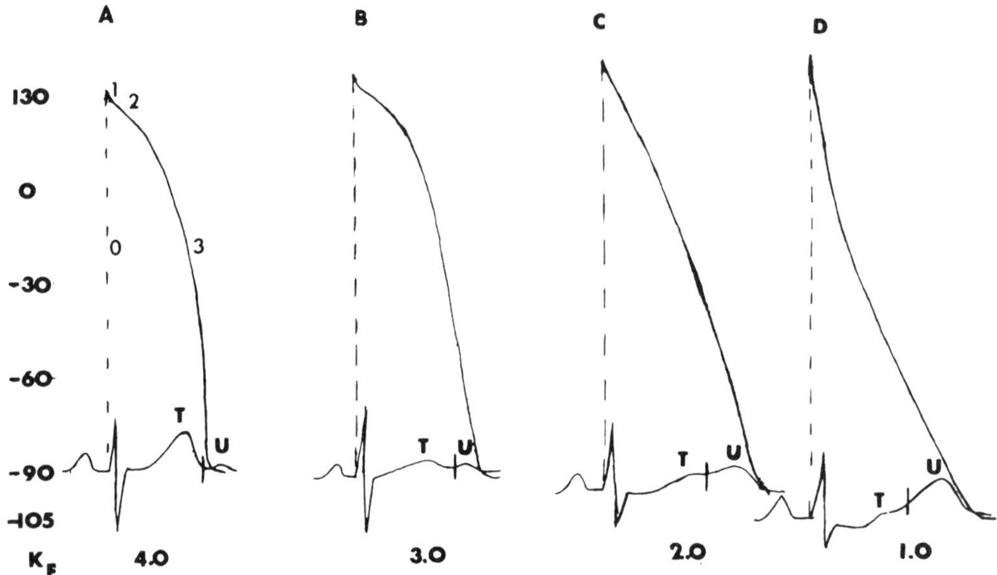

Fig. 11–2 Effect of hypokalemia on the ventricular action potential and ECG. The scale on the left shows the transmembrane potential in millivolts. K_E represents the extracellular potassium concentration in milliequivalents per liter. (Surawicz B: Relationship between electrocardiogram and electrolytes. Am Heart J 73:815, 1967.)

concave. These changes in the action potential are reflected in the ECG, where changes are best seen in the anterior and lateral precordial leads. The T wave decreases in amplitude and becomes wider, and the QTc interval becomes prolonged. These changes may occur at low-normal levels of [K^+] (e.g., 3.5 mEq/L). Low, broad T waves develop, with a double peak due to superimposition of the U wave on the T wave.[1,11,12]

The QT interval may appear prolonged but this may be difficult to determine. The QU interval may be more easily measured and is not prolonged. With decreasing levels of [K^+], T waves become inverted and the U waves more prominent. As potassium levels change, the T and U waves change in opposite fashion; as the T decreases in height, the U wave increases. When both are equal, a camelhump effect is produced. When the U wave is taller than the T, [K^+] is usually less than 2.7 mEq/L. As potassium decreases, the ST segments become depressed and display the sagging appearance characteristic of hypokalemia. The P waves increase in size, and the PR interval becomes prolonged with decreasing K^+ concentration.

Recognition of hypokalemia may be difficult in the presence of a tachycardia because the latter commonly gives rise to ST depression and low-amplitude T waves. Recognition may require the demonstration of an increased U-wave amplitude. However, the U-wave amplitude is generally inversely proportional to the length of the preceding RR interval and therefore may not always be appreciably increased. Also, in tachycardias, fusion of the T, U, and P waves may occur. In such cases, the P wave is tilted because its onset is on the descending limb of the T wave and U wave and farther from the baseline at its onset than at its end. Following correction of hypokalemia, the diastolic potential responsible for the uplifting of the P wave decreases, and the initial portion of the P descends to the baseline.

Digitalis often causes ST and T changes similar to those caused by hypokalemia, but digitalis does not appreciably increase the size of the U wave.[13] Quinidine does increase U-wave amplitude, and the ECG pattern of patients taking both digitalis and quinidine may be indistinguishable from that of hypokalemia.

DYSRHYTHMIAS

Hypokalemia increases the rate of phase 4 depolarization, decreases the threshold potential, and thus enhances automaticity substantially.[9,14] Automatic firing may occur in the SA node and in other tissues of the heart, the most common being the AV junction.

Hypokalemia renders the heart susceptible to any influence likely to elicit dysrhythmias, including catecholamines, hypoxia, hypercarbia, and anticholinergics (e.g., atropine, meperidine, pancuronium). No anesthetic of choice has been identified for the hypokalemic patient.

The rapidity with which hypokalemia develops is also very important. Chronic hypokalemia (as low as 2 mEq/L) is usually well tolerated, whereas acute hypokalemia is often associated with dysrhythmias.

Tachycardias of sinus or atrial origin, as well as frequent ectopic beats, are common. The origin of the ectopic dysrhythmias may be enhanced automaticity of latent pacemaker fibers caused by decreased potassium conductance, because hypokalemia may depress conduction. Thus, hypokalemic dysrhythmias may also be caused by an enhancement of reentry. Patients with hypokalemia have atrial and ventricular extrasystoles three times more frequently than experienced by controls. Facilitation of ectopic beats is attributed to the prolonged duration of phase 3 of the action potential. When the refractory period is over, the repolarization is not yet completed. The membrane potential is therefore closer to the threshold potential, and less current is needed for spontaneous depolarization.

Dysrhythmias commonly associated with hypokalemia include the following:

Ventricular premature contractions
Sinus, atrial, and nodal tachycardia
Ventricular tachycardia
Ventricular fibrillation
AV dissociation
Second-degree AV block with Wenckebach periods

Dysrhythmias in patients with hypokalemia are similar to those produced by digitalis. This is because both increase the automaticity of ectopic supraventricular and ventricular pacemakers and prolong AV conduction, permitting the phenomenon of reentry. Hypokalemia also increases the tissue binding of digitalis glycosides, making more digitalis available for direct cardiac effects. This shift in pharmacokinetics results in a potentiation of digitalis action by hypokalemia. Thus, there is both electrophysiologic synergism of digitalis by hypokalemia as well as potentiation, which may result in digitalis toxicity, even though the total amount of digitalis in the body is normal.

Hypokalemia certainly renders the heart susceptible to any influence likely to produce dysrhythmias, including catecholamines, hypoxia, hypercarbia, and anticholinergics, as well as to digitalis. Vitez et al.[15] reported, however, that chronic hypokalemia does not increase the incidence of dysrhythmias during anesthesia, and these workers have questioned the current practice of acute potassium replacement or surgical postponement in those patients found to be hypokalemic. However, they did not state whether their patients were receiving digoxin.

Excitability Threshold and Potassium

Potassium administration may correct the excitability threshold and restore normal responsiveness to a pacemaker whose function is defective because of decreased stimulus strength or increased tissue resistance. Conversely, the administration of glucose and insulin, which lowers plasma $[K^+]$, may cause a decrease in responsiveness. The lowest excitability threshold may correspond to a plasma $[K^+]$ of 6 mEq/L, whereas both lower and higher concentrations appear to increase the threshold. Measurements of excitability threshold in patients with pacemakers do not distinguish between a lack of response to stimulation and a lack of propagation of the local response.

CALCIUM

Adequate concentrations of ionized calcium are needed for normal cardiac function. Normal serum levels are usually maintained by parathormone, while many calcium effects are dependent on a cytoplasmic modulator, calmodulin.

Hypocalcemia

Causes of hypocalcemia include the following:

Vitamin D deficiency
Parathormone deficiency
Hypoparathyroidism (also pseudo- and pseudopseudohypoparathyroidism)
Pancreatitis
Hyperphosphatemia
Hypomagnesemia
Hyperadrenalism (Cushing's syndrome)
Neoplastic disease
Renal tubular acidosis
Drugs (e.g., EDTA, steroids, chelating agents)
Nephrotic syndrome
Hepatic cirrhosis
Infusion of citrate (large volumes of banked blood), phosphate (used to treat hypercalcemia), or bicarbonate
Alkalosis

EFFECTS ON THE ECG

The main cardiac effect of calcium is on the duration of phase 2 (the plateau phase) of the action potential. Hypocalcemia prolongs phase 2 but does not alter the slope of phase 3. This results in an increased duration of the ST segment and of the QT interval. Hypocalcemia also increases the size of the threshold potential, making it more negative. Reference to Figure 11–3 shows that the end of the ventricular action potential roughly approximates the end of the T wave when $[Ca^{++}]$ is normal or low. Changes in Ca^{++} principally affect the duration of the ST segment without a significant change in the durations of other components of the ECG.

The QT interval represents the time needed for ventricular activation and repolarization and corresponds to mechanical systole. It is measured from the onset of the Q wave to the end of the T wave and is best measured in lead aVL. The QT interval is related to heart rate, age, and sex, the first being the most important. The shorter the RR interval, the shorter will be the QT interval. The corrected interval QTc may be calculated by dividing the actual QT interval by the square root of the duration of one cycle (measured from the peak of one R wave to the peak of the next R wave):

$$\text{QTc} = \frac{\text{QT interval}}{\sqrt{(\text{RR interval})}}$$

The relationship between heart rate and normal QT interval is shown in Table 11–1. While hypocalcemia causes prolongation of the ST and QTc segments, the latter rarely exceeds 1.4 times the normal duration. Therefore, a QTc greater than 1.4 times normal suggests that the U wave is merged with the T and that QU is being measured. Because of these difficulties, some electrocardiographers recommend measurement of QoTC (Q to onset of T wave) or QaTC (Q to apex of T wave) (Fig. 11–4).

In both patients and animals there is a good correlation between QT intervals and hypocalcemia that has been induced by infusions of citrate or EDTA.[16] Progressive changes in QT intervals are obtained during the first 15 minutes of steady-state alterations in Ca^{++}, so that QT measurement is not useful for evaluating $[Ca^{++}]$ during this time.

With severe hypocalcemia, the polarity of the T wave may be altered, becoming flattened or inverted in leads where it is usually upright. This pattern may resemble myocardial ischemia

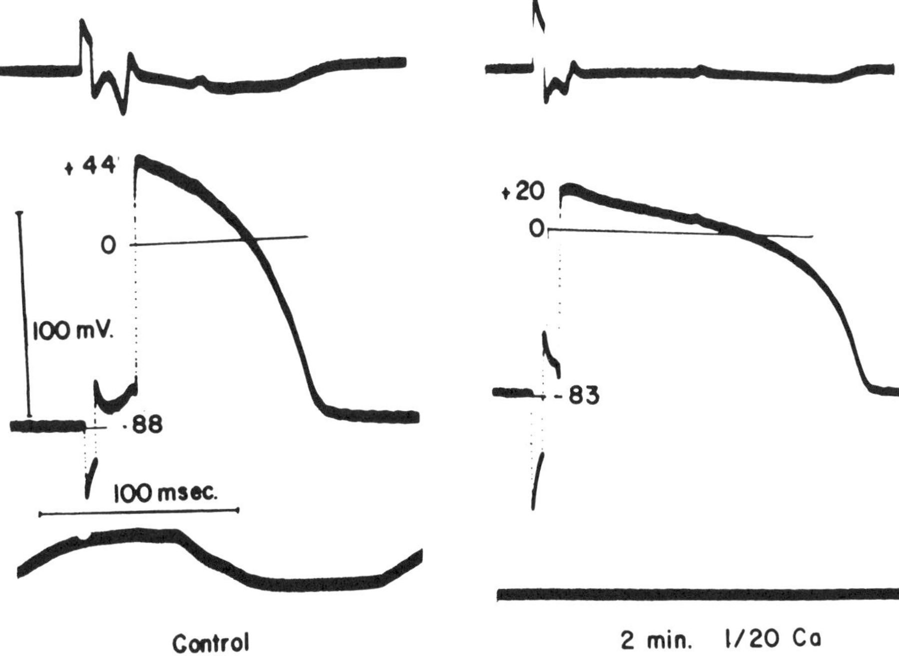

Fig. 11–3 From top to bottom. Electrocardiogram, ventricular action potential, and contractile force of isolated rabbit heart before and during perfusion with low-Ca^{++} (0.25 mM/L) Krebs–Henseleit solution. There is increased duration of the plateau of the action potential and a corresponding increase in the duration of the ST segment. Note the relationship between the end of the T wave and the end of the action potential. Recordable contraction (lowest traces) is abolished during perfusion with the hypocalcemic solution. (Dreifus LS, Likoff W (eds): Mechanisms and Therapy of Cardiac Arrhythmias. Grune & Stratton, Orlando, FL, 1973, by permission.)

(Fig. 11–5). The duration of the T wave is not altered by hypocalcemia.

When hypocalcemia and hypokalemia coexist, the ECG may show prolonged ST and QT segments, but QU is not prolonged. A prominent repolarization wave consisting of T and U waves may be seen. This is the result of prolongation of phases 2 and 3 of the action potential. The administration of IV calcium in this situation will shorten the ST segment and separate T and U waves.

Table 11–1. The QT Interval and Heart Rate

Heart Rate	Normal QT (seconds)
50–60	0.39–0.41
60–70	0.36–0.38
70–80	0.34–0.36
80–90	0.32–0.33
90–100	0.31–0.33

DYSRHYTHMIAS

Within clinically observed variations of Ca^{++} concentration, the ion is without significant effect on the size of the transmembrane resting potential or on phase 4 depolarization, these being the two changes most important in the production of dysrhythmias. By reducing $[Ca^{++}]$ to one-twentieth its normal level, dysrhythmias have been induced in animals. Hypocalcemia will, however, potentiate the dysrhythmogenic effects of hyperkalemia.

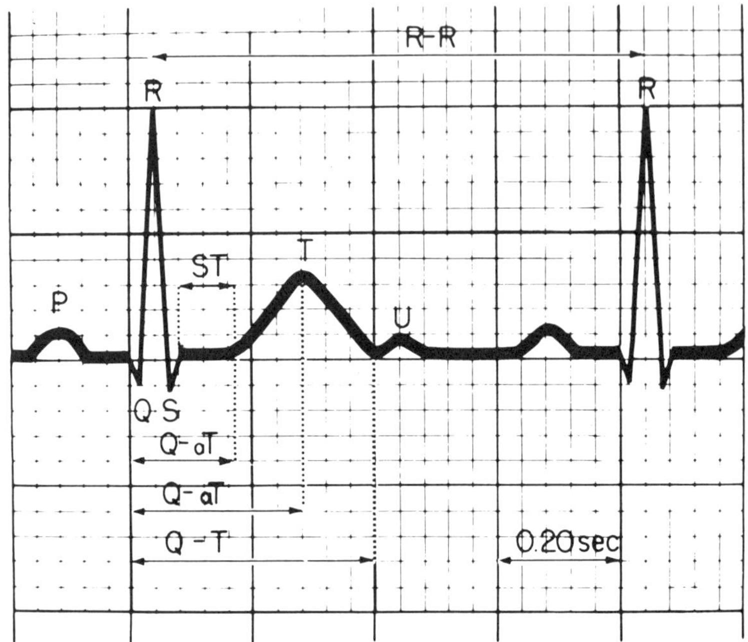

Fig. 11–4 Method of measuring the QoT, QaT, QT, and RR intervals of the ECG. (Nirenberg DN, Ransil BJ: QaTc interval as a clinical indicator of hypercalcemia. Am J Cardiol 44:244, 1979.)

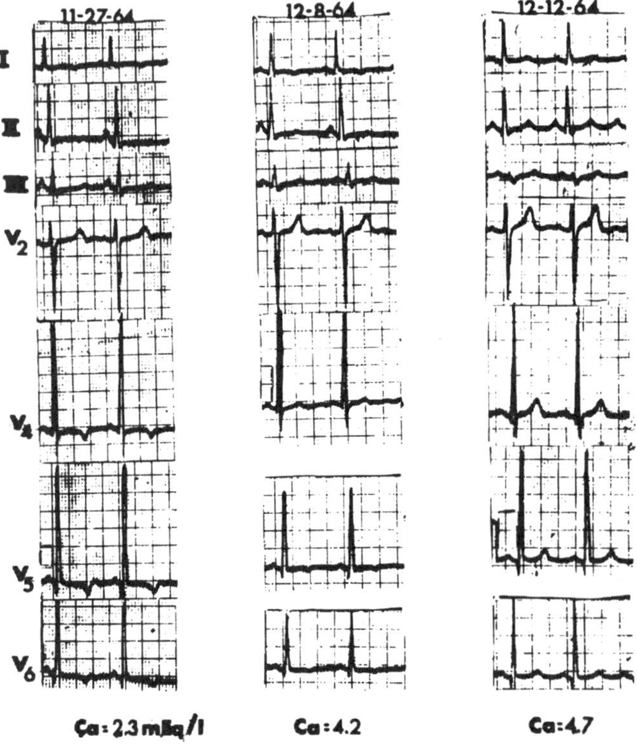

Fig. 11–5 Electrocardiographic pattern of hypocalcemia simulating myocardial ischemia. When the plasma calcium concentration is 2.3 mEq/L pointed inverted T waves are seen in leads I and V_4–V_6. These changes revert to normal when the hypocalcemia is corrected. This patient was an 18-year-old man with hypoparathyroidism but no evidence of heart disease. (Surawicz B: Relationship between electrocardiogram and electrolytes. Am Heart J 73:826, 1967. Reproduced by permission and courtesy of Dr. Lee H. Shields, Camp Hill, Pennsylvania.)

Hypercalcemia

General causes of hypercalcemia include increased absorption and mobilization or decreased excretion. Examples include the following:

Vitamin D excess
Sarcoidosis
Milk-alkali syndrome
Hyperparathyroidism
Osteolytic metastases
Immobilization
Malignant disease
Endocrine disease (e.g., hyperthyroidism)
Diuretics (e.g., thiazides)
Hypervitaminosis A
Calcium exchange resins in hemodialysis
Following renal transplantation
Acute renal failure (diuretic phase)

EFFECT ON THE ECG

Hypercalcemia decreases the duration of phase 2 of the action potential. The ST segment is shorted and QTc interval is decreased. The U-wave amplitude may be normal or increased. As with hypocalcemia, the QU interval is normal. Thus, hypercalcemia shortens ventricular systole and decreases the duration of the effective refractory period.

Of the various QTc indices that are measurable, the QaTc interval is reported to be that most easily and precisely measured at elevated calcium levels, and it exhibits the strongest correlation with serum calcium concentration.[17] The relationship is linear and can be used to estimate serum calcium levels from measurements of QaTc intervals (Fig. 11–6). For a QaTc interval of 0.29 seconds or less (range 0.23 to 0.29 seconds), the serum calcium was estimated

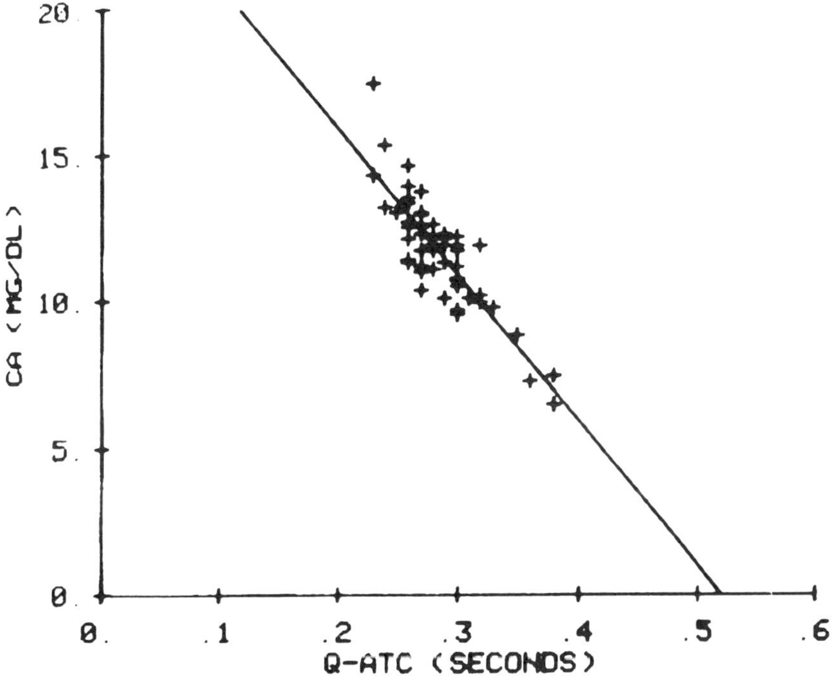

Fig. 11–6 Serum calcium as a function of the QaTc interval with least squares fit. QaTc interval: calcium, 2.7–49.5 (QaTc); standard deviation, ±0.92; F statistic, 166.7, P<0.0001; r, −0.85) (Nirenberg DW, Ransil BJ: QaTc interval as a clinical indicator of hypercalcemia. Am J Cardiol 44:245, 1979.)

to ±1.9 mg/dl with 95 percent confidence.[17] For a QaTc of 0.27 seconds or less, the correspondence with hypercalcemia was 90 percent or better. The equation is as follows:

$$\text{Calcium} = 25.7 - 49.5\ (\text{QaTc}) \pm \text{CL}$$

where CL is the 95 percent (1.9 to 2.0 over the range) or 99 percent (2.5 to 2.7 over the range) confidence limits computed in the usual manner. In this study, the normal range of calcium was given as 8.5 to 10.5 mg/dl. Thus, the ECG may be a useful method of screening for hypercalcemia.

EFFECT ON DYSRHYTHMIAS

Hypercalcemia decreases the size of the threshold potential, making it less negative. In experimental animals, marked hypercalcemia may cause depression of interventricular conduction, ventricular premature systoles, and fibrillation. In patients with severe hypercalcemia, prolongation of the PR interval, higher degrees of AV block, prolongation of the QRS, and bradycardias may be seen.

It has been suggested that hypercalcemia enhances digitalis ectopy because lowering of [Ca^{++}] using EDTA may reverse such dysrhythmias. The antiarrhythmic effect of sodium EDTA has been attributed to a prolongation of the refractory period by lowering [Ca^{++}].

INTERACTIONS OF CALCIUM WITH POTASSIUM

The intraventricular and atrioventricular conduction disturbances and the susceptibility to ventricular fibrillation caused by hyperkalemia may be reversed or prevented by increasing [Ca^{++}]. Conversely, those disturbances caused by hypokalemia can be reversed or prevented by decreasing [Ca^{++}].

SODIUM

Normally, sodium balance is adjusted by the kidney in order to maintain an adequate circulating blood volume. There are no characteristic ECG changes associated with clinical disorders of Na^+ concentration.

Hyponatremia

Causes of hyponatremia include the following:

Hypotonicity and hypovolemia: Burns, diarrhea, vomiting, diuretics, Addison's disease, renal tubular defects
Hypotonicity and normovolemia: Water absorption, early postoperative period, inappropriate secretion of ADH
Hypotonicity and hypervolemia: Edematous conditions (e.g., congestive heart failure, nephrosis, transurethral resection syndrome, hepatic disease)
Hypertonicity and variable volume: Following acute administration of hypertonic solutions which do not contain Na^+

EFFECT ON THE ECG

Hyponatremia decreases the upstroke velocity and amplitude of the action potential. There is no significant effect on transmembrane resting potential or on phase 4 depolarization of pacemaker cells. Consequently, these decreases in sodium concentration, which are compatible with life, cannot be recognized in the ECG and do not cause dysrhythmias.

Hypernatremia

Causes of hypernatremia include the following:

Hypertonicity
Hypovolemia and dehydration (e.g., fever, diabetes insipidus)
Hypervolemia (due to excess salt administration)

EFFECT ON THE ECG

Hypernatremia increases upstroke velocity of the action potential. Increasing the Na^+ concentration may restore normal intraventricular conduction velocity in a situation in which it has been decreased by some condition which had previously decreased the upstroke velocity of the ventricular action potential.

Thus, a widened QRS due to hyperkalemia or quinidine may be normalized by the intravenous administration of NaCl. In the absence of preexisting conduction disturbances, the ECG is not affected by hypernatremia.

MAGNESIUM

The primary cardiovascular effects of Mg^{++} involve myocardial conduction and contraction, but the overall importance of Mg^{++} remains to be established. Mg^{++} promotes the maintenance of a negative resting membrane potential and may oppose the depolarizing effect of K^+ in cardiac cells.

Hypomagnesemia

In the absence of hypocalcemia, the concentration of Mg^{++} within the range encountered in the clinical setting has no significant effect on the action potential.[18] There is a lack of agreement as to what, if any, ECG changes are characteristic of hypomagnesemia. This is because Mg^{++} deficiency is unlikely to occur alone. It is usually dietary in origin. Electrocardiographic changes that have been described include ST segment depression, which does not correlate with Mg^{++} levels, and T wave inversion (Fig. 11–7). In hypomagnesemic children, sharply

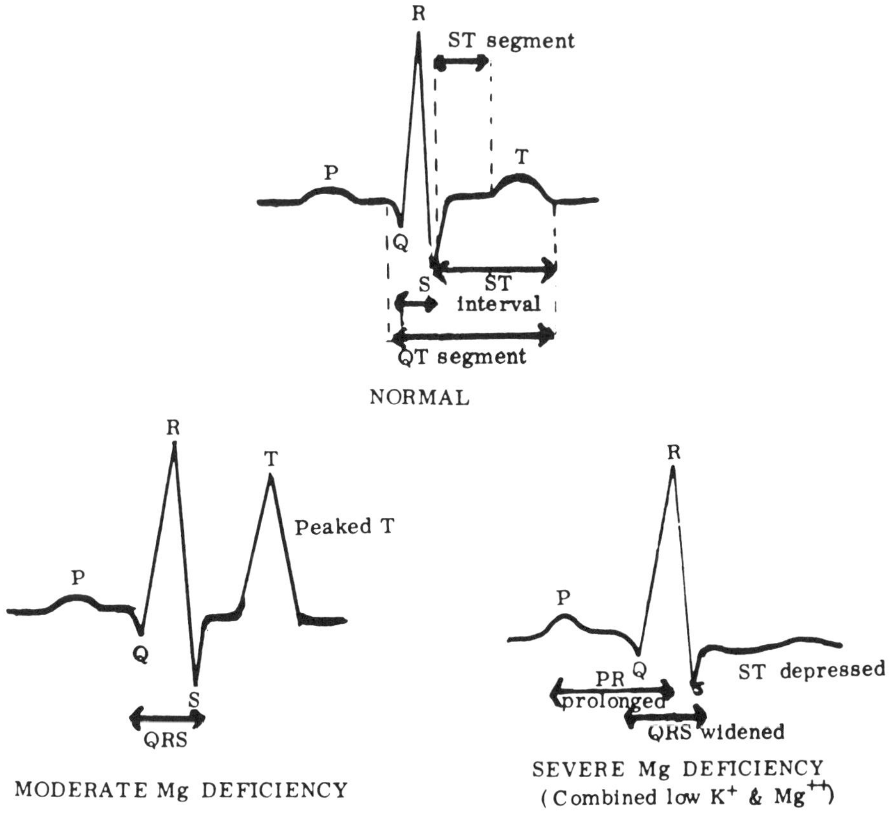

Fig. 11–7 Electrocardiographic changes associated with magnesium deficiency. (Seelig M: Electrocardiographic pattern of magnesium depletion appearing in alcoholic heart disease. Ann NY Acad Sci 162:907, 1969.)

peaked asymmetric T waves and prominent U waves have been reported. Low-voltage P waves and QRS complexes have been recorded in Mg^{++}-deficient patients and were reversed by administration of Mg^{++}. These changes probably reflect in part a relative increase in extracellular $[K^+]$. Late or prolonged Mg^{++} deficiency produces a prolonged PR interval, widened QRS complexes, ST-segment depression, and low T waves. In children with tetany, a lack of QTc prolongation would favor a diagnosis of deficiency of Mg^{++} rather than of $Ca.^{++}$

EFFECT ON DYSRHYTHMIAS

Hypomagnesemia can contribute to dysrhythmia genesis, especially during digitalis administration. Both drugs tend to result in loss of intracellular potassium, and hypokalemia produces electrical instability of the myocardium. Intravenous $MgSO_4$ has been used to treat paroxysmal atrial tachycardia (PAT) and ventricular tachycardia and has been used with limited success in patients with digitalis toxicity.[19] Diuretic therapy may produce both low K^+ and Mg^{++} levels and predisposes to digitalis toxicity. For this reason, Mg^{++} levels as well as K^+ levels should be measured in patients with digitalis toxicity.

Hypermagnesemia

Elevation of Mg^{++} concentration depresses AV conduction, possibly due to slowing of the upstroke of phase 0, and promotes the maintenance of a negative resting potential, which may oppose the depolarizing effect of K^+. Overall, however, hypermagnesemia has no detectable effects on the ECG. Hypermagnesemia has been shown to attenuate the ECG effects of hyperkalemia in canine heart studies.[20]

DEGENERATIVE CHANGES IN THE MYOCARDIUM

These changes have been described in both potassium and magnesium deficiency. In the latter case, the cardiac changes are similar to those of alcoholic cardiomyopathy and may be part of an overall dietary insufficiency syndrome. The ECG changes associated with degenerative changes are nonspecific as regards causative agent.

REFERENCES

1. Surawicz B: Relationship between electrocardiogram and electrolytes. Am Heart J 73:814, 1967
2. Vitez T: Potassium and the anesthesiologist. ASA Refresher Course Lecture #110, ASA, Park Ridge, Illinois, 1982
3. Whang R: Hyperkalemia: Diagnosis and treatment. Am J Med Sci 272:19, 1976
4. Miller RD: Complications of massive blood transfusions. Anesthesiology 39:82, 1973
5. Tolmie JD, Joyce TH, Mitchell GD: Succinylcholine danger in the burned patient. Anesthesiology 28:467, 1967
6. Mazze RI, Escue HM, Houston JB: Hyperkalemia and cardiovascular collapse following administration of succinylcholine to the traumatized patient. Anesthesiology 31:540, 1969
7. Tobey RE: Paraplegia, succinylcholine and cardiac arrest. Anesthesiology 32:359, 1970
8. Kalbian VV: Iatrogenic hyperkalemic paralysis with electrocardiographic changes. South Med J 67:342, 1974
9. Fisch C: Relation of electrolyte disturbances to cardiac arrhythmias. Circulation 47:408, 1973
10. Lindeman RD: Hypokalemia: Causes, consequences and correction. Am J Med Sci 272:5, 1976
11. Schwartz WB, Levine HD, Relman AS: The electrocardiogram in potassium depletion: Its relation to the total potassium deficit and the serum concentration. Am J Med 16:395, 1954
12. Surawicz B, Lepeschkin E: The electrocardiographic pattern of hypopotassemia with and without hypocalcemia. Circulation 8:801, 1953
13. Steiness E, Olesen KH: Cardiac arrhythmias induced by hypokalemia and potassium loss during maintenance digoxin therapy. Br Heart J 38:1678, 1976
14. Kunin AS, Surawicz B, Sims E: Decrease in serum concentrations and appearance of cardiac dysrhythmias during infusion of potassium with glucose in potassium depleted patients. N Engl J Med 266:228, 1962
15. Vitez TS, Soper LE, Wong KC, Soper PG:

Chronic hypokalemia and intraoperative dysrhythmias. Anesthesiology 63:130, 1985
16. Scheidegger D, Drop LJ: The relationship between duration of QT interval and plasma ionized calcium concentration. Anesthesiology 51:143, 1979
17. Nierenberg DW, Ransil BJ: QaTc interval as a clinical indicator of hypercalcemia. Am J Cardiol 44:243, 1979
18. Burch GE, Giles TD: The importance of magnesium deficiency in cardiovascular disease. Am Heart J 94:649, 1977
19. Seller RH, Cangiano J, Kim KE, et al: Digitalis toxicity and hypomagnesemia. Am Heart J 79:57, 1970
20. Kraft LF, Katholi RE, Woods WT, James TN: Attenuation by magnesium of the electrophysiologic effects of hyperkalemia on human and canine heart cells. Am J Cardiol 45:1189, 1980

12

Effects of Drugs on the ECG

Joel A. Kaplan, M.D.
Craig Weinstein, M.D.

A wide variety of pharmacologic agents can have profound effects on cardiac conduction and the myocardium, with resultant changes on the ECG. Usually these ECG effects are expected and predictable, as in the case of digitalis or quinidine; however, there can be other cardiac effects with drugs such as the tricyclic antidepressants that are not always so predictable. Cardiac and noncardiac medications may produce changes in rhythm, conduction, depolarization, or repolarization that may indicate the therapeutic effect and require no change in the pharmacologic regimen. In other cases, the ECG may show impending danger dictating cessation of the drug and/or supportive therapy.

CARDIAC DRUGS

Digitalis

Digitalis preparations have many effects on the ECG. The classic digitalis effect includes (1) PR-interval prolongation, (2) ST-segment flattening, (3) inversion of the T wave, and (4) shortening of the QT interval (Fig. 12–1).[1] The PR interval is lengthened to a first-degree heart block due to the vagal effect of the drug. The shape of the depressed ST segment mimics either a ramplike descent or a hooked-finger pulling down the segment of the ECG.

Digitalis toxicity can occur in up to 25 percent of patients taking the drug. The final diagnosis should be made on the basis of clinical criteria, not the ECG, since almost any type of ECG pattern can be seen with digitalis toxicity. The presence of atrial tachycardia with block in a digitalized patient is highly suggestive of digitalis toxicity, especially if associated with a digitalis plasma level over 2 ng/ml, but should be associated with the appropriate clinical symptoms. Many factors increase the toxicity of digitalis, including hypokalemia, hypercalcemia, hypomagnesemia, hypoxia, alkalosis, catecholamines, and quinidine.[2]

Digitalis toxicity is expressed on the ECG as a combination of suppressant effects on the sinoatrial (SA) and atrioventricular (AV) nodes and excitatory effects on atrial and ventricular tissue. Suppression of the SA node leads to sinus bradycardia or SA block, and effects on the AV node produce first-degree heart block and Mobitz type I second-degree heart block (Wenckebach type) (Fig. 12–2).[3] In patients with atrial fibrillation, digitalis toxicity is often seen as a regularization of an irregularly irregular rhythm due to increased AV block. Excitation leads to increased automaticity of ectopic pacemaker sites with resultant supraventricular (atrial or junctional) and ventricular tachyarrhythmias. Premature ventricular contractions are the most common dysrhythmias seen with

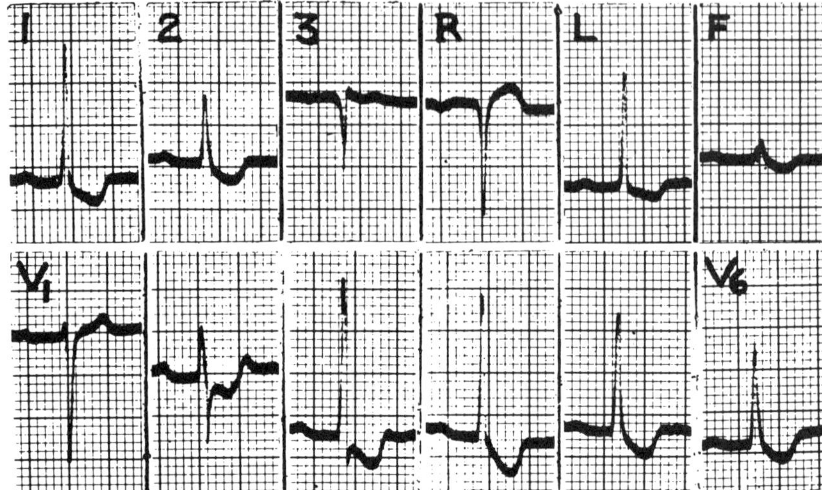

Fig. 12–1 Digitalis effect on the ECG. (Marriott HJ: Practical Electrocardiography. © 1983 The Williams & Wilkins Co., Baltimore.)

digitalis toxicity, and ventricular bigeminy is frequent in these patients.[4] Paroxysmal atrial tachycardia (PAT) with block is a worrisome rhythm often due to digitalis toxicity and combines the suppressant and excitant effects of the drug (Fig. 12–3).

Antiarrhythmic Agents

Antiarrhythmic drugs are grouped into four classes, on the basis of their cellular electrophysiologic effects and resultant ECG changes (Table 12–1).[5,6]

QUINIDINE

The ECG can be a sensitive indicator of the therapeutic and toxic effects of quinidine. At therapeutic plasma levels (2 to 5 μg/ml), there is a prolongation of the QRS and QT intervals due to an increased action potential duration and effective refractory period. These changes are quite dependent on the plasma level of quinidine and become more pronounced as its concentration is increased (Fig. 12–4).[7] Other effects of quinidine can be seen in the T wave, which will flatten and become bifid or double peaked as the levels increase, with appearance of a U

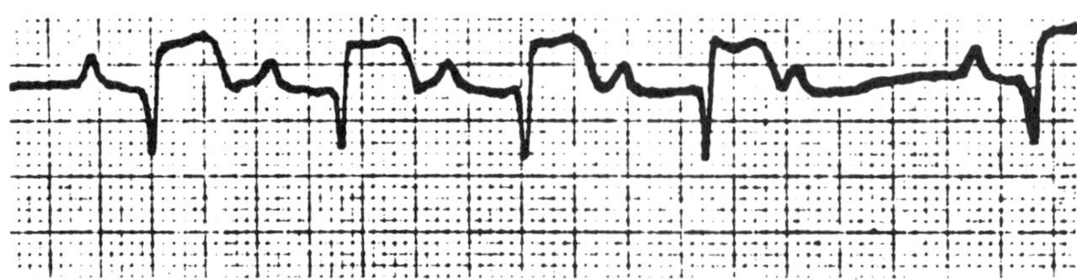

Fig. 12–2 Mobitz-type I heart block in a patient taking digitalis.

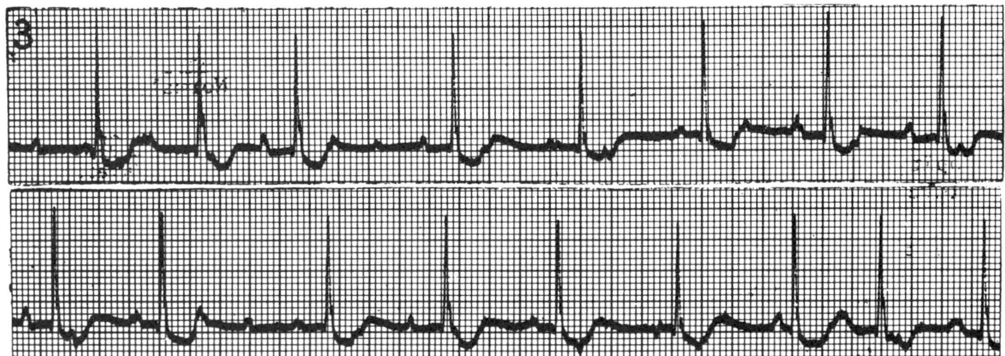

Fig. 12–3 Digitalis intoxication as demonstrated by a patient with multifocal atrial tachycardia with varying AV block. (Marriott HJ: Practical Electrocardiography. © 1983 The Williams & Wilkins Co., Baltimore.)

TABLE 12–1. Antiarrhythmic Drugs and the ECG

		Electrophysiology			Electrocardiogram		
Class	Drugs	CV	ERP	APD	PR	QRS	QT
IA	Quinidine	−	+	+	0+	+	++
	Procainamide	−	+	+	0+	+	++
	Disopyramide	−	+	−	0	0+	+
IB	Lidocaine	0+	−	−	0	0	0
II	Propranolol	−	0	+	0+	0	0−
III	Bretylium	−	0+	+	0+	0	0+
	Amiodarone	−	+	+	0+	0	+
IV	Verapamil	0−	+	+	+	0	0

CV, conduction velocity; ERP, effective refractory period; APD, action potential duration.
−, decrease; +, increase; 0, no change.

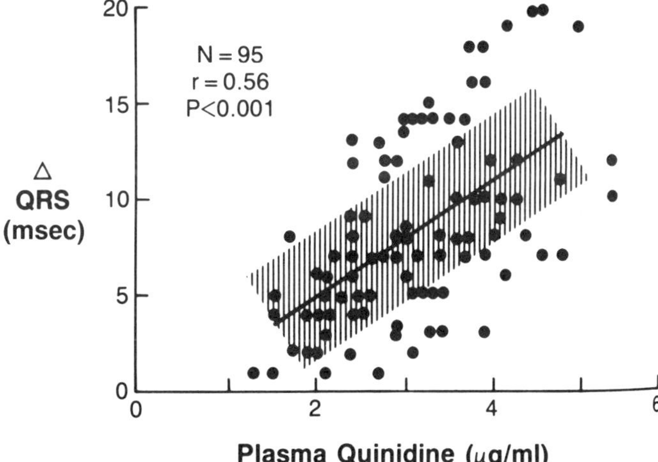

Fig. 12–4 Relationship between changes in QRS duration and plasma quinidine levels. (Hessenbuttel RH, Bigger JT: The effect of oral quinidine on intravenous conduction in man: Correlation of plasma quinidine with changes in QRS duration. Am Heart J 80:453, 1970.)

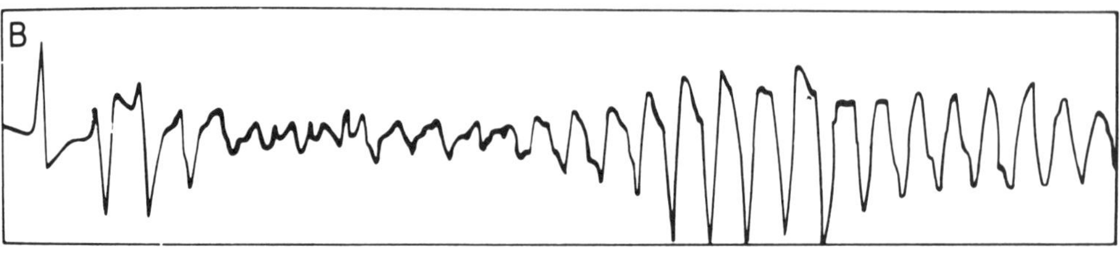

Fig. 12–5 Torsades de pointes ventricular tachycardia. (Atlee JL: Perioperative Cardiac Dysrhythmias. Copyright © 1985 Year Book Medical Publishers, Inc., Chicago. Reproduced with permission.)

wave. As the plasma concentration becomes toxic (greater than 5 μg/ml), there is further widening of the QRS complex (greater than 50 percent), ST-segment distortion, and SA and AV nodal conduction disturbances. Prolongation of the QT interval may precede torsades de pointes, a form of ventricular tachycardia with polymorphic ventricular complexes (Fig. 12–5).[8]

PROCAINAMIDE

The effects of procainamide on the ECG are similar to those of quinidine. At therapeutic levels (4 to 10 μg/ml), the QRS complex may be prolonged (5 to 10 percent) and the PR and QT intervals may also be prolonged.[9] As toxicity supervenes with levels over 12 μg/ml, the above changes are accentuated and occasionally may progress to torsades de pointes.[10] Ventricular dysrhythmias are not as frequent as with an overdose of quinidine.

DISOPYRAMIDE

The electrophysiologic effects of this oral medication are also similar to those of quinidine with a dose-related (therapeutic range 2 to 4 μg/ml) widening of the QRS complex (less than 20 percent) and prolongation of the QT interval. A prominent U wave may also appear. Torsades de pointes may result, usually with a markedly prolonged QT interval; patients who have had this response when given quinidine also have exhibited it when switched to disopyramide.[11] Disopyramide may precipitate or worsen heart block and should therefore be used cautiously in patients with partial AV block. This drug may increase the ventricular rate in nondigitalized patients with atrial fibrillation or flutter in a similar manner to quinidine or procainamide.

LIDOCAINE

In contrast to the three class IA drugs (quinidine, procainamide, and disopyramide), lidocaine causes minimal changes on the ECG. Rarely, the QT interval may shorten, but the QRS complex is not affected.[12] The effective refractory period may shorten in some patients, explaining the increased ventricular rate that can occur in the presence of atrial fibrillation or atrial flutter.[13] Toxicity of lidocaine is usually demonstrated by central nervous system symptoms, not ECG changes. In some patients, however, toxic doses of lidocaine can depress SA nodal function, automaticity, and AV conduction.[14]

β-ADRENERGIC BLOCKING DRUGS

Propranolol, the prototype and most commonly used β-blocker, possesses quinidine-like local anesthetic properties at large doses. The drug slows the sinus rate in humans, but the extent of slowing depends on the resting sympathetic tone. In some patients, the PR interval may be prolonged due to increased AV nodal conduction time and decreased conduction velocity. There are minimal effects on the QRS complex, while the QT interval is often shortened and the T-wave amplitude increased.[15] Other β-adrenergic blocking drugs have similar effects on the ECG. It is important to remember that timolol eyedrops are absorbed systemically and can produce these ECG effects, as well as hemodynamic effects. Toxic doses of β-adrenergic blockers can produce hypotension, congestive heart failure, bradycardia, and heart block.[16] In cases of digitalis toxicity with excitation (increased automaticity) and suppression (block), propranolol should not be used to treat ventricular irritability, since it may produce excessive AV nodal conduction disturbances.

BRETYLIUM AND AMIODARONE

Bretylium is an adrenergic neuronal blocking agent that was introduced during the 1950s as an antihypertensive drug. During the mid-1960s, its antiarrhythmic properties were first demonstrated to be due to adrenergic effects or to a direct myocardial action, or both. At high doses, bretylium initially releases norepinephrine from adrenergic nerve endings, while at lower concentrations it inhibits the release of norepinephrine. The direct myocardial effects include an increase in the action potential duration and the effective refractory period. These effects lead to an increase in the ventricular fibrillation threshold and explain its use in cases of ventricular tachycardia or ventricular fibrillation refractory to standard first-line drugs such as lidocaine.[17] The most common side effect of bretylium is hypotension often associated with sinus tachycardia. The ECG is not primarily affected by the drug, but increases in the PR and QT intervals may be observed.

Amiodarone is a class III drug with antiadrenergic and antiarrhythmic properties.[18] This potent, long-acting drug depresses sinus node automaticity and conduction time, increases refractoriness, and slows AV conduction, which can lead to profound bradycardia. Amiodarone is used to treat refractory supraventricular and ventricular dysrhythmias. Electrocardiographic changes include prolongation of the PR and QT intervals, as well as bradycardia, sinus arrest, and various forms of AV block.

CALCIUM CHANNEL BLOCKERS

The three commonly used calcium channel blockers, verapamil, nifedipine, and diltiazem, have varying effects on cardiac electrophysiology and the ECG. Verapamil, the most useful of this class of drugs as an antiarrhythmic agent, is primarily indicated for supraventricular tachyarrhythmias. It tends to reduce conduction velocity, increases the effective refractory period, and increases the action potential duration in the upper AV nodal region.[19] The primary effect of verapamil on the ECG is to prolong the PR interval by up to 10 percent at therapeutic plasma levels (100 to 300 ng/ml).[20] Heart rate may slow due to the direct effect of the drug or may increase due to reflex sympathetic stimulation. In the presence of sick sinus syndrome or AV block, verapamil can produce severe bradycardia or asystole and should be used cautiously or not at all in these situations.

Diltiazem has similar electrophysiologic effects to verapamil and can slow heart rate and AV conduction. It is currently not approved as an antiarrhythmic drug but may prove useful as such in the future. However, in animal studies, it has been found that a much higher incidence of AV block occurs with diltiazem than with verapamil. Nifedipine has virtually no effect on the AV node, but it usually increases heart rate through a baroreceptor reflex mechanism. It is not useful for treatment of dysrhythmias and is used primarily for therapy of ischemic heart disease. All the calcium channel blockers may intensify the electrophysiologic effects of the β-blockers and/or digitalis.[21]

NONCARDIAC DRUGS

Tricyclic Antidepressants

The tricyclic antidepressants (TCAs) (e.g., imipramine) have electrophysiologic effects similar to quinidine in that they prolong atrioventricular conduction, intraventricular conduction, and repolarization. However, these are usually mild effects and are not important clinically. In addition, they do not correlate well with plasma levels but may exacerbate preexisting conduction disturbances. The ECG can be a sensitive indicator of TCA toxicity, but it is not always reliable, since it can appear normal even in the face of TCA overdose. Therapy with the TCAs is associated with an increased T-wave height and lengthened PR, QRS, and QT intervals. These drugs also have a variety of other cardiovascular effects, including anticholinergic activity, direct myocardial depression, and sympathomimetic activity.[22]

The most common cardiovascular signs of TCA overdosage are hypotension and sinus tachycardia. Electrocardiographic manifestations of TCA toxicity include sinus tachycardia in 71 percent of patients, supraventricular tachycardia in 6 percent, premature ventricular contractions in 34 percent, and prolongation of the PR interval in 11 percent. Widening of the QRS complex was found in 29 percent of cases and prolongation of the QT interval in 86 percent. Ventricular fibrillation, complete AV block, slow idioventricular rhythm, and asystole occur infrequently.[22–24] In the event of TCA toxicity, anesthesia and surgery should be avoided if possible for at least 48 hours, which is the time required to reduce the TCA effects.

Phenothiazines

These drugs also have quinidine-like effects, including reduced membrane responsiveness, decreased amplitude of the action potential, and lengthening of the repolarization time. The QT interval is often prolonged, the ST segment becomes convex, the T wave is flattened and notched, and U waves may appear on the ECG in up to 50 percent of patients receiving these drugs.[25] The QRS interval is not prolonged, however, as it is with quinidine. The phenothiazine that most commonly causes these ECG effects is thioridazine.[26] The ECG changes are less marked with chlorpromazine and least often occur with trifluoperazine.

With toxicity, there may be supraventricular tachyarrhythmias, heart block, or ventricular tachyarrhythmias. Electrolyte imbalance, particularly hypokalemia, may bring out these changes or worsen them if they are already present. Phenothiazines, used in conjunction with TCAs, can produce QRS widening and bizarre QRS complexes.

Lithium

This drug is considered valuable in patients with manic-depressive psychoses. Therapeutic doses rarely cause cardiovascular complications and dysrhythmias are uncommon. T-wave changes similar to hypokalemia occur in almost all patients due to displacement of intracellular potassium by lithium. This is a benign finding on the ECG. The drug has an effect on the SA node, but no effect on the PR interval or QRS complex.[27] Toxic doses produce sinus bradycardia or sinus arrest (Fig. 12–6), second-degree heart block, or premature ventricular contractions.

Xanthines

Compounds such as theophylline, aminophylline, and caffeine produce sinus tachycardia in many patients. If large or toxic doses are administered, supraventricular and ventricular dysrhythmias may result. These drugs should always be considered as possible causative agents of these dysrhythmias, and withdrawal of the drugs will frequently result in cessation of the rhythm disturbances.[28]

In summary, many cardiac and noncardiac drugs can produce dysrhythmias and conduction

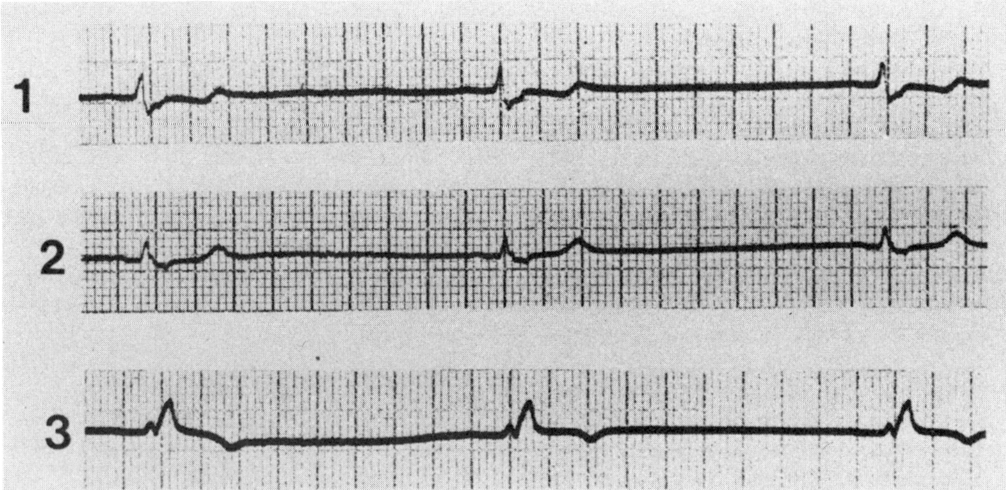

Fig. 12–6 Nodal bradycardia in a patient with a serum lithium level of 1.6 mmol/L. (Commerford PJ: Arrhythmias in patients with drug toxicity, electrolyte and endocrine disturbances. Med Clin North Am 68(5):1066, 1984. Reprinted with permission from WB Saunders Co.)

abnormalities. Electrocardiograph changes are often due to the drug itself but may be augmented by changes secondary to respiratory and CNS effects. Therapy should include drug withdrawal and cardiovascular support as indicated for each individual situation.

REFERENCES

1. Marriott HJL: Practical Electrocardiography. 7th Ed. Williams & Wilkins, Baltimore, 1983
2. Smith TW: Digitalis toxicity: Epidemiology and clinical use of serum concentration measurement. Am J Med 58:470, 1975
3. Surawicz B, Lasseter KC: Effect of drugs on the ECG. Prog Cardiovasc Dis 13:26, 1970
4. Chung DC: Anesthetic problems associated with the treatment of cardiovascular disease. I. Digitalis toxicity. Can Anaesth Soc J 28:6, 1981
5. Atlee JL: Perioperative Cardiac Dysrhythmias. Year Book Medical Publishers, Chicago, 1985
6. Nestico PF, Depace NL, Morganroth J: Therapy with conventional antiarrhythmic drugs for ventricular arrhythmias. Med Clin North Am 68:1295, 1984
7. Hessenbuttel RH, Bigger JT: The effect of oral quinidine on intraventricular conduction in man: Correlation of plasma quinidine with changes in QRS duration. Am Heart J 80:453, 1970
8. Smith WM, Gallagher JJ: "Les Torsades de Pointes." An unusual ventricular arrhythmia. Ann Intern Med 93:578, 1980
9. Greenspan AM, Horowitz LN, Spielman SR, et al: Large dose procainamide therapy for ventricular tachycardia. Am J Cardiol 46:453, 1980
10. Strasberg B, Sclarovsky S, Erdberg A, et al: Procainamide-induced polymorphous ventricular tachycardia. Am J Cardiol 47:1309, 1981
11. Wald RW, Waxman MB, Colman JM: Torsade de pointe ventricular tachycardia: A complication of disopyramide shared with quinidine. J Electrocardiol 3:301, 1981
12. Josephson ME, Caracta AR, Lau SH, et al: Effects of lidocaine on refractory periods in man. Am Heart J 84:778, 1972
13. Adamson AR, Spracklen FH: Atrial flutter with block: Contraindication to the use of lignocaine. Br Med J 2:223, 1968
14. Gupta PK, Lichstein E, Chadda KD: Lidocaine-induced heart block in patients with bundle branch block. Am J Cardiol 33:487, 1974
15. Wit AL, Hoffman BF, Rosen MR: Electrophysiology and pharmacology of cardiac arrhythmias. IX. Cardiac electrophysiologic effects of beta-adrenergic receptor stimulation and blockade. Am Heart J 90:665, 1975

16. Slogoff S: Beta-adrenergic blockers. p. 181. In Kaplan JA (ed): Cardiac Anesthesia. Vol II. Cardiovascular Pharmacology. Grune & Stratton, Orlando, Florida, 1983
17. Cardinal R, Sasyniuk BI: Electrophysiological effects of bretylium tosylate on the heart. J Pharmacol Exp Ther 183:264, 1972
18. Bennett DR (ed): Antiarrhythmic drugs. p. 623. In AMA Drug Evaluations. 5th Ed. American Medical Association, Chicago, 1983
19. Mangiardi LM, Hariman RJ, McAllister RG, et al: Electrophysiologic and hemodynamic effects of verapamil. Circulation 57:366, 1978
20. Sung RJ, Elser B, McAllister RG: IV verapamil for termination of reentrant supraventricular tachycardias. Ann Intern Med 93:682, 1980
21. Fleckenstein A: Calcium Antagonism in Heart and Smooth Muscle. John Wiley & Sons, New York, 1983
22. Marshall JB, Forker AD: Cardiovascular effects of tricyclic antidepressant drugs: Therapeutic usage, overdose, and management. Am Heart J 103:401, 1982
23. Goldberg RJ, Capone RJ, Hunt JD: Cardiac complications following tricyclic antidepressant overdose. JAMA 254:1772, 1985
24. Vohra J, Burrows G, Hunt D, et al: The effect of toxic and therapeutic doses of tricyclic antidepressant drugs on intracardiac conduction. Eur J Cardiol 3:219, 1975
25. Ban TA, St. Jean A: The effect of phenothiazines on the ECG. Can Med Assoc J 91:537, 1964
26. Kelly HG, Fay JE, Laverty SG: Thioridazine hydrochloride (Mellaril): its effect on the ECG. Can Med Assoc J 89:546, 1963
27. Wellens HJ, Cats VM, Duren DR: Symptomatic sinus node dysfunction following lithium carbonate therapy. Am J Med 59:285, 1975
28. Stirt JA, Berger JM, Ricker SM, et al: Arrhythmogenic effects of aminophylline during halothane anesthesia in experimental animals. Anesth Analg 59:410, 1980

13

The Pediatric ECG

Ivan Dimich, M.D.

In spite of the increasing use of more sophisticated methods in pediatric cardiology, the ECG remains an essential tool in the cardiac evaluation of a child. Indications for obtaining a preoperative ECG in the pediatric age group include (1) presence of congenital or rheumatic heart disease, (2) unexplained significant heart murmurs, (3) cardiomegaly found on routine chest x-ray, (4) cyanosis, (5) irregular heart rate, (6) systemic hypertension, (7) infant with respiratory distress of unknown cause or failure to thrive, (8) child with chromosomal abnormalities (i.e., Down's syndrome), (9) presence of neuromuscular or metabolic-related disease, (10) electrolyte disturbances, or (11) an older child with a history of significant easy fatigue or shortness of breath on exercise.[1]

TECHNIQUES TO OBTAIN THE PEDIATRIC ECG

Special techniques are required to obtain a suitable ECG from the infant and young child.

1. A small electrode (½-inch in diameter) should be used, especially for the precordial leads.
2. The voltage standardization mark should be on each lead tracing of the ECG, especially in young children who tend to have such high voltage that one-half the standard voltage may be required in some leads.
3. Electrode paste should be wiped off before moving to the next location. Failure to do so will result in a large diphasic deflection, almost identical throughout the precordial leads, which might be interpreted as combined ventricular hypertrophy.
4. A wide ECG exploration of the heart is advised in children and especially in infants. In addition to conventional precordial leads V_1–V_6, leads V_4R and V_3R over the right chest should be taken routinely for adequately assessing right ventricular predominance. Leads V_3 and V_5 can be omitted in very small infants.

INTERPRETATION OF THE PEDIATRIC ECG

Interpretation of the pediatric ECG is not easy for those who do not analyze them frequently. Pediatric ECGs are more complex because of the significant changes that occur in early childhood. It should be emphasized that available criteria for the normal pediatric ECG have been obtained by statistical data with standard deviations, so there is necessarily an overlap between normal and abnormal findings. Therefore, a systematic approach to interpretation of the pediatric ECG is essential. The ECG should not

Table 13–1. Heart Rate and Age in Pediatric Group

Age	Heart Rate (Beats/min)
Newborn	110–150
2 years	85–125
4 years	75–115
6 years	65–100
>6 years	60–100

(Park MK, Guntheroth W: How to Read Pediatric ECG's. © 1981. Year Book Medical Publishers, Chicago. Reproduced with permission.)

be interpreted unless the age of the patient, clinical diagnosis, and current therapy are known. Previous ECGs should always be available for comparison.[2-4]

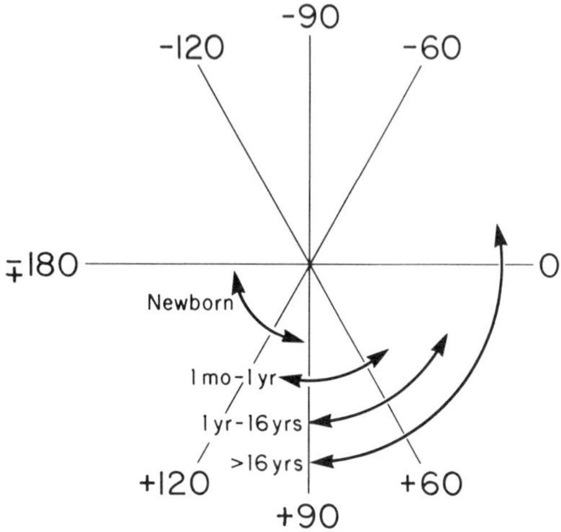

Fig. 13–1 Electrical axis of the ECG in pediatric patients.

Heart Rate and Rhythm

The heart rate of pediatric patients varies with age. Children with fever, anemia, or hypovolemia can have a significant sinus tachycardia. Normal heart rates according to age are as shown in Table 13–1.[2]

Because of numerous extraneous factors influencing the heart rate in children, the sleeping pulse rate should be used to assess the normal or resting rate. In children, sinus tachycardia exists when the rate is more than 150 beats/min; and in infants when the rate is more than 180 beats/min. In infants, a sinus rate of 100 beats or less, and, in children, a rate less than 80 beats/min, is considered a sinus bradycardia.

Sinus dysrhythmia is a common finding in the pediatric age group. This variation is nearly always recognized clinically without an ECG; however, it may occasionally be confused with other dysrhythmias, including ectopic atrial dysrhythmias or atrial fibrillation. Fast rates tend to abolish a sinus arrhythmia, and slow rates predispose to it.

Electrical Axis

The QRS axis represents the mean vector of the ventricular depolarization process. The newborn infant normally has a right axis compared with adult standards (Fig. 13–1). The newborn QRS axis is usually about +125 degrees, but up to +180 degrees is considered normal. An axis of less than +60 degrees in the newborn period would be considered abnormal. With increasing age, the vector moves to the left and by the time an infant is 3 months of age, a mean QRS axis of +90 degrees is reached. As the child grows the vector continues to move farther to the left, and at 3 years of age approaches the adult mean value of +60 degrees.[5]

A right axis deviation is normally found in young infants. It is also observed in conditions associated with right ventricular (RV) hypertrophy, hence in most cyanotic congenital heart lesions. A left axis deviation occurs in a small percentage of normal children and is also associated with left ventricular (LV) hypertrophy or certain types of congenital heart disease, that is, atrioventricular (AV) canal and tricuspid atresia.[6]

P Wave

In children, the P wave does not normally exceed 0.10 seconds; however, in the newborn and infant it is even shorter. The P-wave amplitude should not exceed 2.5 mm.[2]

A negative P wave in lead I indicates either an ectopic atrial beat or dextrocardia, provided there are no technical errors or reversal of the right- and left-arm electrodes. Peaked or tall, but not prolonged P waves in leads II and III, coupled with pointed P waves in chest leads V_1 and V_2, usually indicate right atrial hypertrophy (P pulmonale). Left atrial enlargement is present if the P wave is broad and notched in leads I and II and V_5 and V_6. Left atrial enlargement can also be recognized by a prominent negative component of a biphasic P wave in leads V_1 or V_3R.[2,4] Bilateral atrial enlargement is presumably present when P waves are both broad and tall.

PR Interval

The PR interval is dependent on both heart rate and age, decreasing with increased rate and increasing with advanced age. The upper limits of the PR interval in infants is 0.14 seconds, in children under 14 years 0.16 seconds, and in adolescents 0.18 seconds.[2]

Prolongation of the PR interval may be seen in acute myocarditis (i.e., rheumatic or viral), congenital heart disease (i.e., atrial septal defect, Ebstein's anomaly), and digitalis administration. When the PR interval is shorter than normal, either an ectopic atrial beat or Wolff–Parkinson–White syndrome is present.

QRS Complex

The QRS complex reflects depolarization of the ventricular myocardium. The maximum duration of the normal QRS interval during the first year of life is 0.065 seconds, while at 4 years it is 0.08 seconds and thereafter, it is 0.09–0.10 seconds.[7] A QRS complex of more than 0.12 seconds in duration with slurred and notched complexes and discordant T waves indicates a bundle branch block. In infants and young children, a bundle branch block may be present with a QRS complex of only 0.08 seconds, depending on age.[4,8] Right bundle branch block (RBBB) is commonly seen in children following open heart surgery (i.e., tetralogy of Fallot) or in certain congenital heart diseases (i.e., Ebstein's anomaly). By contrast, left bundle branch block (LBBB) is extremely uncommon in children.[9]

Q Waves

The Q wave has no great significance in the pediatric age group. It is commonly found in leads II, III, aVF, and V_5 and V_6. However, a Q wave followed by an R wave is never found normally in V_3R or V_1. Deep and wide Q waves in leads I, aVL, V_5, and V_6 in an infant usually indicate an anomalous origin of the left coronary artery. This anomaly produces left lateral myocardial ischemia at a very early age.[4]

ST Segment

The normal ST segment is horizontal and isoelectric. In children the ST segment may be displaced 1 to 2 mm in the standard leads and up to 3 mm in the right precordial leads. Greater displacement of the ST segment indicates myocardial or pericardial disease, early myocardial ischemia, or digitalis effect.

QT Interval

The QT interval varies with heart rate, but not with age, except in infancy. Many formulas have been described to calculate the QT interval. Prepared tables of expected normal values for age or rate can be used, or the corrected QT interval can be calculated by using Bazett's formula:

$$QTc = \frac{\text{QT interval}}{\sqrt{\text{RR interval}}}$$

The average QTc in the pediatric age group is 0.38 seconds ±0.04 seconds.[2,10]

Prolongation of the QT interval occurs with electrolyte alterations (i.e., hypocalcemia, hypokalemia), myocarditis, and drug effects (i.e., procainamide, quinidine). It has also been described in a rare type of congenital perceptive deafness associated with syncopal attacks called the Jervell and Lange-Nielsen syndrome. It is important to mention that sudden death may occur in this syndrome even at an early age, possibly due to an extrasystole developing on the T wave of a preceding beat that may trigger ventricular fibrillation.[5] Shortening of the QT interval is also found with electrolyte alterations (i.e., hypercalcemia, hyperkalemia) and following digitalization.

The T Wave

The normal T wave, the terminal portion of ventricular activity, is always positive in lead I, except in dextrocardia. Low-voltage or negative T waves can be seen in myocarditis, myocardial ischemia, and electrolyte disturbances (i.e., hypocalcemia, hypokalemia). Inverted T waves in V_1–V_3 are a normal finding in infants and young children. Tall, tent-shaped peaked T waves are characteristic of potassium intoxication.[11]

The U Wave

The U wave is a small upright deflection following the T wave. Its practical importance is unknown, but these waves are frequently observed in normal children. Unusually prominent U waves are seen in hypokalemia or as a drug effect (i.e., digitalis, epinephrine).[5]

NORMAL ECG IN NEWBORNS, INFANTS, AND CHILDREN

Since recognition of an abnormal ECG must be based on a departure from criteria that set normal limits, a brief summary of normal ECG findings in the pediatric age group is reviewed.

There is no time in life when such significant hemodynamic changes occur as in the newborn period. Full understanding of these circulatory developments is necessary for proper interpretation of ECGs in infancy. The circulatory changes after birth are primarily reflected in the anatomic relationship between the right and left cardiac chambers. In utero, resistance to flow into the systemic circulation is lower than into the pulmonary vascular bed. Because of the very high pulmonary vascular resistance, the right ventricle hypertrophies, and at full term the myocardial weight ratio of right-to-left ventricle is about 1.3:1. Therefore, RV preponderance is a normal finding in ECGs of the newborn. Following birth, the systemic vascular resistance increases in contrast to the pulmonary vascular resistance which falls. Furthermore, the sudden large increase of pulmonary venous blood flow into the left atrium greatly increases the work of the left ventricle. By the end of 1 month of age, the pressure in the pulmonary artery falls to the normal adult levels. At the same time, the LV myocardial weight becomes greater than the right, and by the time of adolescence the ratio of left-to-right ventricle is about 2.5:1.[12,13]

Hemodynamic events in the neonatal period are reflected in T-wave changes on the ECG. T waves are upright in V_3R and V_1 in newborns for 24 hours before gradually turning negative by 3 to 4 days of age.[6] In general, an upright T wave in V_3 R and V_1 in a newborn over 4 days of age is considered abnormal, although the entire ECG must be considered. In older infants and children, an inverted T wave is a common finding in leads V_3R or V_1. In V_5 and V_6, the T waves are inverted for the first 24 hours but then become upright.[12]

In contrast to the T-wave alterations that represent acute hemodynamic events in the early newborn period, QRS changes reflect slower reversal in the ventricular thickness secondary to circulatory changes. Precordial chest leads in the newborn reflect RV preponderance by prominent R waves in V_3R and V_1, with small S waves, and a large R/S ratio. This is complete reversal of the adult R/S progression. The R wave in the right precordial leads may be up to 15 to 20 mm high. Similarly, the S wave in the left precordial leads (V_5 and V_6) may be quite deep. Usually by 4 or 5 years of age, the R and S waves are approximately equal in

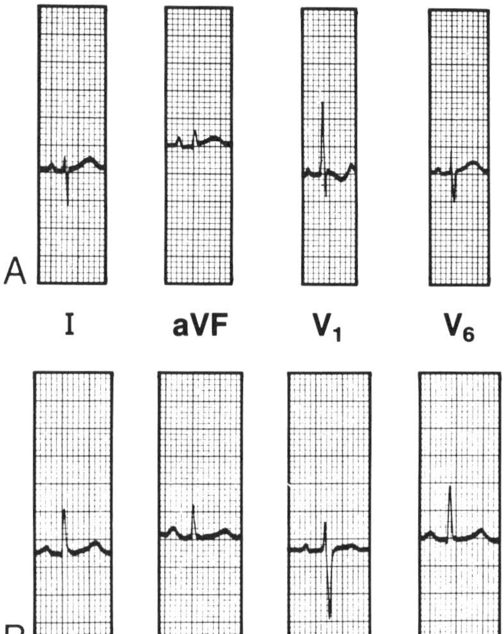

Fig. 13–2 (A) The normal neonatal ECG; **(B)** the normal adolescent ECG. (Garson A Jr: The Electrocardiogram in Infants and Children. Lea & Febiger, Philadelphia, 1983.)

the right precordial leads.[4,12,13] After 5 years of age, the R wave gradually decreases in the right precordial leads until the adult pattern is reached by age 6 to 8. In summary, changes in ECG patterns in the pediatric age group represent normal progression from RV dominance in the newborn to LV predominance seen in late childhood. Typical ECG tracings of a neonate and an adolescent are shown in Figure 13–2.

VENTRICULAR HYPERTROPHY

One of the most important uses of the ECG in pediatrics is in the diagnosis of ventricular hypertrophy. The most common cause is congenital heart disease. In general, two types of hypertrophy are seen in congenital heart disease: (1) concentric ventricular hypertrophy–systolic overload, seen in lesions with increased resistance to flow (e.g., pulmonary or aortic valvular stenosis); and (2) eccentric ventricular hypertrophy–diastolic overload, present in anomalies associated with a large left-to-right shunt or valvular incompetence (e.g., atrial or ventricular septal defect, mitral or aortic insufficiency).[14]

Right Ventricular Hypertrophy

Pressure work overload of the right ventricle occurs whenever there is increased resistance to the emptying of this chamber. The increased pressure work of the right ventricle results in muscular hypertrophy of the chamber (e.g., pulmonary valvular or infundibular stenosis or pulmonary hypertension). This is reflected in the right precordial leads by increasingly tall R waves and the ST segment later becoming depressed (Fig. 13–3). In contrast, eccentric ventricular hypertrophy (diastolic overload) is characterized by an RSR[1] pattern in the right precordial leads (Fig. 13–4). It should be emphasized that in evaluation of RV hypertrophy in

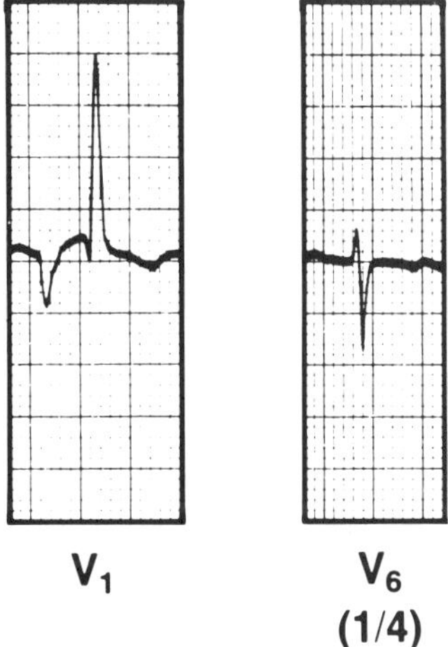

Fig. 13–3 Part of an ECG in a patient with right ventricular hypertrophy due to pulmonary atresia. The tall R wave in lead V_1 is shown. The duration of the R wave in V_1 is 0.07 seconds. (Garson A Jr: The Electrocardiogram in Infants and Children. Lea & Febiger, Philadelphia, 1983.)

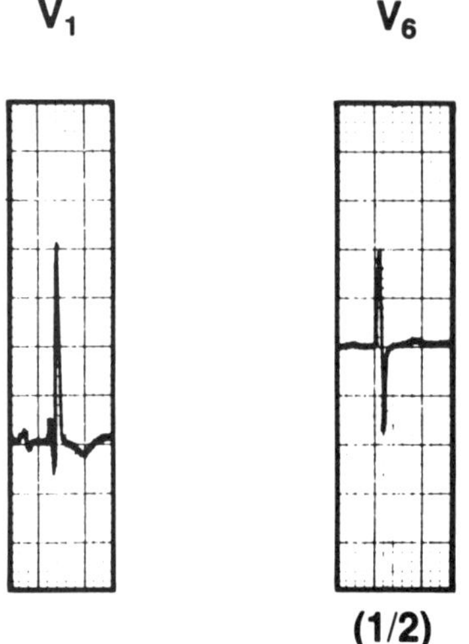

Fig. 13–4 Leads V_1 and V_6 of an ECG in a child with right ventricular hypertrophy due to diastolic overload. An RSR^1 pattern is present in lead V_1. (Garson A Jr: The Electrocardiogram in Infants and Children. Lea & Febiger, Philadelphia, 1983.)

infants and young children, the age of the patient must be taken into consideration.

There is general agreement that right ventricular hypertrophy (RVH) exists if one of the following criteria is present:

1. Tall R waves in the right precordial leads (An R wave in V_1 of more than 20 mm is abnormal in infants over three months of age.)
2. Q wave in the right precordial leads followed by dominant R wave
3. RSR^1 complex in V_1 in older children (if the R^1 is more than 10 mm in height)
4. S wave greater than 6 mm in V_6

Supporting evidence of RVH includes the following:

1. Upright T wave in V_3R or V_1, after 4 days of age
2. Electrical axis greater than 135 degrees (except in the neonate)
3. Depressed ST segment in the right precordial leads preceded by a tall R wave and followed by a deeply inverted symmetrical T wave strain pattern[4,8,15]

Left Ventricular Hypertrophy

In contrast to RVH diagnostic criteria for left ventricular hypertrophy (LVH) do not clearly differentiate systolic from diastolic overload. Criteria for LVH include the following (see Fig. 13–5)[6]:

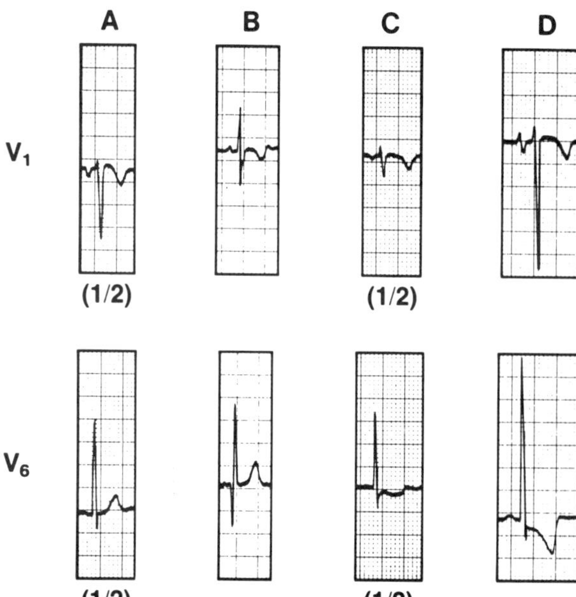

Fig. 13–5 Left ventricular hypertrophy. **(A)** Voltage criteria with deep S wave in V_1 and tall R wave in V_6. **(B)** Deep Q wave in lead V_6. **(C)** Absent Q wave in lead V_6. **(D)** T-wave inversion in lead V_6 with ST depression. (Garson A Jr: The Electrocardiogram in Infants and Children. Lea & Febiger, Philadelphia, 1983).

1. Left axis deviation to the left of +60° degrees during the first week of life, to the left of +20° degrees in the first 3 months of life, and negative subsequently.
2. R in aVL or an aVF greater than 25 mm
3. Precordial leads
   a. R in V_6 greater than 30 mm
   b. S in V_1 greater than 20 mm
   c. R in V_6 plus S in V_1 greater than 45 mm
   d. Depressed ST segment and negative T wave in V_5 or V_6
   e. Q greater than 4 mm in V_6 with a tall symmetric T wave
4. An intrinsicoid deflection greater than 0.04 seconds in children in leads aVL, aVF, V_5, and V_6[8,15,16]

Biventricular Hypertrophy

Biventricular hypertrophy can be diagnosed if one of the following criteria is present (see Fig. 13–6)[4]:

1. Independent criteria for the diagnosis of RVH and LVH
2. Signs of LVH by previous criteria plus
   a. Sizable R wave in V_1 ($\geq$10 mm)
   b. S greater than R in V_6
3. Signs of RVH plus
   a. Q wave of 3 mm in V_5 and V_6
   b. Sizable R wave with a tall positive T wave in V_5 and V_6
4. Approximately equiphasic RS deflection across the precordial leads

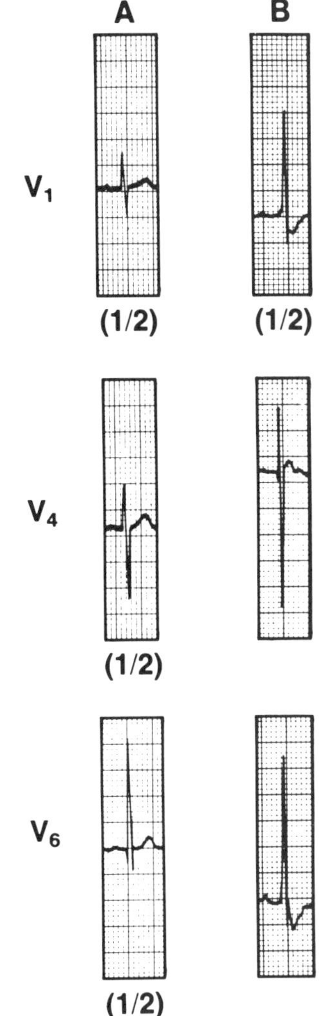

Fig. 13–6 Biventricular hypertrophy. **(A)** R wave in V_6 is 42 mm (left ventricular hypertrophy, LVH) and R wave in V_1 is 15 mm (right ventricular hypertrophy, RVH). **(B)** Another example of tall R waves in a neonate, making the diagnosis. (Garson A Jr: The Electrocardiogram in Infants and Children. Lea & Febiger, Philadelphia, 1983.)

THE ELECTROCARDIOGRAM IN CONGENITAL HEART DISEASE

When the ECG is used in conjunction with a good clinical history, careful physical examination, and good-quality chest x-ray, sufficient information is usually present to make the diagnosis of a congenital heart disease. Further sophisticated diagnostic studies (i.e., echocardiography and cardiac catheterization) may be required to define the precise nature of the defect. A wide variety of congenital malformations may occur either as a single anomaly or in combination with other anomalies. In the rest of this chapter, brief anatomic and hemodynamic characteristics of the most common anomalies are presented and related to their ECG findings (Fig. 13–7A–C).

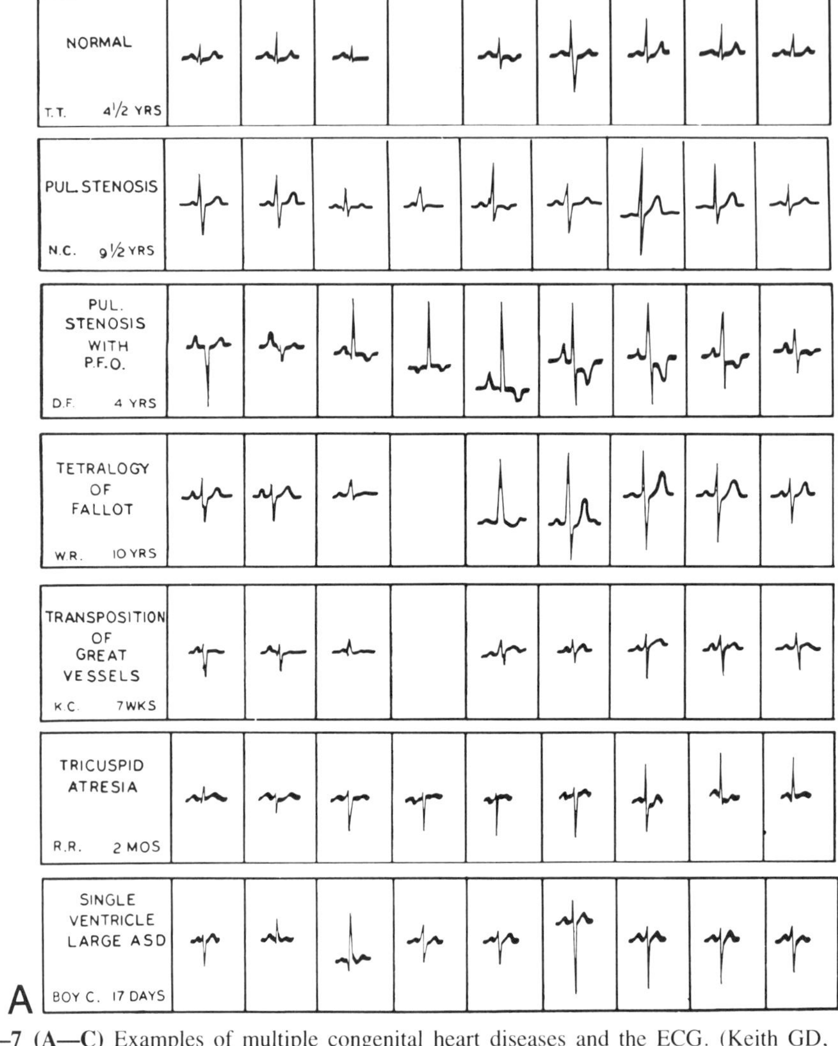

Fig. 13–7 (A—C) Examples of multiple congenital heart diseases and the ECG. (Keith GD, Rowe RD, Vlad P: Heart Disease in Infancy and Childhood. 3rd Ed. Copyright © 1978 by Macmillan Publishing Company, a Division of Macmillan, Inc.)

Acyanotic Congenital Heart Disease

VENTRICULAR SEPTAL DEFECT

A normal ECG is the rule with a small ventricular septal defect. In moderate-sized ventricular septal defects (L-R shunt less than 2:1), a greater hemodynamic load is placed on the left ventricle, resulting in LVH. In large ventricular septal defects (L-R shunt more than 2:1), a definite LVH pattern is seen with variable degrees of RVH (biventricular hypertrophy). In addition, in patients with advanced pulmonary hypertension and increased pulmonary vascular resistance (Eisenmenger's syndrome), RV pres-

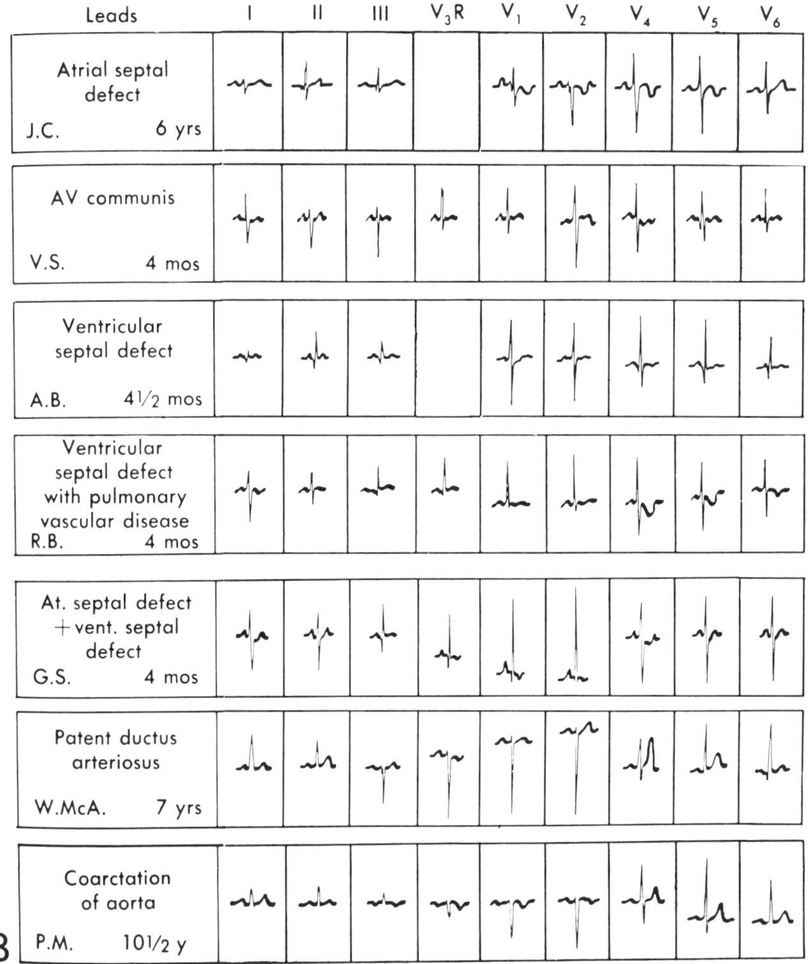

Fig. 13–7(B) (*Continued*).

sure exceeds LV pressure, the shunt becomes reversed, and, characteristically, the RVH becomes more prominent.[17,18]

ATRIAL SEPTAL DEFECT—SECUNDUM TYPE

The ostium secundum type of atrial septal defects are large openings associated with normal AV valves. A large L-R shunt at the atrial level results in enlargement of the right atrium and ventricle and dilatation of the pulmonary arteries. The ECG shows an RSR[1] pattern in aVR and the right chest leads in practically all cases of atrial septal defect. A prolonged PR interval is noted in about 10 percent of patients. Severe RVH is uncommon in children with this anomaly.

ENDOCARDIAL CUSHION DEFECTS (Ostium Primum Atrial Septal Defect)

This anomaly is characterized by an ostium primum atrial septal defect plus a high ventricular septal defect and malformed mitral or tricus-

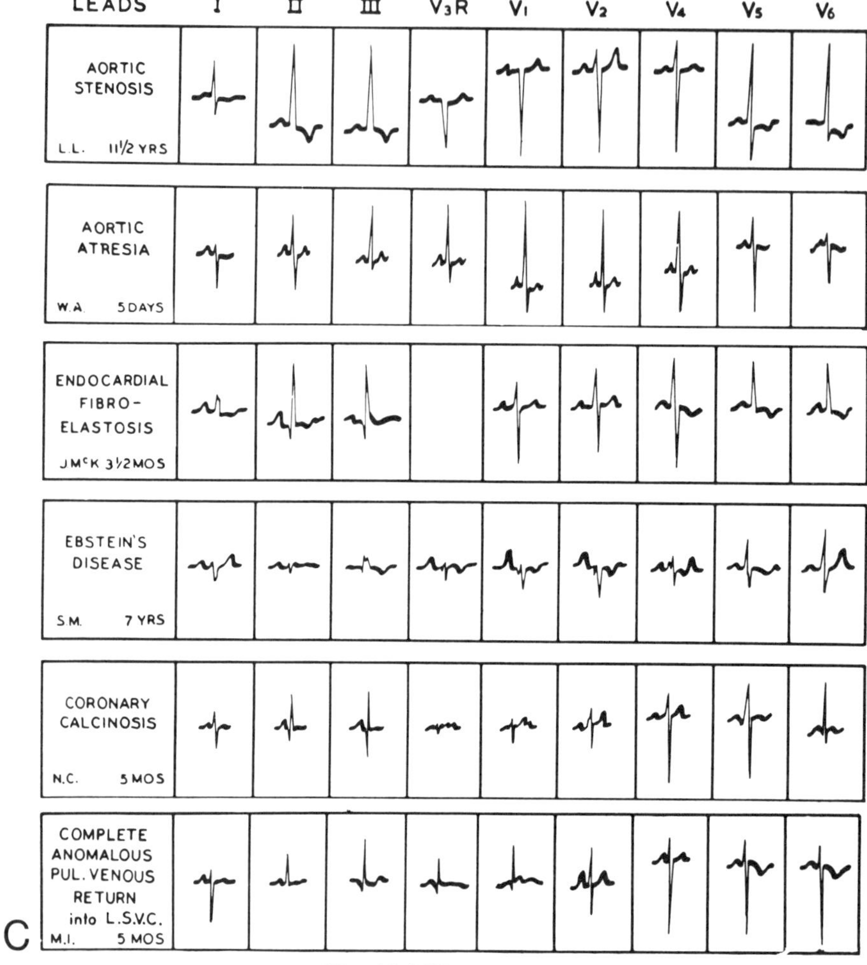

Fig. 13–7(C) (*Continued*).

pid valvular rings. The anomaly is commonly encountered in Down's syndrome. Patients with an endocardial cushion defect have the combined features of a left-to-right shunt at the ventricular and atrial levels with those of atrioventricular valve regurgitation, and, commonly, pulmonary hypertension. The ECGs have fairly consistent patterns and are frequently diagnostic. The abnormalities consist of (1) prolongation of the PR interval, (2) left superior axis due to aberration of the left bundle branch systems, (3) biventricular hypertrophy, and occasionally (4) left atrial enlargement.[19]

PATENT DUCTUS ARTERIOSUS

A patent ductus arteriosus (PDA) forms an arteriovenous shunt between the aorta and the pulmonary artery leading to increased pulmonary blood flow, increased pulmonary artery pressure, and greater pulmonary venous return to the left side of the heart. For this reason, an uncomplicated PDA causes diastolic overloading of the left ventricle with LVH and left atrial enlargement. If, however, severe pulmonary hypertension occurs, systolic overloading of the right ventricle takes place and RVH becomes more prominent on the ECG.[20]

COARCTATION OF AORTA

Anatomically and hemodynamically there are two types of coarctation of the aorta, the infantile type and the adult type.

Infantile Type

There is a markedly elongated narrowing of the aortic segment between the origin of the left subclavian artery and the opening of the PDA. This anomaly is frequently associated with other complex cardiac malformations, such as mitral or aortic valvular disease, and a large ventricular septal defect. Congestive heart failure and pulmonary hypertension occur very early. Ventricular hypertrophy is usually present on the ECG.

Adult Type

This is the more common type of coarctation, occurring as a localized stricture just below the origin of the left subclavian artery and about twice as often in males than females. Because of the mechanical obstruction of the aorta, the blood pressure is elevated in the vessels arising proximal to the coarctation (upper extremities.) The ECG is commonly normal in these children but may reveal evidence of LVH or, rarely, LBBB.[15]

Pulmonary Stenosis

The obstruction may be valvular, supravalvular, or infundibular. The ventricular septum is intact. There is a relatively high degree of correlation between the RVH seen on the ECG (amplitude of the R wave in the right precordial leads) and the degree of obstruction. In patients with mild pulmonary stenosis (RV pressure less than 90 mmHg), the ECG may be normal or show only slight RVH (R pattern in V_3R, V_1). In moderate pulmonary stenosis (RV pressure between 90 and 130 mmHg), the R wave is tall and the T waves are frequently positive in the right precordial leads. In severe pulmonary stenosis (RV pressure over 130 mmHg), the right precordial leads show a strain pattern with a QR pattern, inverted T waves in V_1, and prominent, tall P waves.[8]

AORTIC STENOSIS

The obstruction may also be valvular, supravalvular, or subaortic. In contrast to pulmonary stenosis, the ECG in aortic stenosis is only a crude indicator of the severity of the lesion. In mild aortic stenosis the ECG is frequently normal. In moderate and severe aortic stenosis, LVH becomes more obvious on the ECG.[4]

Cyanotic Congenital Heart Disease

TRANSPOSITION OF THE GREAT ARTERIES

In this condition, the aorta arises from the right ventricle and the pulmonary artery from the left ventricle. The systemic venous return is to the right atrium, and the pulmonary venous return is to the left atrium. Thus, blood from the right side of the heart passes to the aorta, and the pulmonary venous blood is returned to the lungs. The two independent circulations cannot support life unless there is a significant shunt at the atrial or ventricular level or a PDA exists to permit some mixture of blood. This condition accounts for the majority of deaths in infants with cyanotic congenital heart disease. Early atrial septostomy is often life saving. The ECG in most cases shows RVH, commonly associated with tall P waves.[20]

TETRALOGY OF FALLOT

This is one of the most common cyanotic heart diseases seen in childhood. The anomaly consists of infundibular pulmonary stenosis, RVH, and a large ventricular septal defect. Pressure in the right and left ventricles is balanced.[15] The ECG usually indicates moderate RVH. Signs of severe RVH are uncommon in this anomaly.

TRICUSPID ATRESIA

Patients with this relatively uncommon congenital heart disease exhibit no direct communication between the right atrium and the right ventricle because of the atretic valve. The atrial blood is shunted to the left side through a foramen ovale or an atrial septal defect. From the left side, the blood is partially shunted back to the right side through a patent ductus arteriosus or ventricular septal defect. The left ventricle is hypertrophied in contrast to a hypoplastic right ventricle. The combination of findings on an ECG of left axis deviation, atrial enlargement, and LVH in a cyanotic child are almost always diagnostic of tricuspid atresia.[17]

SUMMARY

There are several practical points in pediatric electrocardiography that may be helpful to the anesthesiologist:

1. The ECG should always be interpreted with knowledge of the patient's age, clinical diagnosis, and current therapy.
2. Sinus dysrhythmias, as well as shifting pacemakers, are normal findings in this age group.
3. Right axis deviation is normally present in newborns and infants. By contrast, left axis deviation at this early age indicates LVH.
4. A negative P wave in lead I is an abnormal finding and requires that the ECG be repeated preoperatively to exclude technical errors.
5. Deep Q waves are commonly observed in leads II, III, aVF, and V_5 and V_6 and do not indicate myocardial ischemia.
6. Precordial complexes are frequently very prominent in infants and young children with thin chests, and by themselves are not diagnostic of ventricular hypertrophy.
7. T waves are inverted in V_1 to V_3 in the pediatric age group.
8. Right ventricular preponderance is normally observed in newborns and infants. A normal adult R-wave progression in the precordial leads of the newborn and infant ECG is abnormal and indicative of LVH. The adult ECG pattern is reached at 6 to 8 years of age.
9. Prominent U waves are frequently seen in normal children.
10. A normal ECG does not exclude the presence of congenital heart disease.

REFERENCES

1. Moss A, Emanoulidos G: Practical Pediatric Electrocardiography. JB Lippincott, Philadelphia, 1973
2. Park MK, Guntheroth W: How to Read Pediatric ECGs. Year Book Medical Publishers, Chicago, 1981
3. Harris LC, Ferstain E: Understanding the ECG in Infants and Children. Little, Brown, Boston, 1979
4. Nadas A: Pediatric Cardiology. WB Saunders, Philadelphia, 1973
5. Garson A: The Electrocardiogram in Infants and Children. Lea & Febiger, Philadelphia, 1983
6. Alimurung MM, Joseph LG, Nadas AS: The unipolar precordial and extremity electrocardiogram in normal infants and children. Circulation 4:420, 1951
7. Ziegler RF: Electrocardiographic Studies in Normal Infants and Children. Charles C Thomas, Springfield, Illinois, 1951
8. Cassels DE, Ziegler RF: Electrocardiography in Infants and Children. Grune & Stratton, Orlando, Florida, 1981
9. Moller Z: Heart Disease in Infancy. Appleton-Century-Crofts, East Norwalk, Connecticut, 1981
10. Alimurung MM, Joseph LG, Nadas AS: QT interval in normal infants and children. Circulation 4:420, 1951
11. Lipman B, Dun M, Moss E: Clinical Electrocardiography. Year Book Medical Publishers, Chicago, 1984

12. Liebman J: The normal electrocardiogram in newborns and infants. p. 79. In Cassels DE, Zieger RF (eds): Electrocardiographs in Infants and Children. Grune & Stratton, Orlando, Florida, 1969
13. Walsh SZ: The electrocardiogram in the neonate and infants. p. 263. In Cassels DE (ed): The Heart and Circulation of the Newborn Infant. Grune & Stratton, Orlando, Florida, 1966
14. Cabrera E, Monroy TR: Systolic and diastolic loading of the heart. Am Heart J 43:661, 1952
15. Keith JD: Heart Disease in Infancy and Childhood. Macmillan, New York, 1978
16. Gasul B, Arcilla R, Lev M: Heart Disease in Children. JB Lippincott, Philadelphia, 1966
17. DuShane TW, Weidman WH, Brandenburg RO et al: The electrocardiogram in children with ventricular septal defect and severe pulmonary hypertension. Circulation 22:49, 1960
18. Vince DT, Keith TD: The electrocardiogram in ventricular septal defect. Circulation 23:225, 1961
19. Borkan AM, Pieroni PR, Varghese PT et al: The superior QRS axis in ostium primum ASD. Am Heart J 90:215, 1975
20. Burch GE, DePasquale NP: Electrocardiography in the Diagnosis of Congenital Heart Disease. Lea & Febiger, Philadelphia, 1967

14

The ECG Following Cardiac Surgery

George Silvay, M.D., Ph.D.
Jonathan L. Halperin, M.D.

Interpretation of the ECG following cardiac surgery depends greatly on comparison with preoperative recordings. Differences are to be expected, depending on the form of organic heart disease, type of surgical procedure, anesthetic technique, and other clinical factors. Abnormalities range from routine consequences of operative intervention to critical derangements of myocardial physiology reflecting complications of surgery. The reader is referred to Chapters 1 through 6 for a review of basic electrocardiography. The commentary that follows assumes familiarity with interpretation of ECG rate, rhythm, axis, conduction, and repolarization and with identification of patterns indicating myocardial ischemia, infarction, hypertrophy, and metabolic imbalance. This discussion isolates two broad categories of ECG abnormalities—distortions of waveform morphology and disturbances in cardiac rhythm.

ABNORMALITIES OF THE ECG WAVEFORM

Upon completion of any cardiac operation, the ECG should be monitored continuously as the patient is transported to the recovery area. Shortly after transfer, the rhythm monitor should be supplemented by a standard 12-lead ECG, which provides a vectorial transcript of three-dimensional cardiac electrical activity. A single ECG lead monitored on the oscilloscope permits fairly accurate diagnosis of cardiac rhythm, but changes in waveform morphology must be interpreted hesitantly, since this lead configuration provides only a glimpse of cardiac electricity from a poorly defined vantage point. Changes in the ECG pattern other than dysrhythmias, such as widening or narrowing of the QRS complex, upward or downward shifts of the ST segment, peaking or inversion of T waves, or development of U waves, may reflect equally acute disturbances of myocardial physiology. Since sternotomy and anterior thoracotomy incisions hinder intraoperative recording of precordial leads, the postoperative ECG provides the first thorough opportunity to judge the impact of surgery on the amplitude and direction of cardiac electrical forces reaching the body surface.

Differences between the preoperative and early postoperative ECGs reflect a combination of mechanical and metabolic factors. It is frequently impossible to differentiate ischemia from metabolic imbalance or myocardial strain, particularly when the underlying organic disease has resulted in hypertrophy of one or more cardiac chambers, yet certain diagnostic characteristics can be discerned. Interpretation should proceed systematically, considering first the clinical situation and preoperative ECG pattern, then sequentially assessing the rate, rhythm, axis, and duration of the dominant complexes (P, QRS and T), accounting for deviations of the intervening segments of the ECG waveform (PR and ST) and, finally, identifying pathologic waves (abnormal U, J, Δ, t_a).

The P Wave

The P wave represents depolarization of the atria, normally initiated from the sinoatrial node in the posterior–superior aspect of the right atrium near the inlet of the superior vena cava. The normal P wave of the ECG recorded from the body surface is less than 120 msec in duration and less than 0.3 mV in amplitude, but considerably greater force is detectable within the mediastinum. It consists of two components derived from right and left atrial activation that fuse into a single wave with a mean electrical axis in the frontal plane (limb leads) between 0 and +90 degrees—making the P wave upright in the standard inferior leads II, III, and aVF and inverted in lead aVR. The tall, peaked P waves designated P pulmonale or broad waves termed P mitrale (also characterized by prominent late negative deflection in lead V_1) actually reflect abnormalities of right and left atrial conduction.[1] These do not usually revert toward normal after surgical treatment of the valvular, endocardial, or cardiac skeletal defect that produced the abnormal P-wave appearance, at least during the first postoperative days. A shift in the atrial depolarization pattern, however, may indicate that the cardiac impulse no longer has its origin in the sinus node (Fig. 14–1). The so-called coronary sinus rhythm reflects such an alteration in the intrinsic cardiac pacemaker activity. This is but one variety of ectopic atrial rhythm in which each cardiac cycle is heralded by a uniform P wave inscribed as a negative deflection in the inferior leads. Its cause may be trauma inflicted on the SA tissue during venous cannulation resulting in exit block or atrial

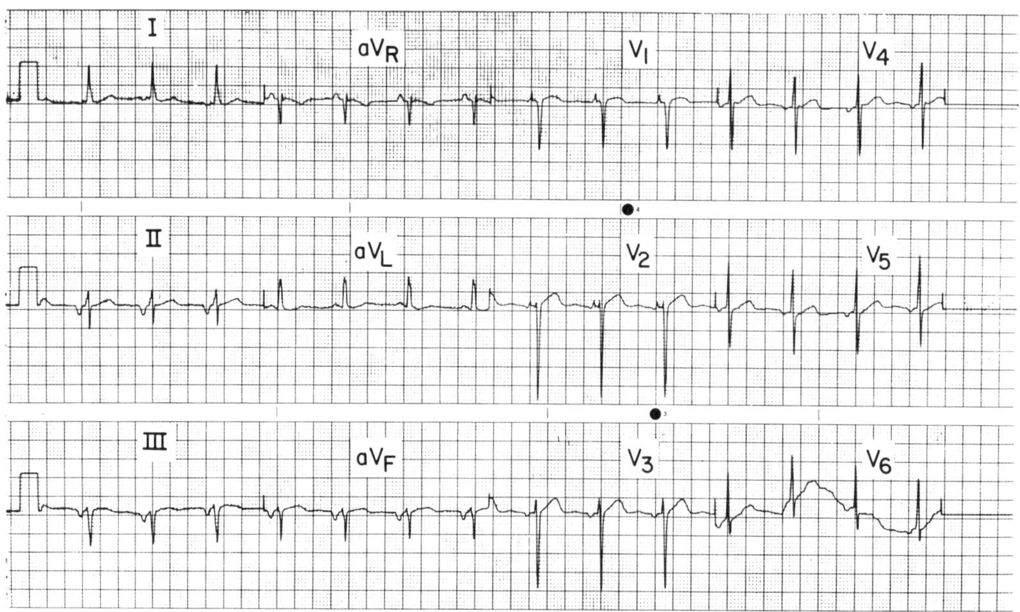

Fig. 14–1 Ectopic atrial rhythm in a patient with a left axis deviation. The rhythm is also termed coronary sinus rhythm. Note the inverted P waves in leads II, III, and aVF.

quiescence, toxic–metabolic disturbances or acceleration of a subsidiary atrial pacemaker. A major shift in the direction of atrial depolarization, without an accompanying change in the QRS axis to suggest a mechanical disruption of cardiac position, usually indicates atrial electrical dysfunction. This may be the harbinger of more serious atrial dysrhythmias. Following cardiac transplantation, changes in the atrial depolarization vector (P-wave axis) reflect the interruption of atrial electrical continuity along the suture margin and the recipient SA tissue, which is usually left intact in the form of atrial cuffs.

The PR Segment

Strictly defined, this stage of the ECG cycle incorporates the delay in impulse propagation related to refractoriness of tissues in the region of the atrioventricular (AV) node. Actually, the delay may occur in proximal internodal tissues or within the bundle of His. Paranodal, accessory pathways of conduction may distort the PR segment in certain electrophysiologic variants called the preexcitation syndromes (e.g., Wolff–Parkinson–White, Lown–Ganong–Levine) by shortening the PR interval to less than 120 msec. Upward or downward shifts of the PR segment—indeed, displacement of all segments of the ECG—are defined with reference to the baseline T-P segment, that portion of the waveform between cardiac cycles (a period of normal electrical silence except when diastolic injury has been sustained). At rapid rates engendering T-P fusion, this baseline becomes effaced and uncertain.

The PR segment incorporates the onset of atrial repolarization (sometimes designated the t_a wave), but this is seldom identified as a discrete entity. Elevation of the PR segment above the baseline signifies acute irritation or injury of endocardial or epicardial atrial surfaces. On the standard ECG, PR-segment elevation occurs in acute atrial infarction. This is not often recognized unless the right atrium is affected. Atrial infarction may accompany acute right ventricular (RV) infarction if there has been interruption of blood flow in the right coronary artery near its origin. Hypotension commonly attends the syndrome, a result of both the impaired atrial contribution to ventricular filling and RV dysfunction.[2,3] Volume loading is essential in acute management, yet it is typical for hemodynamic instability to resolve over several hours or days. Atrial tachyarrhythmias and bradyarrhythmias should be anticipated over a longer period, and these may be poorly tolerated. Atrial infarction may also render temporary right atrial epicardial pacing electrodes malfunctional because of increased impedance to current flow at the electrode–myocardial interface. In some cases, application of electrodes to the left atrium and ventricle should be entertained while these chambers remain accessible during surgery.

Vastly more common than elevation of the PR segment is depression, usually a manifestation of the pericardial/epicardial inflammation that accompanies virtually every operation on the heart.[4,5] In other settings, clinically significant pericarditis is usually accompanied by tachycardia, but this is not invariably the case during the first 8 to 12 hours following cardiac surgery. Ectopic atrial dysrhythmias frequently develop in patients with pericarditis; depression of the PR segment provides an ECG marker of the inflammatory process (Fig. 14–2).

Prolongation of the PR interval beyond 200 msec (first-degree AV block) may occur as a consequence of myocardial inflammation or as a result of sundry metabolic or autonomic factors. The finding develops relatively often in patients who undergo repair of atrial septal defect, transposition of the great vessels, Ebstein's anomaly, tetralogy of Fallot, and following operations involving the mitral valve apparatus. Shortening of the PR interval has been described as an early ECG sign of cardiac transplant rejection.[6]

The QRS Complex

Changes in the morphology of the QRS complexes on the postoperative ECG rank among the most meaningful findings, since this portion of the tracing is less subject to variation on

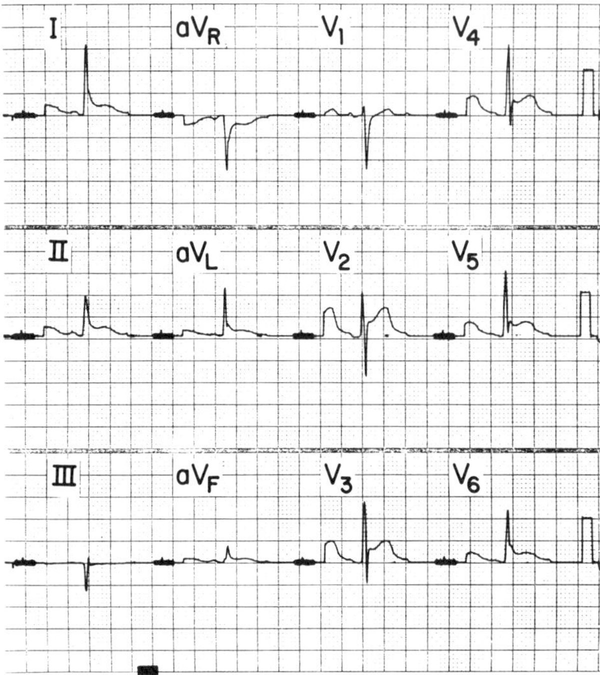

Fig. 14–2 Acute pericarditis in a patient in the early postoperative period following coronary artery bypass graft surgery. The ST origins are elevated above the baseline defined by the TP segment, and the PR segments are depressed.

the basis of metabolic or irritative phenomena than the PR or STU phases. Changes in QRS configuration may result from alterations in Purkinje system conduction or from structural changes in the myocardium. In practice, the concepts of velocity and pathway of conduction merge with one another, since depolarization of the ventricles is intimately dependent upon impulse propagation. The first step in QRS analysis is, therefore, measurement of the QRS duration, which is normally less than 120 msec. The second step is determination of the polarity, or axis, of the mean QRS vector, normally between −30 and +90 degrees in the frontal plane. QRS duration in excess of 120 msec implies delayed intraventricular conduction, and usually the configuration of right or left bundle branch block (RBBB or LBBB) can be discerned, but lesser delay does not exclude conduction abnormalities. The causes of conduction delay are varied, but certain surgical procedures are frequently associated with specific forms of conduction block. RBBB often accompanies repair of septal defects at the ventricular level, especially when accompanied by pulmonary outflow tract obstruction (tetralogy of Fallot), and more advanced grades of heart block may be late sequelae. RBBB is a common perioperative finding in patients with isolated pulmonic stenosis and Ebstein's anomaly, as it is with other disorders associated with RV hypertrophy. LBBB frequently follows aortic valve replacement because of the proximity of the left bundle branch to the aortic valve annulus. Left bundle branch conduction delay is also seen in cases of idiopathic hypertrophic subaortic stenosis, congenital coronary anomalies, and tricuspid atresia. Incomplete forms of LBBB may be encountered whenever severe LV hypertrophy is present.

When they develop alone, RBBB and LBBB do not displace the mean frontal plane QRS vector outside the normal range. Axis deviation either toward the right (positive) or the left (negative) should prompt consideration of additional abnormalities. Delay in anterior or posterior hemifascicular conduction commonly shifts the QRS axis to the left or right, respectively, prolonging ventricular activation without necessarily lengthening the total QRS duration. Left anterior hemiblock is by far the most common of these, frequently developing during myocardial revascularization procedures in patients with atherosclerosis involving the left coronary artery. The left anterior hemiblock pattern has the following features: (1) left axis deviation more negative than −30 degrees; (2) greater R-wave amplitude in lead aVL than in lead I; (3) terminal S waves in leads II, III, and aVF; (4) terminal R waves in lead aVR; (5) initial Q waves in leads I and aVL; and (6) prolongation of the ventricular intrinsicoid deflection (from onset of Q to peak of R) in lead aVL beyond 40 msec (Fig. 14–3). Not infrequently, the left anterior hemiblock pattern is accompanied by retarded precordial R-wave development or even minute initial Q waves in the right precordial leads V_1 and V_2, producing a pattern that might be mistaken for anteroseptal myocardial infarction, right atrial enlargment or preexcitation. As an isolated abnormality postoperatively, left anterior hemiblock seldom progresses to AV dissociation (complete heart block), so prophylactic cardiac pacing is not required. The diagnosis of left posterior hemiblock is less common, is more difficult to establish with certainty, and more frequently implies damage to or irritation of the specialized conducting tissues of the heart, since the posterior hemifascicle has earlier branching and richer blood supply than the anterior tract. The acute right axis deviation characteristic of left posterior hemiblock (to or beyond +120 degrees) must be distinguished from other causes, such as acute right heart pressure overload due to pulmonary embolism or pneumothorax or lateral wall myocardial infarction.

The preexcitation syndromes may distort the inception of the QRS complex on an intermittent basis, producing a Δ wave, as the ventricles are electrically activated by an accessory pathway of AV conduction. These conditions may be suggested by either the clinical history or the appearance of the ECG. The Wolff–Parkinson–White type B configuration is commonly encountered in patients with Ebstein's anomaly (Fig. 14–4). Here the pattern of RBBB present preoperatively may give way to that of LBBB with a prominent S wave in lead V_1.[7] Particular

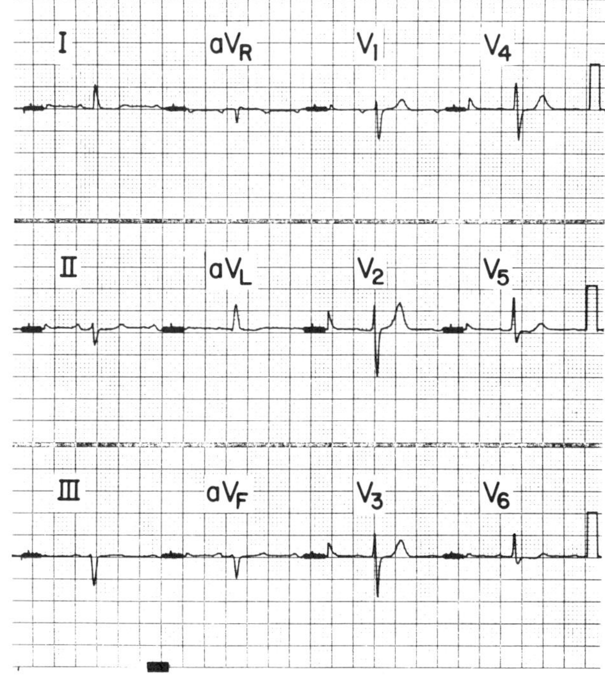

Fig. 14–3 Left anterior hemifasicular block developing in a patient following coronary artery bypass graft surgery. Note the left axis deviation (−45 degrees), terminal S waves in leads II, III, aVF, terminal R wave in aVR, and prolonged ventricular activation time in lead aVL.

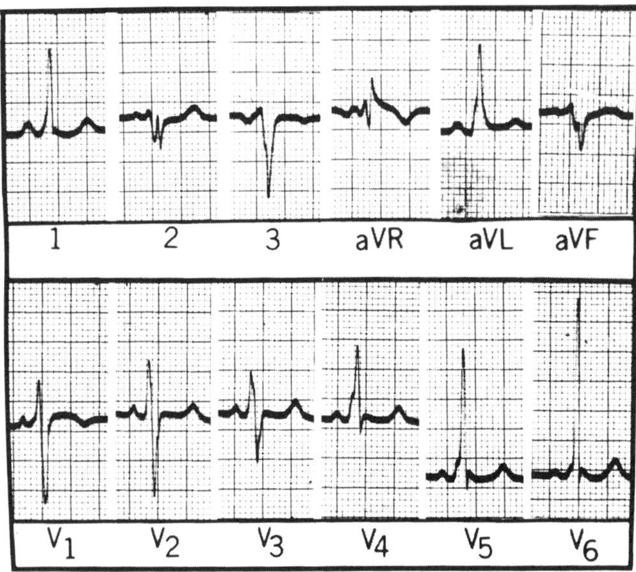

Fig. 14–4 Electrocardiogram from a 17-year-old boy with Ebstein's anomaly. The tracing exhibits the Wolff–Parkinson–White, type B pattern with short PR intervals and delta waves best seen in leads I, aVL, and V4–V6. Note the rS pattern in lead V_1. The Δ wave is directed to the left and superior so the frontal leads show left axis deviation. (Reprinted with permission from Perloff JK: Ebstein's anomaly of the tricuspid valve. p. 239. In Perloff JK (ed): The Clinical Recognition of Congenital Heart Disease. 2nd Ed. WB Saunders, Philadelphia, 1978.)

attention should be given to the possibility of developing reentrant tachyarrhythmias in the early postoperative period, when metabolic and autonomic imbalances predispose to this type of complication. These dysrhythmias are troublesome because of the extremely rapid heart rates they sometimes induce and the special pharmacologic insight they demand for safe control.

Aside from conduction defects, changes in QRS morphology should bring to mind the possibilities of myocardial infarction as an acute perioperative event or direct surgical violation of myocardial integrity. The diagnosis of myocardial infarction in the cardiac surgical patient is fraught with difficulty, but fairly firm evidence of this development is found in the appearance of new pathologic Q waves in leads corresponding to a myocardial segment subserved by a single coronary vessel. Septal infarction is represented in leads V_1 and V_2; anterior infarction in leads V_3 and V_4; inferior infarction in leads II, III, and aVF; and extensive anterior infarction from leads V_2–V_5 or beyond. In the inferior, anterior, or lateral leads, Q waves may have formed by the time of the first postoperative ECG without the intervening changes of the ST segments and T waves commonly associated with the evolution of acute myocardial infarction in nonoperated patients. Inferior infarction may shift the QRS axis leftward and simulate the pattern of left anterior hemiblock, while lateral infarction may shift the axis toward the right, as discussed within the context of left posterior hemiblock. Anterior infarction may have little impact on the frontal plane leads and therefore may go quite unnoticed in the operating room (if only lead II is monitored) until precordial lead changes are revealed on the postoperative ECG. The ECG diagnosis of posterior infarction presumes that the precordial lead patterns represent mirror images of posterior configurations. Hence, abnormally tall and/or broad R waves in the right precordial leads V_1–V_3 may be the reflection of Q waves, which are invisible without posterior thoracic leads.

Patients with old myocardial infarctions may have lost all ECG features of the previous coronary event on the preoperative ECG (quite common in cases of past inferior myocardial infarction), only to have Q waves reappear on the postoperative tracing without other evidence of an acute ischemic event. The mechanisms by which the cardiac surgical procedure (usually coronary artery bypass grafting) unmasks the ECG pattern of established infarction remain somewhat speculative. The diagnosis of perioperative myocardial infarction in patients subjected to surgical procedures involving ventriculotomy or reconstruction of the ventricular walls is a rather moot point. In cases of LV aneurysmectomy, infarctectomy, aneurysm plication, pseudoaneurysm repair, or closure of a ventricular septal defect, for example, the surgery itself can properly be considered the explanation for appearance of pathologic Q waves on the postoperative ECG.

The simple observation of lower QRS amplitude on the postoperative ECG may indicate one of several problems. Before interpretation proceeds, however, it is essential that the sensitivity of ECG recording be first verified by noting the deflection produced by the standard 1-mV calibration pulse artifact. Reduced R-wave voltage may occur when abnormal fluid accumulates in the pericardium, pleural spaces, or subcutaneous tissues and raises the electrical impedance to signal transmission. It may also develop as a consequence of myocardial disease in cases of infarction or transplant rejection.[6,8,9]

The ST Origin, or J Point

Much of the difficulty in interpreting changes in the ST segment of the ECG may be eliminated if one considers the ECG manifestations of ventricular repolarization in two categories. The moment repolarization begins is designated the ST origin (or J point) and the remainder, formed by the ventricular electrical gradient, is designated the T wave. Since it has no duration, the instant transcribed as the ST origin can be only elevated, depressed, or normally aligned with the baseline TP segment. Minor shifts of the ST origin on postoperative ECGs following cardiac surgery may reflect the epicardial irritation, which is part and parcel of such procedures, but deviations of more than 2 mV raise the possibility of acute ventricular epicardial irritation, transmural myocardial ischemia, or perioperative myocardial infarction. Marked elevation of the ST origin raises the possibility of acute injury or transmural ischemia characteristic of severe coronary vasospasm or other causes of sudden epicardial coronary obstruction. Major depressions of the ST origin may occur under conditions of even subendocardial myocardial ischemia. Severe ventricular hypertrophy may lead to chronic shifts of the ST origin, but these tend to be less pronounced than distortions of T-wave morphology.

The TU Complex

Directional changes of the T wave normally parallel those of the QRS complex, so that the difference between their respective vectors does not exceed 75 to 90 degrees. Segmental inversion of T waves may bespeak subendocardial myocardial infarction, while widening of the QRS–T angle is a feature of the strain pattern associated with ventricular hypertrophy. While the patient is in a state of hypothermia, if the heart is not fibrillating, the Osborne complex may develop, in which an abnormal J wave is inscribed as an upward deflection of the ST origin followed by a descending T wave culminating in inversion of its terminal component (Fig. 14–5). Hypokalemia is characterized on the electrocardiogram first by lowering of T-wave amplitude, then by heightening of the U wave, lengthening of the QTU interval, and finally prolongation of the PR and QRS durations. In hyperkalemia, the T waves first become tall and peaked, followed by conduction delay and protracted repolarization. Hypocalcemia may become manifest during the immediate postoperative period as a function of hemodilution and transfusion. Under these circumstances, the TU complex is heralded by a long, early horizontal segment followed by relatively late inscription of the repolarization deflection. Hypercalcemia may produce foreshortening of early repolarization, lowering of T waves, and heightening of U waves; the appearance of ectopic activity is a common correlate.[10] In cardiac transplant rejection, T-wave inversion is a fairly frequent finding.[8]

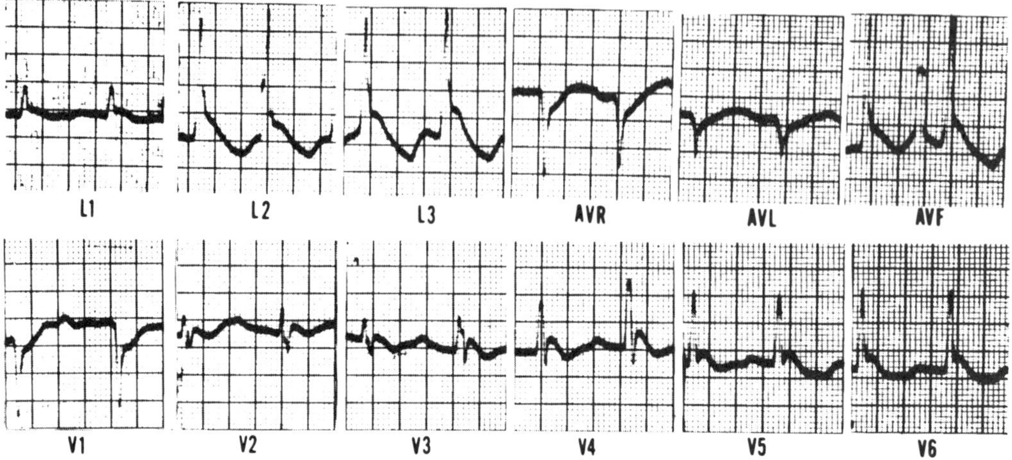

Fig. 14–5 Recorded during hypothermia, the PR interval is prolonged and the QRS complex is lengthened in its final portion by the superimposed Osborne wave. The ST origin is elevated and the T wave is inverted. (Reprinted with permission from Fisch C: Electrocardiography and vectrocardiography. p. 235. In Braunwald E (ed): Heart Disease: A Text Book of Cardiovascular Medicine. 2nd Ed. WB Saunders, Philadelphia, 1984.)

CARDIAC RHYTHM DISTURBANCES

Cardiac dysrhythmias are among the most frequent complications of open heart surgery and often the earliest problems to arise during the postoperative period. Many are benign sequelae of the surgical procedure, while others are potentially life threatening and capable of converting a routine operative procedure into a disaster. The present discussion should be integrated with previous chapters, which describe the classic ECG approach to the diagnosis of cardiac dysrhythmias. A pragmatic clinical approach to the diagnosis of dysrhythmias in the patient following cardiac surgery is presented emphasizing the use of ancillary information provided by the epicardial atrial and ventricular electrodes affixed to the heart at the conclusion of many cardiac operations. The routine application of two temporary electrodes to the right atrial and two to the RV epicardial surfaces is recommended in almost every patient, since neither the occurrence of dysrhythmias preoperatively nor the nature of the surgical procedure is sufficient to predict the incidence or type of dysrhythmias postoperatively. Complications arising from the use of these electrodes can be kept to a minimum. The method of installation of temporary electrodes and their care during the postoperative period is extensively discussed elsewhere.[11] These wires have application in both the diagnosis and management of postoperative cardiac dysrytmias. Dysfunction of the electrodes when it occurs as a result of mechanical dislodgement, fracture, or increased impedance at the electrode–epicardial interface may be a crippling development to the patient with postoperative tachyarrhythmias or bradyarrhythmias, and under these circumstances substitution of transvenous endocardial electrodes may be appropriate.

The general approach to the patient with postoperative cardiac dysrhythmias begins with full consideration of the clinical setting in which they arise. This includes recognition of the nature of organic heart disease, the specific surgical procedure, anesthetic technique, and associated metabolic factors described earlier. It proceeds from evaluation of the rhythm monitor through examination of the 12 standard ECG leads, recalling the value of multiple leads in establishing the predominant rhythm responsible for cardiac impulse generation. Identification of atrial activity and determination of its rate and regularity is often the most difficult step in the analysis of tachyarrhythmias. Identification of ventricular activity helps evaluate the electrophysiologic relationship between atrial and ventricular events, and this leads to an understanding of the functional status of the myocardial conducting system. The standard ECG does not always clearly reveal the nature of atrial activity. In these cases, special leads may be employed in the postoperative period. In the absence of atrial electrodes, the transsternal Lewis lead may help expose occult atrial activity. This lead is configured by placing the right arm and left arm leads across the sternum (attaching Welsh-type suction cup electrodes to the tip of each wire) and recording lead I on the ECG. Another approach is transesophageal recording. This can be done by attaching the unipolar precordial electrode to one end of a small-gauge insulated transvenous pacing electrode and passing the other end of the wire through the lumen of a Levine-type nasogastric tube to a point where the distal electrode tip is at approximately the level of the left atrium. This is frequently convenient in the patient who already has a nasogastric tube in place. The best technique in patients who are still intubated is to pass the Portex cardioesophagoscope (Chapter 2). At many centers, cardiac surgical patients are routinely evaluated by atrial electrograms using temporary epicardial electrodes. When one or both of these electrodes is connected to the precordial lead of the ECG and the V lead is selected for recording, unipolar atrial electrography is accomplished, characterized by high-amplitude atrial (P wave) activity and prominent ventricular (QRS) activity as well. In certain dysrhythmias, particularly the various forms of atrial flutter, it is often difficult to be sure whether additional atrial activity is superimposed on ventricular complexes. To evaluate this possibility, bipolar atrial electrograms may be recorded by connecting one atrial wire to the right arm electrode of the ECG and another to the left arm electrode and selecting lead I for recording. This will reveal prominent epicardial P waves, while the relatively far-field QRS complexes are vastly diminished in relative amplitude (Fig. 14-6A,B). A case could be made for recording the unipolar atrial electrogram, bipolar atrial electrogram and surface ECG in any patient with a tachyarrhythmia postoperatively to avoid misdiagnosis resulting from inapparent atrial activity on the ECG. In patients with a multipurpose pacing Swan Ganz catheter in place, similar information can be obtained by this invasive ECG technique (Chapter 2).

The ventricular electrodes are mainly of therapeutic value for cardiac pacing, as ventricular activity is usually evaluated from the appearance of the QRS complex on surface ECG leads. The relationship between atrial and ventricular activation is inferred after each complex has been identified individually; again, this frequently depends on clear identification of P waves, which may require atrial electrography. QRS complex duration helps determine the physiology of myocardial conduction; it is also useful in the evaluation of anomalous ventricular beats. Prolongation of this complex where it was previously narrow implies aberrant conduction of supraventricular rhythms or development of a ventricular dysrhythmia. The value of physiologic correlates of cardiac rhythm disturbances should not be discounted during the postoperative period. Frequently, evaluation of atrial or venous pressure waveforms will give important clues to the diagnosis of the rhythm abnormality, as when cannon A waves suggest AV discoordination. Finally, the response to certain therapeutic maneuvers may also be important from a diagnostic standpoint. This involves not only the suppression of dysrhythmias by antiarrhythmic medications, but the variations that occur after carotid sinus massage, cardiac pacing, countershock, or administration of drugs affecting the sympathetic nervous system, as well as digitalis glycosides or calcium channel antagonists. The remainder of this chapter reviews specific cardiac dysrhythmias that may arise in the cardiac surgical patient postoperatively.

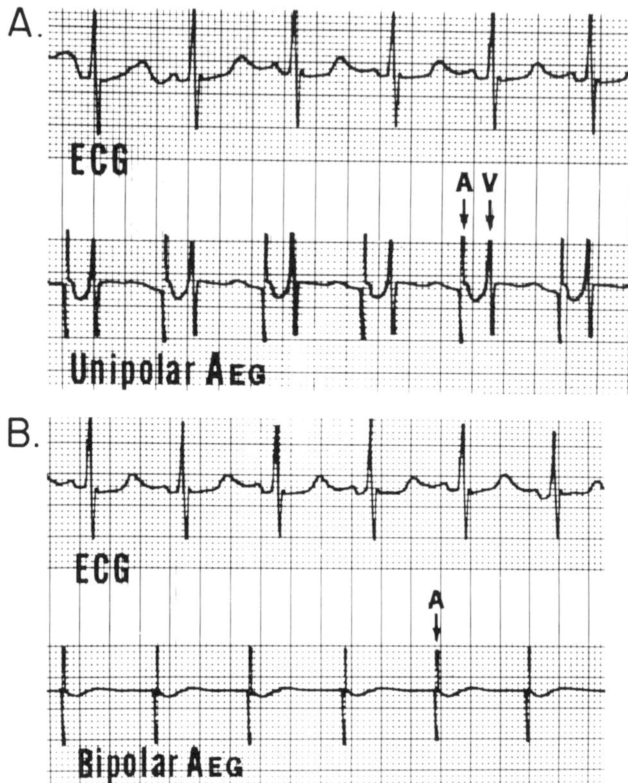

Fig. 14–6 **(A)** Monitor ECG lead recorded simultaneously with a unipolar atrial electrogram during normal sinus rhythm. Although the atrial (A) and ventricular (V) complexes in the unipolar atrial electrogram are approximately the same amplitude in this tracing, this is not a constant finding. Rather, there is considerable variation, in that the atrial complex may be larger or smaller than the ventricular complex. **(B)** Monitor ECG lead recorded simultaneously with a bipolar atrial electrogram during normal sinus rhythm in the same patient described in (A). Although the atrial complex (A) is the only discrete deflection recorded in the bipolar atrial electrogram, a small ventricular complex may also be recorded. (Waldo AL, MacLean WA: Diagnosis and Treatment of Cardiac Arrhythmias Following Open Heart Surgery. Futura, Mt. Kisco, New York, 1983.)

Abnormal Sinus Rhythms

Sinus tachycardia and sinus bradycardia are certainly the most common dysrhythmias on any surgical service. P-wave morphology on the ECG is almost always normal in these sinus rhythms, a helpful feature in differentiating them from ectopic supraventricular rhythms such as the coronary sinus rhythm or the abnormal supraventricular tachyarrhythmias. Again, it is emphasized that upright P waves are the rule in the inferior leads II, III, and aVF. Sinus tachycardia following surgery seldom exceeds rates of 150 to 170 bpm unless the patient is receiving chronotropic drugs such as atropine or catecholamines. Pancuronium also produces increases in heart rate, probably on a vagolytic basis. The diagnostic approach leans heavily toward the identification of the basis for accelerated SA activity, with common factors being volume depletion, fever, anemia, hemodilution, catecholamine excess, acute pulmonary pathology (e.g., pneumothorax, hydrothorax, or pulmonary embolism), and restriction of cardiac filling due to pericardial tamponade. Indeed, the therapy of sinus tachycardia depends almost exclusively on the withdrawal of chronotropic stimuli, although rate-retarding drugs such as propranolol or verapamil are occasionally employed in acute management. Circumspection about this pharmacologic approach is appropriate in most cases, in which the tachycardia is compensatory and hypotension may result if it is eliminated. The diagnosis of sinus tachycardia is sometimes more difficult than one would imagine, particularly at very rapid rates, when it must be differentiated from reentrant paroxysmal atrial tachycardia (PAT) and automatic ectopic atrial tachycardia. The response to atrial pacing or carotid sinus massage may sometimes be helpful in the differential diagnosis.

Sinus bradycardia may be induced by hypothermia or β-adrenergic antagonist drugs. Succinylcholine can produce slowing of heart rate, usually through cholinergic mechanisms. Sinoatrial trauma related to venous cannulation for cardiopulmonary bypass may inhibit SA activity from depolarizing atrial tissues, resulting in marked fluctuation in sinus rate (sinus dysrhythmia) linked with the respiratory cycle, sinus pauses, sinus exit block, or complete atrial quiescence. It is worth remembering that occult atrial extrasystoles blocked at the AV node are among the most common causes of pauses. These hidden premature atrial depolarizations may or may not penetrate and reset the SA pacemaker cells. Atrial electrography effectively discloses these events and should be performed whenever sinus pauses are identified on the surface ECG. Disturbances of sinus node function—in fact, all atrial dysrhythmias—tend to develop in patients subjected to atriotomy, particularly on the right side of the heart, as in repair of atrial septal defects, sinus venosus defects, endocardial cushion defects, correction of anomalous pulmonary venous drainage, and total cardiac transplantation.

Premature Atrial Depolarizations

Atrial premature beats may arise during the postoperative period as a consequence of mechanical or metabolic abnormalities. The former are of the sort just described; the latter involve electrolyte disturbances, such as hypokalemia, hypercalcemia, alkalemia, or the process of rewarming in the first few hours following systemic hypothermia. These extrasystoles are characterized by the prematurity and ectopic nature of atrial impulse formation and may be uniform in appearance or arise from multiple foci within the atria. Like ventricular extrasystoles, they may show coupling with normal beats at intervals leading to atrial bigeminy, trigeminy, or quadrigeminy, or they may occur at the AV node in relationship to prematurity, becoming a fairly frequent cause of pulse lapse. When conducted, atrial extrasystoles may result in aberrant ventricular depolarization with wide QRS complexes commonly displaying a RBBB configuration. If P-wave morphology can be recognized from the surface ECG, this alone is sufficient to establish the diagnosis and distinguish premature atrial from ventricular or junctional ectopic activity; otherwise, esophageal or atrial electrography is required. The chief importance of atrial extrasystoles is that they may herald or precipitate supraventricular tachycardias such as PAT, atrial flutter, ectopic atrial tachycardia, or atrial fibrillation. The appearance of frequent premature atrial depolarizations therefore requires a search for etiology, careful monitoring of the cardiac rhythm, and an attempt at suppression either by correcting causal factors, prophylactic overdrive pacing, or drug administration.

Paroxysmal Atrial Tachycardia

This reentrant rhythm is characterized by a rate between 150 and 200 bpm and a 1 : 1 AV relationship. In most cases, reentry occurs within the AV node, but at least one-third may also involve an accessory bypass tract with or without other manifestations of ventricular preexcitation. In these cases, the accessory pathway is usually concealed, implying that only retrograde ventriculoatrial conduction is possible and that anterograde conduction occurs through the AV node itself. Frequently during PAT, the atria and ventricles are simultaneously depolarized, so that P waves are difficult to discern on the surface ECG. Under these circumstances, bipolar atrial or esophageal electrography can be helpful in establishing the diagnosis, while unipolar electrography is not so useful. When P waves are visible on the surface ECG, they are often directed superiorly, producing negative deflections in leads II, III, and aVF. The most important diagnostic considerations involve distinction from sinus tachycardia or ectopic atrial tachycardia resulting from acceleration of an automatic, nonreentrant focus in the atria. Although the atrial rate and regularity and its relationship to ventricular activation permit the diagnosis of PAT to be suspected by ECG means alone, atrial pacing provides more definitive identification. Atrial pacing has both diagnostic and therapeutic value, as it is effective in terminating the tachyarrhythmia. Several pacing methods are effective in interrupting PAT, the simplest of which is to initiate pacing slightly faster than the spontaneous rate of the dysrhythmia. Upon establishment of atrial capture, pacing may be interrupted and a spontaneous rhythm, usually of sinus origin, will recover. Single premature atrial stimuli may also be effective in terminating PAT, permitting asychronous pacing at slower rates. Since PAT is by definition reentrant and dependent on a 1 : 1 relationship between atrial and ventricular activation, any interruption of this sequence terminates the tachycardia (Fig. 14–7).

Ectopic Atrial Tachycardia

Like PAT, ectopic atrial tachycardia is a rapid rhythm initiated in the atria, with atrial rates generally between 150 and 230 beats/min. Unlike the reentrant tachycardia, this dysrhythmia behaves as though there were an automatic focus discharging in the atrial tissue outside the sinus node. A fairly constant rate may be maintained

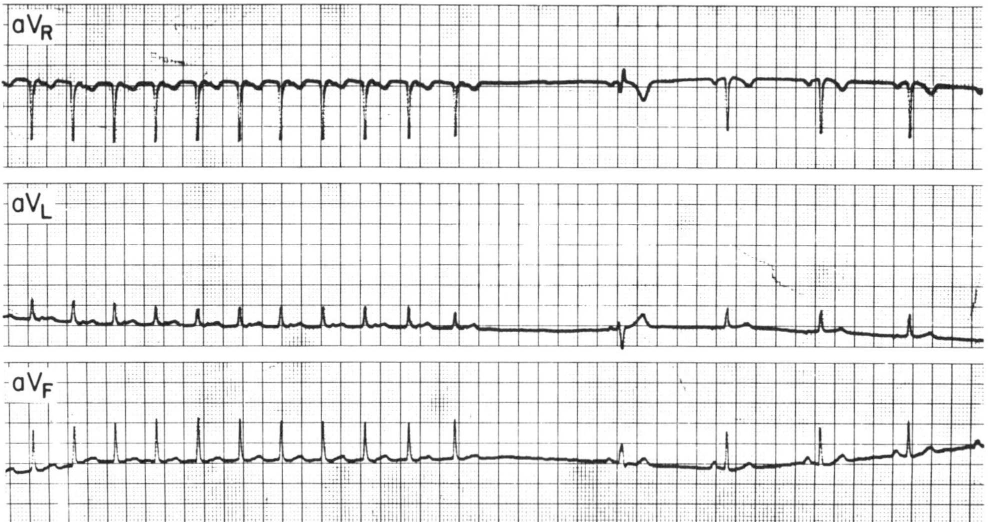

Fig. 14–7 Paroxysmal supraventricular tachycardia with P waves visible in the ST segment. Vagal tone induced by carotid sinus massage resulted in momentary slowing, interruption of the reentrant circuit, and termination of the tachycardia. This is followed by an escape complex and then by restitution of sinus rhythm.

minute by minute, but some fluctuation in speed can be observed over longer intervals. While PAT is obligated to 1 : 1 AV conduction, ectopic atrial tachycardia may be accompanied by AV block, resulting in 2 : 1, 3 : 1, 4 : 1 or higher ratios of impulse retention. Indeed, the designation of PAT with block associated in the older literature with digitalis toxicity is best regarded electrophysiologically as a form of ectopic atrial tachycardia. This is not to say that digitalis therapy is contraindicated in patients with ectopic atrial tachycardia, since the glycoside drugs may be effective in controlling the ventricular response, but one should be alert to the possibility of digitalis excess when ectopic atrial tachycardia is associated with AV block. The differential diagnosis of ectopic atrial tachycardia includes sinus tachycardia, PAT, atrial flutter (particularly when the atrial rate has been modified by drug therapy), and atrial fibrillation (which, at rapid rates, can appear rather regular). Atrial electrography may help make the distinction from flutter or fibrillation, but PAT and sinus tachycardia are best excluded by noting the response to atrial pacing. Overdrive suppression does not usually occur with rapid atrial pacing, although this is not invariably the case. Management may involve either rapid atrial pacing techniques that take advantage of physiologic AV block or drug therapy with digitalis, β-adrenergic antagonists, or verapamil.

Multifocal Atrial Tachycardia

A relatively uncommon dysrhythmia in the early period following cardiac surgery, multifocal atrial tachycardia is usually encountered in patients with cor pulmonale. It is characterized by rapid rates, constantly changing P-wave morphology, and variable PR intervals, indicating advanced atrial electrical disorganization short of fibrillation. This form of tachycardia is resistant to therapy unless the arterial blood gas (ABG) picture can be improved through respiratory care but verapamil and, less commonly, digitalis may sometimes help control ventricular rate by producing AV block.

Atrial Flutter

This rhythm disturbance represents one of the most common tachyarrhythmias following many types of cardiac surgery for ischemic, valvular, congenital, or pericardial heart disease. When the atrial rate is at or near the classic 300 beats/min and sufficient AV block is present to disclose the sawtooth pattern of the ECG baseline in the inferior leads, the diagnosis is not difficult to establish from the standard ECG. As is more often the case, however, the atrial rate may range from 230 to 430 beats/min in atrial flutter and 2 : 1 AV conduction may be maintained, obscuring the atrial pattern on the ECG. In these cases, recording of atrial electrograms, particularly in the bipolar configuration, is extremely useful in establishing the diagnosis of atrial flutter (Fig. 14–8). Moreover, the response to rapid atrial pacing helps distinguish two types of flutter. Both types (I and II) are thought to have reentrant mechanisms, but in the first the response to rapid atrial stimulation is that of a macroreentry circuit in that the tachyarrhythmia is interrupted, while in type II flutter more localized circus atrial depolarization behaves as an electrically isolated or protected focus resistant to overdrive inhibition. Hence, type I atrial flutter is distinguished by its termination after pacing the atria in excess of the flutter rate, while type II flutter permits capture of the atria at more rapid rates without interrupting the flutter mechanism, which dominates once pacing is terminated. When the pacing apparatus, including electrode function, is adequate, both types of atrial flutter permit fibrillation if the atria are stimulated in excess of about 450 pulses per minute and, in cases in which the rhythm is refractory to pharmacologic therapy, fibrillation may be maintained while the ventricular response is slowed by drug action.

Atrial Fibrillation

Atrial fibrillation is electrophysiologically the most variable of the atrial tachyarrhythmias, and it may be thought of as involving atrial electrical chaos. Several morphologic varieties

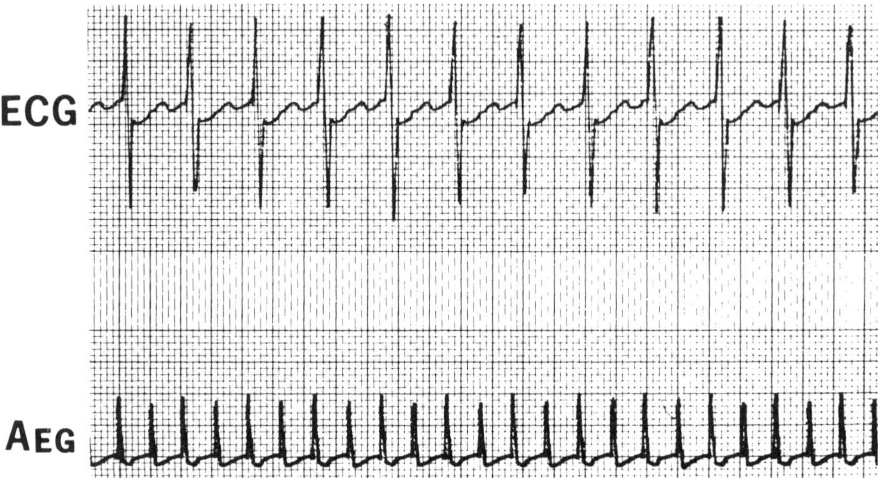

Fig. 14–8 Monitor ECG lead recorded simultaneously with a bipolar atrial electrogram during a episode of type I atrial flutter. The atrial rate is 280 beats/min, and there is 2 : 1 AV conduction. Note that the atrial complexes are not readily discerned from the surface ECG alone, but the bipolar atrial electrogram clearly establishes the nature of atrial activation and its relationship to ventricular activation. (Waldo AL, MacLean WA: Diagnosis and Treatment of Cardiac Arrhythmias Following Open Heart Surgery. Futura, Mt. Kisco, New York, 1983.)

have been identified by atrial electrography, but atrial pacing is totally ineffective in the presence of atrial fibrillation. This dysrhythmia represents the most advanced form of atrial electrical disorganization, although it occurs very commonly both as a function of underlying heart disease and as a complication of anesthesia and surgery. Factors predisposing to the development of this rhythm disturbance include atrial enlargement or hypertrophy, electrolyte imbalance such as hypokalemia or hypercalcemia, and other metabolic derangements such as alkalosis. Both adrenergic and cholinergic stimuli may provoke atrial fibrillation because of their influence on electrical refractoriness of atrial tissue. Atrial fibrillation is common following hypothermic cardioplegia and, accordingly, is frequent in the early phases of recovery from cardiac surgery. In this setting, while the myocardium is still cool and quite noncompliant from the standpoint of diastolic ventricular filling, the hemodynamic consequences of atrial fibrillation may be greater than at other times. During the first few hours following cardiac surgery in a patient not previously in atrial fibrillation, the development of this dysrhythmia may call for electrical cardioversion. Patients with preoperative atrial fibrillation may be restored to sinus mechanism during the surgical procedure; in these cases, atrial dysrhythmias are to be expected during the early postoperative period. The culmination is often degeneration back into atrial fibrillation within 3 days of surgery. The likelihood that sinus rhythm can be maintained longer relates to the duration of preoperative fibrillation, and return to this rhythm postoperatively is almost invariably well tolerated. In these cases, control of the ventricular response may be attained with digitalis glycosides, β-adrenergic antagonists, or verapamil. Patients in preoperative sinus rhythm who develop late (beyond 72 hours) postoperative atrial fibrillation may respond to digitalis and quinidine, procainamide, or disopyramide.

Premature Ventricular Depolarizations

Common in all patients subjected to general anesthesia, ventricular irritability is particularly frequent in patients with underlying or surgically induced abnormalities of ventricular myocardium. In the postoperative setting, the major concern in the face of ventricular extrasystoles is the enhanced potential for the development of malignant ventricular dysrhythmias such as ventricular tachycardia, ventricular flutter, or ventricular fibrillation. The circumstances leading to malignant potential are similar to those that give rise to acutely appearing ventricular ectopic activity, namely, hypokalemia, hypercalcemia, digitalis excess, hypoxemia, ischemia, alkalemia, rewarming following hypothermia, myocardial infarction, and mechanical factors. The most important features distinguishing ventricular from supraventricular extrasystoles are the dissociation of the former from atrial activity and prolongation of the QRS complex beyond 120 msec. From a practical standpoint, it is difficult if not impossible to distinguish junctional extrasystoles conducted with aberration from ventricular premature depolarizations using surface ECG or epicardial atrial or ventricular electrography, which do not display activation of the bundle of His. When ventricular irritability does occur, it is important to exclude readily reversible causes while the patient is monitored closely for patterns associated with malignant degeneration, such as early-cycle extrasystoles arising within the T wave of the preceding repolarization, coupled or tripled extrasystoles, or frequent multiform appearance. Lidocaine often provides prompt suppression, and other antiarrhythmic agents may be required. In patients with atrial fibrillation, occasional aberration may be difficult to distinguish from ventricular extrasystoles unless the Ashman phenomenon is evident, characterized by wide QRS complexes, usually in RBBB configuration, arising early in the first cycle following a long interventricular interval.

Ventricular Tachycardia

This potentially lethal dysrhythmia arises in the ventricles, usually on a reentrant basis. Diagnosis depends on identification of a wide QRS tachycardia, usually quite regular, which is dissociated from atrial activity. The last feature may require confirmation by atrial electrography, but often time is not available for this as hypotension and systemic hypoperfusion rapidly ensue, requiring prompt cardioversion. Rates range from less than 100 to more than 250 beats/min, and it is sometimes difficult to distinguish this dysrhythmia from a supraventricular tachycardia with aberrant ventricular conduction. The latter is unlikely when the QRS duration exceeds 140 msec or the frontal plane QRS axis is directed superiorly. Ventricular tachycardia occurs with relative frequency, following surgery for obstructive hypertrophic cardiomyopathy (idiopathic hypertrophic subaortic stenosis), ventricular septal defect, coronary arterial anomalies, ventricular aneurysm, and tetralogy of Fallot. It is not infrequent in the first few hours after many cardiac surgical procedures, particularly if these involve ventriculotomy or myocardial infarction. Antiarrhythmic drugs such as lidocaine may be effective in suppressing the dysrhythmia, but overdrive pacing from the atria or ventricles is another useful modality.

Ventricular Flutter and Torsades-de-Pointes

These transient but very dangerous ventricular dysrhythmias may be regarded as a variety of ventricular tachycardia in which the vulnerable period of repolarization is virtually simultaneous with the subsequent depolarization of the ventricles. This leads to accelerating tachycardia and rapid degeneration to ventricular fibrillation and is therefore an immediate harbinger of sudden death. Prompt cardioversion using asynchronous DC countershock is indicated, and the cause of the dysrhythmia should be carefully sought. Potential precipitants include excessive exposure to certain antiarrhythmic drugs such as procainamide, quinidine, flecainide, or disopyramide, or cardiomyopathy and ventricular aneurysm.

Ventricular Fibrillation

Although this rhythm occurs during cardiopulmonary bypass, it represents the most disastrous of cardiac rhythm disturbances in the intensive care unit (ICU). The ultimate in electrical instability, the rhythm (if sustained for more than a few minutes) is incompatible with life. Pacing is invariably ineffective in the setting of fibrillation since the ventricular myocardium may be considered both continuously depolarized and continuously refractory. Electrical defibrillation is mandatory on an immediate basis, following which a search for causes should be made and adequate suppressive therapy instituted. Since ventricular fibrillation is a medical emergency, recording of the electrocardiogram is limited to documentation of the dysrhythmia.

Junctional Tachycardia

This automatic or nonreentrant dysrhythmia is initiated in the region of the AV node and produces a regular, narrow QRS tachycardia dissociated from atrial activity or accompanied by retrograde atrial depolarizations, often manifest as negatively inscribed P waves in the inferior leads immediately preceeding or following the QRS complex (Fig. 14–9). The rhythm may be a manifestation of digitalis excess, but in cardiac surgical situations it arises most commonly in pediatric patients following repair of congenital lesions, such as the Mustard procedure for repair of transposition of the great arteries with intact ventricular septum or procedures designed to correct Ebstein's anomaly, atrial septal defect, or tricuspid atresia. In these cases, sustained tachycardia may produce progressive hemodynamic deterioration, since the dysrhythmia is often not amenable to pharmacologic control. In these cases, some success has been achieved with the technique of ventricular paired pacing in which dual ventricular stimuli are applied at a combined rate more rapid than the

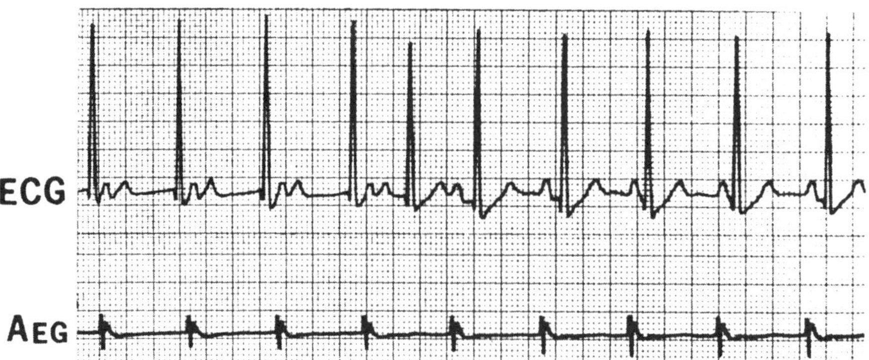

Fig. 14–9 Junctional tachycardia. ECG monitor lead recorded simultaneously with a bipolar atrial electrogram showing a narrow QRS tachycardia dissociated from atrial activity. In other cases retrograde atrial activation results in negatively inscribed P waves in the inferior leads of the surface ECG. The fourth atrial complex results in antegrade atrioventricular conducting capturing the ventricles. (Modified from Waldo AL, MacLean WA: Diagnosis and Treatment of Cardiac Arrhythmias Following Open Heart Surgery. Futura, Mt. Kisco, New York, 1983.)

tachycardia, but the second stimulus is timed early after the first, so that the effective pulse rate is reduced by half. This form of pacing can be sustained over surprisingly long periods, sometimes days, until the AV junctional tachycardia subsides spontaneously.

Asystole and Atrial Quiescence

These electrical disturbances, truly arrhythmias, may occur as a result of trauma to the SA node or injury to its blood supply. They may occur in patients undergoing cardiopulmonary bypass but are most common in the setting of preexisting sinus node dysfunction (sick sinus syndrome) in the elderly, in the Mustard procedure, and in the repair of lesions associated with congenitally corrected transposition of the great arteries. Antiarrhythmic drugs such as procainamide may produce atrial quiescence as well. Even an atrial electrogram in this setting fails to disclose atrial electrical activity. In true atrial quiescence, the atria are inexcitable, and therefore atrial pacing therapy cannot be effectively employed. Ventricular pacing may be used if the spontaneous ventricular rate is suboptimal.

Exit Block

The concept of exit block involves depolarization of cells within the sinus node or an ectopic focus without transmission of a wave of depolarization to surrounding myocardial cells. In the postoperative cardiac surgical patient, exit block most commonly involves the SA nodal tissue itself, leading to the appearance of slow atrial rhythms and sinus dysrhythmia as manifestations of second- and third-degree exit block. Wenckebach periodicity may be observed, while a relationship of P waves to QRS complexes is constant; this form of SA block is usually characterized by progressive shortening of the cardiac cycles leading to a short pause (Fig. 14–10A,B). The etiology, again, is usually ischemia or trauma to atrial tissue, although in surgery for congenital heart disease such as Ebstein's anomaly or tricuspid atresia, internodal pathways in the atria may also be involved. Digitalis glycosides may also produce SA exit block or exit block from other foci. In general, drugs with negative chronotropic properties should be used with great caution when exit block is suspected.

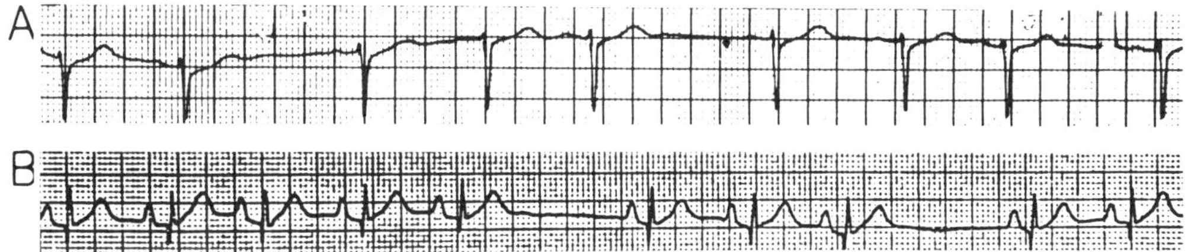

Fig. 14–10 Sinoatrial nodal exit block. **(A)** Sinus node exit block demonstrating Mobitz type I physiology. The P-P interval shortens from the first to the second cycle in each grouping, followed by a pause. The duration of the pause is less than twice the shortest cycle length, and the cycle length after the pause exceeds the cycle before the pause. The PR interval is normal and constant. Lead V_1. **(B)** Sinus node exit block demonstrating Mobitz type II physiology. The P-P interval varies slightly because of sinus dysrhythmia. The PR interval is normal and constant. Lead III. (Reproduced with permission from Zipes DP: Specific arrhythmias: Diagnosis and Treatment. p. 691. In Braunwald E (ed): Heart Disease: A Textbook of Cardiovascular Medicine. 2nd Ed. WB Saunders, Philadephia, 1984.)

Electrically Isolated Ventricular Foci

This disturbance requires special consideration in the diagnosis of ventricular extrasystoles and tachyarrhythmias because of their unexpectedly benign or malignant potential. Ventricular parasystole is a form of ventricular extrasystole characterized by protection of an ectopic focus displaying entrance block. This means that a single site in the ventricular myocardium outside the Purkinje system is depolarized at a fairly constant rate that is relatively uninfluenced by the native rhythm. These myocardial cells discharge repeatedly, resulting in myocardial depolarization when the surrounding myocardial tissue is not refractory. The diagnosis may be suspected when uniform ventricular ectopic complexes display variable coupling intervals to preceding beats and is confirmed when the interectopic interval is shown to be a multiple of some fixed rate of depolarization from the parasystolic focus (Fig. 14–11). These rhythms are almost invariably benign in that they seldom degenerate into ventricular tachycardia or fibrillation. On the other hand, certain forms of accelerated idioventricular rhythm, often designated slow ventricular tachycardia, may display the property of exit block. In these cases, usually accompanying acute myocardial infarction, seemingly stable rhythms characterized by wide QRS complexes dissociated from atrial activity yet occurring at nominal rates may suddenly double or quadruple in speed as the ectopic focus (sometimes reentrant) becomes less impeded in depolarizing the ventricular myocardium. In this setting, therefore, pharmacologic suppression should be carefully considered, particularly when ventricular pacing electrodes are affixed and available postoperatively.

Atrioventricular Block, Atrioventricular Dissociation, and Complete Heart Block

Prolongation of conduction across the internodal pathways or AV node commonly occurs in the repair of lesions associated with congenitally corrected transposition of the great vessels, although the incidence of this complication has been reduced by intraoperative electrophysiologic mapping. Heart block also complicates the partition of a single ventricle and the Mustard operation in some cases, and it frequently develops late postoperatively in patients undergoing

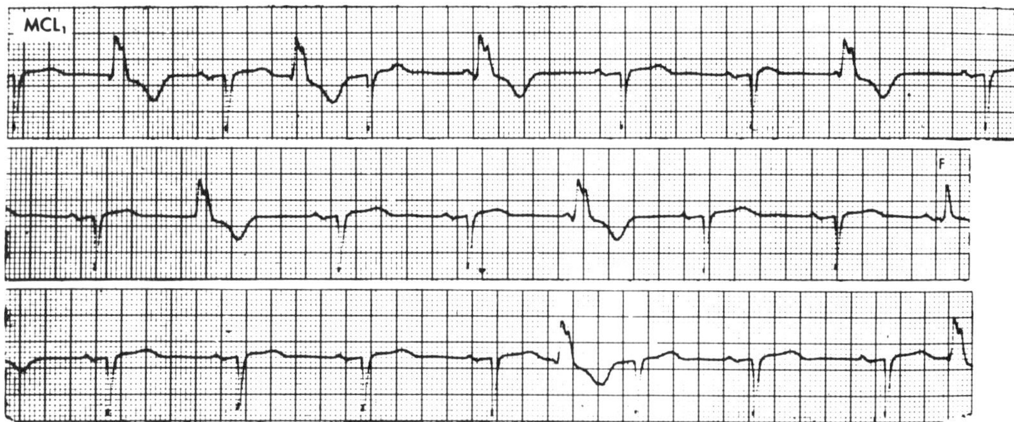

Fig. 14–11 Ventricular parasystole. Unifocal ectopic complexes with varying coupling intervals to the preceding QRS. The first three ectopic beats indicate the shortest manifest interectopic intervals. All subsequent interectopic intervals are multiples of this cycle length. (Marriott HJ: Advanced Concepts in Arrhythmias. CV Mosby, St. Louis, 1983.)

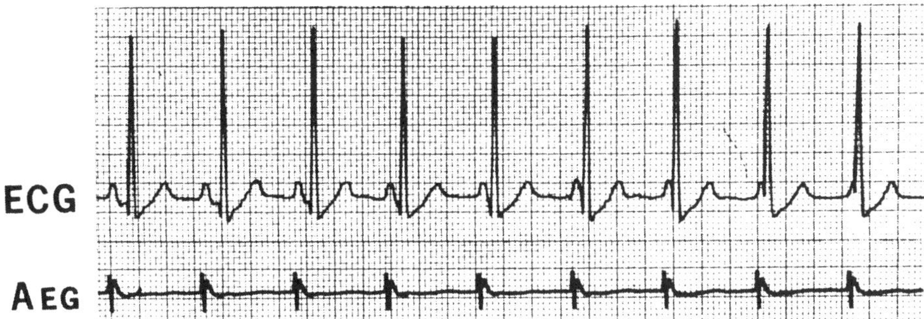

Fig. 14–12 Isorhythmic atrioventricular dissociation mimicking the appearance of normal sinus rhythm. The derangement is increasingly apparent toward the right hand portion of the tracing. (Modified from Waldo AL, MacLean WA: Diagnosis and Treatment of Cardiac Arrhythmias Following Open Heart Surgery. Futura, Mount Kisco, New York, 1983.)

repair of tetralogy of Fallot. Drugs such as digitalis, propranolol, verapamil, and quinidine may depress conduction across these pathways, leading to advanced forms of heart block. Impaired conduction must be distinguished from accelerated junctional rhythms without block at the AV node. It is also important to recognize the occurrence of isorhythmic AV dissociation, which may have the appearance of normal sinus rhythm, except that close inspection of long portions of the ECG reveals that the P waves and QRS complexes bear a close but not fixed relationship (Fig. 14–12). Mobitz type I (Wenckebach) block is usually reversible and is related to tissues proximal to the bundle of His, while Mobitz type II block more frequently progresses to complete dissociation for which cardiac pacing, even permanently, may be required[11] (Fig. 14–13A,B).

ACTIONABLE ISSUES IN POSTOPERATIVE ECG

The foregoing remarks emphasize the importance of considering clinical context in interpreting ECG patterns following cardiac operations. The same may be said of the actionable issues in electrocardiography—namely, when and how to treat the patient who has evolved important variations in waveform morphology or cardiac rhythm. When the ECG gives clues to the presence of major mechanical, ischemic, or metabolic derangement from the expected surgical course, appropriate management begins with confirmatory testing and careful observation for hemodynamic and electrophysiologic sequelae.

Electrical Cardioversion

In the case of cardiac rhythm disturbances, a decision must often be rapidly made about pharmacologic or resuscitative therapy, including cardioversion by DC countershock. This technique should be considered in cases of tachyarrhythmias accompanied by hypotension, acute congestive cardiac failure, or active myocardial ischemia thought to be related to the rhythm disturbance. In other cases, these features of hemodynamic compromise may be lacking immediately, but there is a high degree of likelihood that decompensation will occur. One typical example is the patient with preoperative sinus rhythm who develops atrial fibrillation (even with an acceptable rate of ventricular response) while still in a state of systemic hypothermia during the first few hours after myocardial revascularization surgery. Suboptimal systemic perfusion and progressive acceleration of the ventricular rate may be anticipated, and R-wave synchronized electrical cardioversion

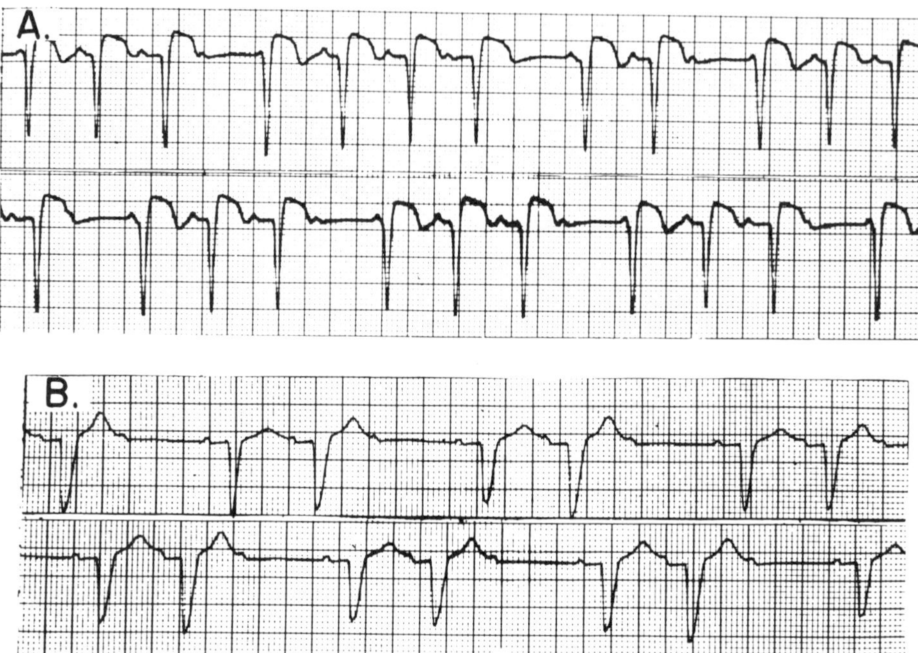

Fig. 14–13 Sinus tachycardica with Mobitz type I (Wenckebach) atrioventricular block. **(A)** The increment in PR interval generally shortens before the dropped beat and the PR interval after the dropped beat is shorter than the PR interval preceding the dropped beat. **(B)** A 3 : 2 AV block characterized by consecutive atrial impulses conducted by the same PR interval immediately before the dropped beat. The PR interval after the dropped beat is the same as the PR interval before: the PR interval is of normal duration, and there is a bundle branch block. (Marriott HJ: Advanced Concepts in Arrhythmias. CV Mosby, St. Louis, 1983.)

is appropriate once normal serum electrolytes have been verified. Another example is the situation with ventricular tachycardia occurring at only a mildly accelerated rate with satisfactory blood pressure when rapid administration of antiarrhythmic medication has failed to terminate the tachyarrhythmia. Since this dysrhythmia is apt to degenerate into more rapid ventricular beating or fibrillation, definitive therapy is in order. DC countershock, like all therapeutic antiarrhythmic measures, is therefore appropriate either when a dysrhythmia is producing hemodynamic decompensation or is likely to lead to this form of clinical deterioration. Electrical cardioversion should generally not be employed when the ECG reveals periods of normal sinus mechanism punctuating a tachyarrhythmia. Patients with this type of intermittent atrial fibrillation, for example, will almost invariably show recurrence of the rhythm disturbance whether sinus rhythm is momentarily reestablished spontaneously or by therapeutic means, unless causal factors are diminished or pharmacologic agents are employed.

Digitalis

Some mention should be made of the ECG significance of the digitalis glycosides, which are electrophysiologically unique by virtue of their opposite impact on myocardial conduction and automaticity. The diagnosis of digitalis excess takes account of these features of drug action in combination with an understanding of the patient's clinical characteristics. Virtually all cardiac dysrhythmias have been reported in association with glycoside toxicity, but it must be particularly suspected whenever sufficient amounts of the drug have been given and the ECG reveals evidence of conduction block (at the atrial, nodal, or ventricular level) and/or accelerated discharge of ectopic foci. It is intriguing that halothane, which affects phase 4 of the cardiac action potential, significantly reduces digitalis glycoside cardiotoxicity and may thus mask the condition until the postoperative period. Management may involve antiarrhythmic medication, cardioversion, or cardiac pacing, all of which bear increased risks of complications in the presence of excessive (but not therapeutic) concentrations of digitalis. Since the drug cannot be removed from plasma or tissue by conventional means including hemodialysis, careful monitoring of the ECG may be required for periods of several days.

REFERENCES

1. Morris JJ, Estes EH, Whalen RE, et al: P wave analysis in valvular heart disease. Circulation 29:242, 1964
2. Gardin JM, Singer DH: Atrial infarction: importance, diagnosis and localization. Arch Intern Med 141:1345, 1981
3. Cushing EH, Feil HS, Stanton EJ, Wartman WB: Infarction of the cardiac auricles (atria): Clinical, pathological and experimental studies. Br Heart J 4:17, 1942
4. Jurado RA, Osborn JJ: Patient surveillance and general care. p. 123. In Litwak RS, Jurado RA (eds): Care of the Cardiac Surgical Patient. Appleton-Century-Crofts, East Norwalk, CT, 1982
5. Spodick DH: Pathogenesis and clinical correlations of the electrocardiographic abnormalities of pericardial disease. p. 201. In Rios JC (ed): Cardiovascular Clinics: Clinical–Electrocardiographic Correlations. Vol. 8. FA Davis, Philadelphia, 1977
6. Scheuer J, Shaver JA, Harris BC, et al: Electrocardiographic findings in cardiac transplantation. Circulation 40:289, 1969
7. Perloff JK: Ebstein's anomaly of the tricuspid valve. p. 239. In Perloff JK (ed): The Clinical Recognition of Congenital Heart Disease. 2nd Ed. WB Saunders, Philadelphia, 1978
8. Griepp RB, Stinson EB, Dong E, et al: Acute rejection of the allografted human heart. Ann Thorac Surg 12:113, 1976
9. Reitz BA, Dong E, Baumgartner WA, Shumway NE: Heart and lung transplantation. p. 1598. In Sabiston DC, Spencer FC (eds): Gibbon's Surgery of the Chest. 4th Ed. WB Saunders, Philadelphia, 1983
10. Nirenberg DW, Ransil BJ: Q–atc interval as a clinical indicator of hypercalcemia. Am J Cardiol 44:243, 1979
11. Waldo AL, Maclean WA: Diagnosis and Treatment of Cardiac Arrhythmias Following Open Heart Surgery. Futura, Mt. Kisco, NY, 1983

OTHER RECOMMENDED READING

Chung E: Principles of Cardiac Arrhythmias. 2nd Ed. Williams & Wilkins, Baltimore, 1977

Constant J: Bedside Cardiology. 3rd Ed. Little, Brown, Boston, 1985

Constant J: Learning Electrocardiography: A Complete Course. Little, Brown, Boston, 1981

Josephson M, Wellens H (eds): Tachycardias: Mechanisms, Diagnosis and Treatments. Lea & Febiger, Philadelphia, 1984

Marriott HJ: Advanced Concepts in Arrhythmias. CV Mosby, St. Louis, 1983

Marriott HJ: Practical Electrocardiography. 7th Ed. Williams & Wilkins, Baltimore, 1983

Pick A, Langendorf R: Interpretation of Complex Arrhythmias. Lea & Febiger, Philadelphia, 1979

Schamroth L: The Disorders of Cardiac Rhythm. 2nd Ed. Blackwell/Mosby, St. Louis, 1980

Schamroth L: Diagnostic Pointers in Clinical Electrocardiology: Abnormalities of the PQRST Pattern. Charles Press, Bowie, MD, 1978

Wharton MJ, Goldschlager N: Guide to Interpreting 12-Lead EKG's. Medical Economics Company, Oradell, NJ, 1984

15

Pacemakers

Jorge Camuñas, M.D.

GENERAL CONSIDERATIONS

Brief History

A comprehensive history of cardiac pacing would include many experiments that arose from man's fascination with electricity and its effects on skeletal and heart muscle. The application of these principles to cardiac pacemakers as they are known today had to wait until reliable leads and power sources became available.

In 1952, Zoll demonstrated that rhythmic stimulation applied through the chest wall of patients with Morgagni-Adam-Stokes syndrome could be effective in maintaining a cardiac rhythm.[1] The advances of cardiac surgery provided an added stimulus to the development of pacemakers as patients with intraoperative heart block required epicardial electrodes for pacing. In 1957 Lillehei and his group became pioneers in the development of portable external pulse generators.[2]

In 1958, Furman and Robinson used endocardial electrodes and a large external power source to pace the heart without the need for thoracotomy.[3] Elmqvist and Senning used intramyocardial leads with an implantable pulse generator which could be recharged.[4] The next year Chardack et al. were the first to use implantable pulse generators that did not require recharging.[5]

During the next decade, more reliable endocardial leads were developed. Together with longer-lasting power sources such as lithium batteries, these advances in technology ushered in the period of reliable single-chamber pacing systems, which lasted 5 to 10 years.

Soon thereafter, the electronic circuitry was miniaturized. Hybrid circuits and, more recently, integrated chips were substituted for separate components and smaller programmable units became available. During the late 1970s, dual-chamber systems started to be used frequently for patients with intact sinus node function. A brief chronology of the early developments in the history of cardiac pacing is listed in Table 15–1.

Indications for Pacing

A thorough review of the indications for pacing is beyond the scope of this chapter. However, the generally accepted indications are listed below. The Subcommittee on Pacemaker Implantation of the joint American College of Cardiology/American Heart Association Task Force on Assessment of Cardiovascular procedures recently published Guidelines for Permanent Cardiac Pacemaker Implantation.[6] In the following list, symptoms refers to syncope, seizures, dizziness, confusion, or congestive heart failure (CHF).

Table 15–1. Early Developments in the History of Cardiac Pacing

Development	Innovators	Year	Techniques
SA node stimulation	Hyman	1931	Endocardial glass cannula
	Shafiroff, Linder	1957	Transesophageal lead
Asynchronous pacing	Zoll, Belgard, Zarsky	1952	Transthoracic, esophageal chest wall stimulation
External pulse generators	Lillehei, Bakken	1956	Intramyocardial leads, compact external pulse generator
	Furman, Robinson, Schwedel	1958	Endocardial right ventricular lead, external pulse generator
Implantable pulse generators	Senning, Elmqvist	1958	Rechargeable generator, intramyocardial leads
	Chardack, Greatbatch	1959	Battery-driven pulse generator
	Kantrowitz, Zoll	1960	Similar devices
	Abelson, Samet, Rand	1962	Temporary endocardial lead, external generator
	Lagerqueer, Johnson	1962	Reliable endocardial leads

Sick sinus syndrome
- Severe persistent or episodic sinus bradycardia
- Sinus arrest
- Episodes of tachyarrhythmias alternating with normal sinus rhythm or sinus bradycardia
- Sinoatrial block without drug toxicity

Acquired complete heart block with symptoms
Congenital complete heart block with severe bradycardia and symptoms
Chronotropic incompetence (inappropriate slow supraventricular rate in presence of CHF and limited stroke volume or atrial fibrillation with slow ventricular response)
Mobitz type II second-degree AV block with symptoms attributable to intermittent complete heart block
Carotid sinus hypersensitivity
Bifascicular and trifascicular block with symptoms

The precise indications must be clearly documented by a careful history with specific reference to the symptoms listed. The physical examination should include a search for signs of congestive heart failure and for carotid bruits or decreased pulsations. The laboratory examinations must include an ECG and rhythm strip in patients with constant or frequent symptoms. In those with intermittent symptoms or unexplained syncope, an ambulatory electrocardiogram (Holter monitor) is very helpful in documenting the rhythm disturbance. Patients with symptoms and normal ECG studies may require electrophysiologic testing to obtain the proper diagnosis. It is also important to note whether the observed dysrhythmia is primary or due to underlying heart disease and not a transient phenomenon due to drugs or electrolyte abnormalities. The indications for temporary pacing are listed in Table 15–2.

Table 15–2. Indications for Temporary Pacemaker Insertion

Ventricular or dual chamber pacing
Complete heart block secondary to acute myocardial infarction
Mobitz type II second-degree AV block and anterior myocardial infarction
Bradyarrhythmias secondary to drug toxicity
Mobitz type I second-degree AV block and inferior myocardial infarction if emergency surgery is indicated
Atrial pacing
To terminate frequent episodes of supraventricular tachycardia

Pacing Modes

It is necessary to know precisely how a given pacemaker is supposed to interact with the patient's underlying heart rhythm in order to be able to determine whether it functions properly. To simplify the nomenclature, in 1974 the Intersociety Commission for Heart Disease Resources developed a three-position pacemaker identification code. This code was expanded in 1981 to five positions and incorporates more recent advances in pacemaker design[7] (Table 15–3).

The first position identifies the chamber that is *paced*. The second position refers to the chamber that is *sensed*. The third position indicates the *mode* of response of the pulse generator. Inhibited is a mode in which the output of the generator is blocked by a sensed signal. Triggered indicates a mode in which a sensed signal elicits the output. Double, in this position, indicates that the unit can respond in both inhibited and triggered modes. Reverse indicates a mode in which there is no response to slow rates, but output is elicited by rapid rates, as in certain antitachycardia devices.

The fourth position describes the programming capability of the pulse generator. *P* refers to programmability of one or two parameters, usually rate and output. *M* indicates multiprogrammability of more than two programmable parameters such as rate, output, hysteresis, mode, sensitivity, and refractory period for single-chamber units and the AV delay for dual-chamber units. *C* indicates a communicating or telemetry function and implies multiprogrammability. *O* indicates that there is no programmability; it is used only if there is a designation in the next column.

The fifth position refers to special antitachycardia features. *B* designates bursts of impulses such as in rapid atrial pacing. *N* indicates normal rate competition as in the dual demand pacemaker. *S* stands for a scanning response such as timed extrasystoles. *E* stands for external control either by application of a magnet or radiofrequency. The control may be patient or physician activated. Recently it has been proposed that for simplicity the letter *A* should be used in this position when antitachycardia features are present.

Table 15–4 shows some examples of commonly used pacemakers and their ICHD designation.

Pacemaker Identification

Before the proper function of a pacemaker can be evaluated, the pacemaker model and its particular mode of operation must be known. For most VVI pacemakers this is not as crucial, since they are all very similar in their mode of operation. For dual-chamber pacemakers it

Table 15–3. ICHD Five-Position Pacemaker Code

Position				
I	II	III	IV	V
Category				
Chamber(s) Paced	Chamber(s) Sensed	Mode of Response(s)	Programmable Functions	Special Tachy-arrhythmia Functions
Letters used				
V = Ventricle	V = Ventricle	T = Triggered	P = Programmable (rate and/or output)	B = Bursts
A = Atrium	A = Atrium	I = Inhibited	M = Multiprogrammable	N = Normal rate competition
D = Double	D = Double	D = Double[a]	C = Communicating	S = Scanning (telemetry)
	O = None	R = Reverse	O = None	O = None
		O = None		E = External

[a] Atrial triggered, atrial and ventricular inhibited.

Table 15–4. Intersociety Commission for Heart Disease Codes of Commonly Used Pacemakers

ICHD Code	Generic Description	Previously Used Description
VVI	Ventricular pacing and sensing, inhibited mode, not programmable	Ventricular demand, standby, R-wave inhibited
VOO	Ventricular pacing, no sensing function	Fixed rate, asynchronous
VVI, MO	Ventricular pacing and sensing, inhibited mode, multiprogrammable	Ventricular demand, adjustable
AAI	Atrial pacing and sensing, inhibited mode	Atrial demand, P inhibited
AOO	Atrial pacing, no sensing	Atrial fixed rate, asynchronous
DVI, MO	AV pacing, ventricular sensing, inhibited mode, multiprogrammable	AV sequential, bifocal
DDD, MO	Atrial and ventricular pacing, atrial and ventricular sensing, atrial triggered, atrial inhibited, ventricular inhibited, multiprogrammable	Fully automatic, universal dual chamber
VDD, MO	Ventricular pacing, atrial and ventricular sensing	Atrial sensing, ventricular inhibited pacing, (ASVIP)
AOO, OE	Atrial spacing, no sensing function, externally activated antitachycardia feature	Rapid atrial pacer
AAR, ON	Atrial pacing and sensing, activated by fast atrial rates normal rate competition at fast rates	

AV, atrioventricular.

is absolutely necessary to know the model, the last programmed settings, and certain other peculiarities in order to determine proper function.

The simplest way to obtain this information is to check the patient identification card given to every recipient of an implantable pulse generator (IPG). This card contains information about the model, the date of implant, leads used, and the rate. If the IPG is programmable, the card often says so. It may also have a space for the last programmed parameters.

When this information is not readily available, a chest x-ray usually shows enough of the IPG to identify its manufacturer and possibly its model (Fig. 15–1). If faced with an unfamiliar model, the reference book "A Guide to Cardiac Pacemakers" may help with precise identification.[8]

When a patient with a pacemaker is prepared for a surgical procedure, it is important to determine whether the IPG is of unipolar or bipolar configuration. The unipolar generator has a lead with a stimulating electrode (the cathode) in the chamber being paced. The ground or anode in this system is the case of the generator. The bipolar generator has both stimulating and ground electrodes within the paced chamber. This type of configuration is much less susceptible to electromagnetic interference from outside sources or from myopotentials.[9–11] In procedures that may involve use of electrocautery or nerve stimulators it is important to know which type of pacing configuration is being used so that there is no risk of inhibiting the pacemaker output when the patient is pacemaker dependent.

The ECG can also be used to confirm the pacing configuration (Fig. 15–2). In the unipolar type, the amplitude of the pacing stimulus is usually larger than that of the resulting ventricular complex (in a ventricular pacemaker). The bipolar generators, with both electrodes within the heart, has a pacing stimulus of much smaller amplitude which may not be noticeable in some leads of the surface electrocardiogram. The appearance of the lead on the chest x-ray will reveal whether it is unipolar or bipolar (Fig. 15–3). In some instances a bipolar lead may

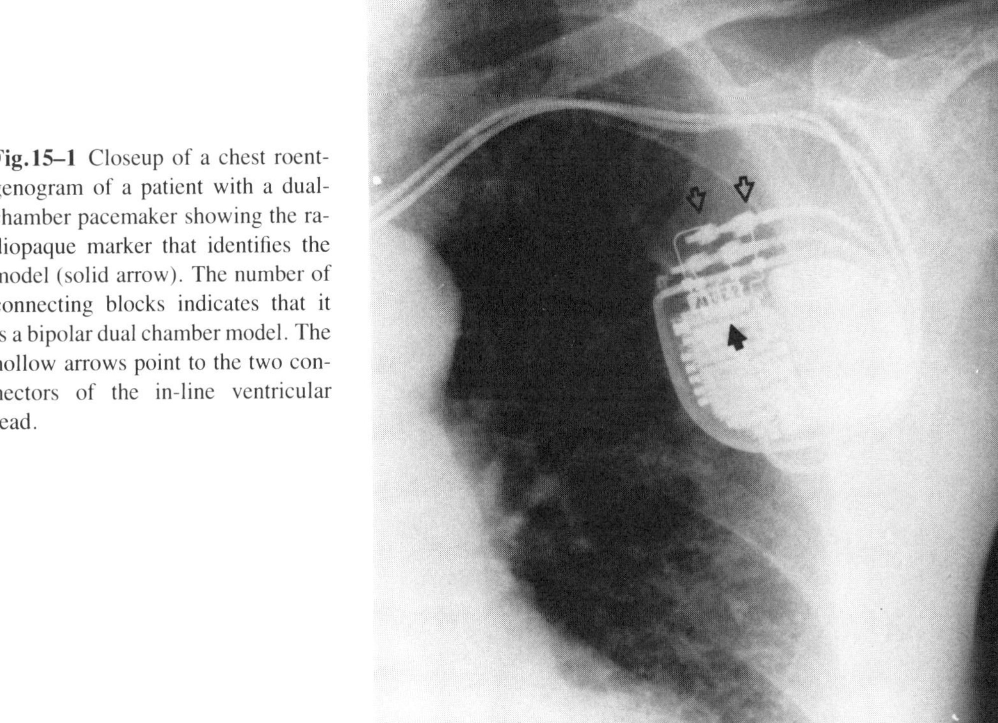

Fig. 15–1 Closeup of a chest roentgenogram of a patient with a dual-chamber pacemaker showing the radiopaque marker that identifies the model (solid arrow). The number of connecting blocks indicates that it is a bipolar dual chamber model. The hollow arrows point to the two connectors of the in-line ventricular lead.

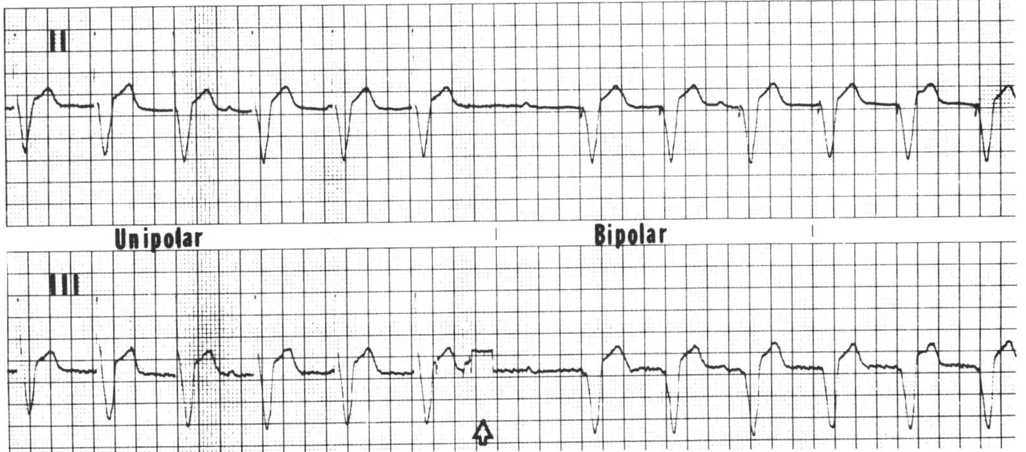

Fig. 15–2 Simultaneous lead II and III ECG of a patient with a pacemaker that can be programmed to the unipolar or bipolar configuration. The left-hand side shows the large pacing artifact produced on the surface ECG with unipolar pacing. The pacemaker was programmed to the bipolar mode (arrow). The bipolar pacing artifact is very small in lead II and is not noticeable in lead III.

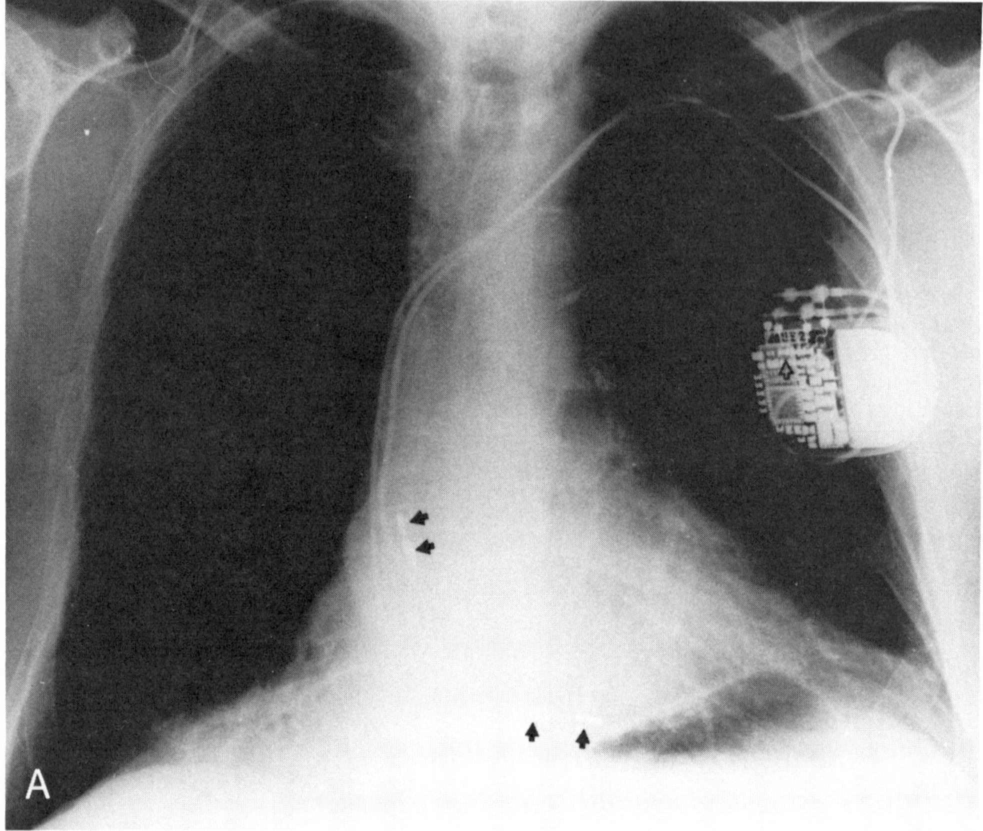

Fig. 15–3 Radiographic appearance of a bipolar dual-chamber pacemaker in (**A**) PA and lateral (**B**) views. The solid arrows point to the two electrodes of the atrial lead located in the right atrial appendage and the two electrodes of the ventricular lead near the right ventricular apex. The hollow arrow points to the identifying radiographic marker. (*Figure continues.*)

be unipolarized, which means that the tip or marked electrode is used as the cathode and the unmarked or proximal electrode is not used and capped. This may give the radiographic appearance of a loose wire.

Programmable Parameters

Most of the pacemakers in use today are programmable. They permit prescribing the precise settings that will give a good safety margin and best suit the patient's particular indication for pacing.[12]

Each individual pacemaker manufacturer has a programming device for use with its pacemakers. The programmer must be matched to the pacemaker, as currently no universal programmer is available. These devices emit a coded radiofrequency message to the pacemaker changing one or several parameters at a time. Telemetry-equipped IPGs will directly confirm that programming has occurred. Others depend on a specific signal or an ECG obtained during pacing for confirmation of programming. For safety, programming should always be done while observing the ECG. The most common programmable parameters are as follows:

Rate
Output

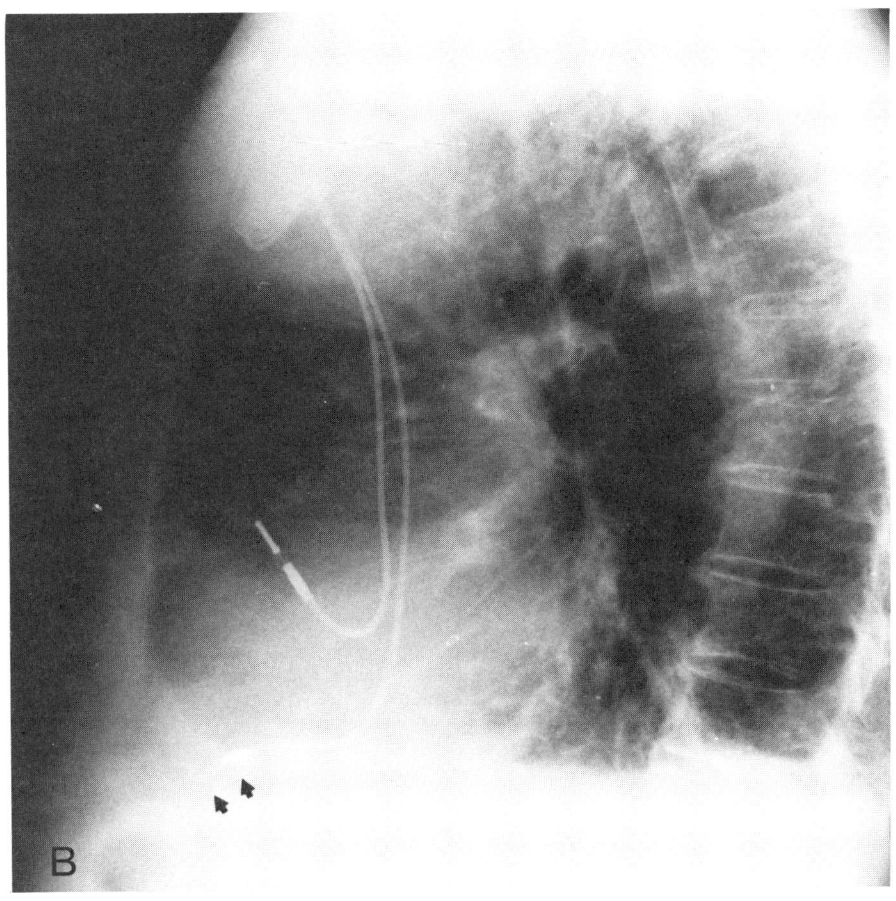

Fig. 15–3 (**B**) (*continued*).

Mode
Sensitivity
Refractory period
Hysteresis
AV delay

Some of the situations in which these parameters may require programming are briefly reviewed.

RATE

The rate may be increased:

1. To improve cardiac output especially during the perioperative period[13]
2. To override the patient's intrinsic rhythm and confirm capture of the pacing stimulus
3. To suppress ectopic rhythms
4. For rapid atrial pacing to terminate atrial flutter and supraventricular tachycardias[14]

The rate may be decreased:

1. To evaluate the underlying rhythm
2. To check for pacemaker dependency
3. To allow the patient to remain in sinus rhythm and restore AV synchrony. This can be the initial treatment for patients who develop the pacemaker syndrome or intolerance to ventricular pacing during the postimplant period

In some models the rate may be transiently decreased to zero by programming the IPG to

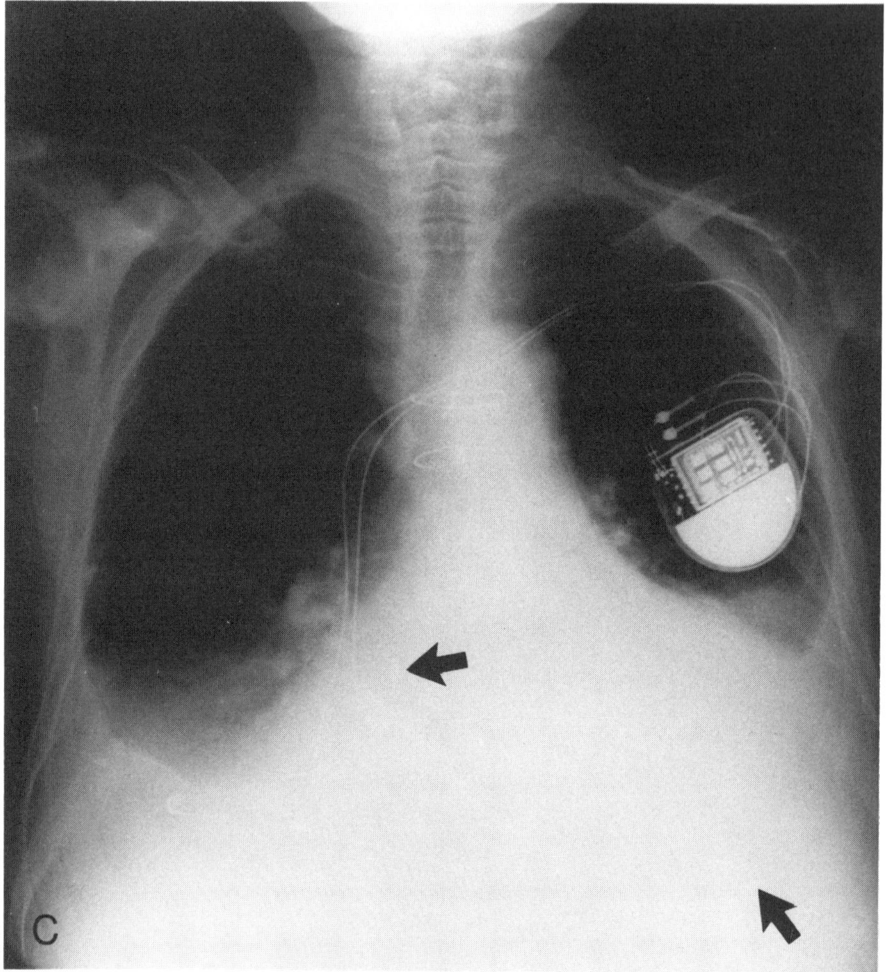

Fig. 15–3 (C) (*continued*) Radiographic appearance of a unipolar dual-chamber pacemaker. The arrows point to the atrial and ventricular electrodes within the heart. Note the single connecting blocks for each lead in the pacemaker generator.

an off mode or by inhibiting the output. Most pacemakers have a lower rate limit of 30 or 40 ppm.

Dual-chamber pacemakers working in the DDD mode have both a lower rate and maximum tracking rate. The lower rate indicates that both atrial and ventricular pacing will occur if there is no intrinsic activity and no AV conduction. If the atrial intrinsic rhythm is between these two limits, the atrial activity is sensed, it inhibits atrial output and starts timing an AV interval. If there is no ventricular activity by the end of this interval, ventricular pacing occurs. This is commonly referred to as atrial tracking and ventricular pacing (Fig. 15–4). If, on the other hand, the atrial activity is above the maximum tracking rate, the rate of ventricular pacing is limited either by a Wenckebach phenomenon, a fall-back rate or a variable (4 : 3, 3 : 2, or even 2 : 1) AV block, depending on how the pacemaker is designed and programmed.[15]

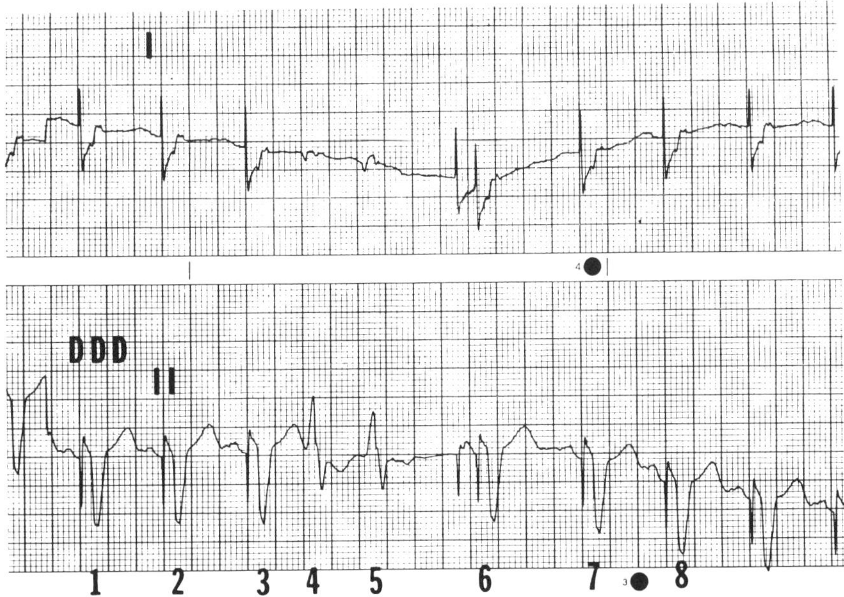

Fig. 15–4 Simultaneous lead I and II ECGs of a patient with a dual-chamber (DDD) pacemaker. For most complexes the pacemaker is sensing the atrial activity and pacing the ventricle after the appropriate AV delay (complexes 1, 2, 3, 7, and 8). P waves are not easily detectable in lead I, showing that it is preferable to have a simultaneous multiple-lead tracing for interpretation. Ventricular premature events inhibit the atrial and ventricular outputs (complexes 4 and 5). After an escape interval determined by the lower rate minus the AV delay, there is atrial and ventricular sequential pacing (complex 6).

OUTPUT

The output can be modified by controlling one or more of the variables that control the energy of the pacing stimulus: pulse width, current, and voltage. In simple programmable pacers only the pulse width can be modified. Multiprogrammable units permit current or voltage modification in addition to the pulse width. This gives greater flexibility in adjusting the energy of the pacing stimulus.

The output may be increased:

1. To provide a greater margin of safety for capture (a margin of 3 : 1 is adequate in the acute implant situation)
2. To regain capture, if it has been lost or is intermittent
3. To check for diaphragmatic or pectoral muscle stimulation

It may be decreased:

1. To conserve battery charge and prolong the useful life of the IPG
2. To check stimulation thresholds noninvasively (Fig. 15–5)
3. To diminish pectoral or diaphragmatic stimulation
4. To inactivate the pacemaker or one of its channels

MODE

Almost all pacemakers will revert to the asynchronous mode (AOO, VOO, DOO) when a magnet is placed over them. This is one method of programming, which can be done without a specific programming device. Applying a magnet or programming to the asynchronous mode will allow for testing of capture when the pa-

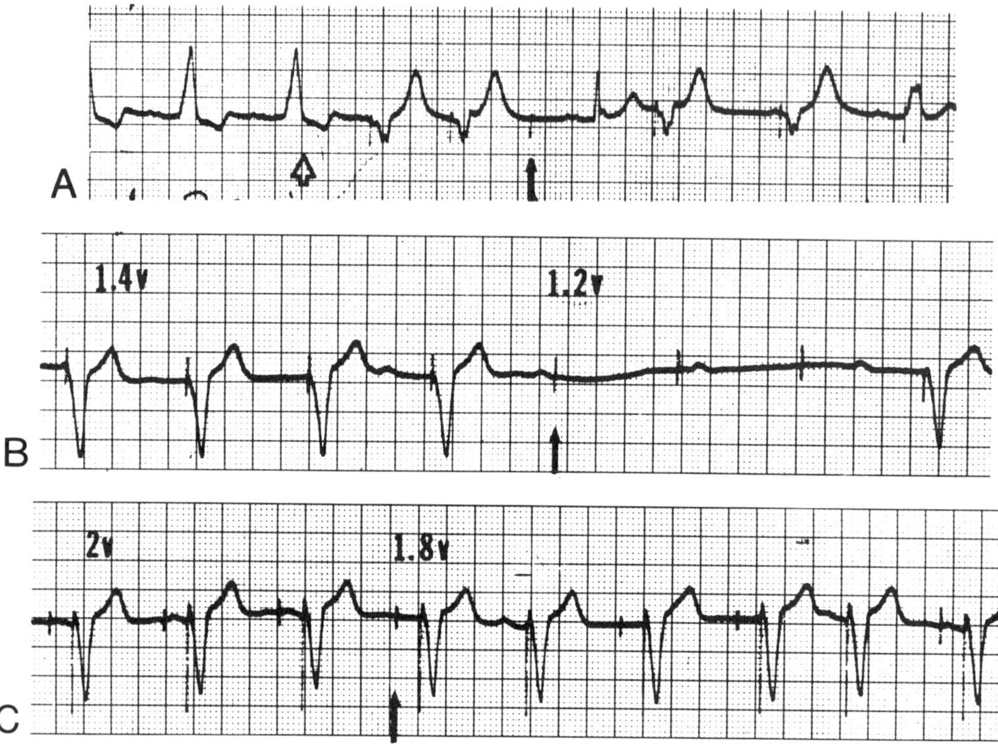

Fig. 15–5 (**A**) Application of a magnet (hollow arrow) to this VVI pacemaker starts asynchronous pacing at a rate of 100 ppm. The third impulse at this rate is at a 25 percent lower output. In this case, as the pacemaker output was very close to the stimulation threshold, the reduction of 25 percent caused loss of capture (solid arrow). The pacemaker continues pacing asynchronously at the programmed rate with the full output. (**B**) The ouput is decreased in a threshold testing sequence. At 1.4 volts, there is complete capture. As the output is decreased to 1.2 volts, there is loss of capture (arrow) until a higher output is restored (last complex). The stimulation threshold is 1.4 volts at the pulsewidth used. (**C**) Atrial thresholds are similarly measured by decreasing the atrial output. At 2 volts, there is complete capture and P waves are seen between the A and V pacing stimuli. At 1.8 volts, the AV interval is isoelectric, denoting loss of atrial capture. The atrial threshold is 2 volts. After atrial capture is lost, intrinsic P waves are occasionally observed (complexes 5 and 8). This is sensed and elicits ventricular pacing after the AV delay. Atrial capture is restored in the last complex.

tient's intrinsic rate is faster than the set lower rate of the IPG and the pacemaker is thus inhibited (Fig. 15–6).

In patients with a unipolar pacemaker who may be pacemaker dependent, the IPG should be programmed to the asynchronous mode at an appropriate rate during operations in which electrocautery is to be used. This is safer than the temporary use of a magnet, which may lose its position with movement. A moving magnet may also temporarily inhibit some IPGs.

Programming to a triggered mode (VVT) is useful to assess the sensing function of the IPG (Fig. 15–7). As a permanent setting it can be used when a high sensitivity setting is needed, but the patient should not be left unprotected against inhibition by electromagnetic interference from myopotentials or outside sources.

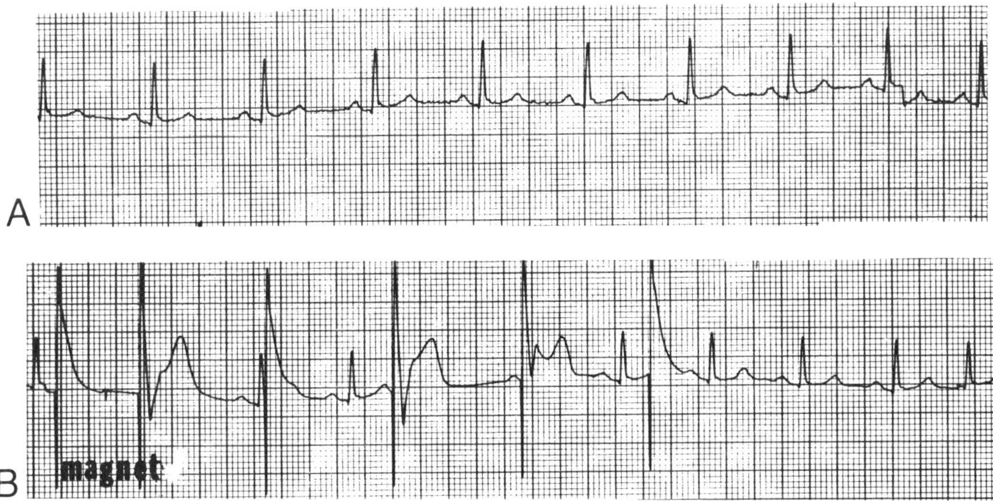

Fig. 15–6 (**A**) The pacemaker is in the VVI mode and the intrinsic rate is faster than the programmed lower rate. There are no pacing artifacts. It could be inferred that the pacer was sensing properly. However, an IPG with no output would give a similar picture. (**B**) A magnet was applied. The pacemaker is now in the VOO mode (asynchronous) so there is no sensing. Capture is noted in the second and fourth complexes. The first and last pacing artifacts fall within the absolute refractory period and do not produce capture. In this unipolar pacemaker there is distortion of the baseline (afterpotential), which could be mistaken for capture. The third and fifth complexes are pseudofusion and fusion beats, respectively.

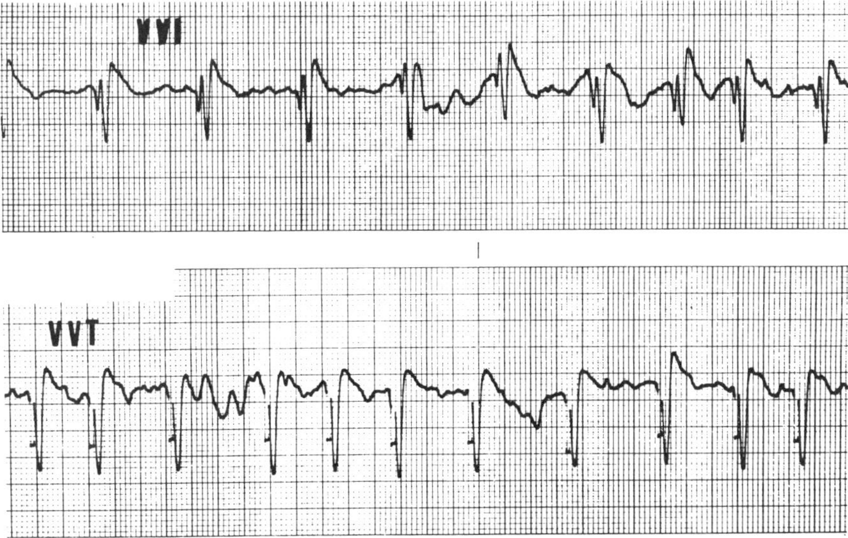

Fig. 15–7 Patient with atrial fibrillation at a fast rate. There are no pacing artifacts in the VVI mode. Application of a magnet (not shown) produced complexes with large afterpotentials similar to those seen in the preceding figure; capture was documented. To help assess sensing, the pacer was programmed to VVT mode. Sensed ventricular complexes elicited pacing artifacts. Note that the pacing interval is very irregular, as it is triggered by the patient's intrinsic rhythm.

DVI pacing has been advocated to prevent rapid tracking rates in dual chamber systems when the patient is prone to have rapid atrial tachyarrhythmias. However, setting a maximum tracking rate while in the DDD mode is probably more effective, as it maintains AV synchrony and avoids competition in the atrial channel, which can produce atrial fibrillation.[16]

SENSITIVITY

This setting (programmable parameter) refers to the lowest-amplitude signal that will be detected by the sensing amplifier and interpreted as a cardiac event. The pacemaker sensing circuitry depends on a signal from the endocardial or epicardial electrogram of sufficient amplitude (millivolts) and slew rate (volts/second) to be considered an intrinsic deflection (R wave or P wave). Signals of lesser amplitude or insufficient slew rate will be rejected. In this way only true P waves and R waves will be sensed, and T waves, myopotentials, or other electromagnetic signals are less likely to interfere with pacemaker function.

A higher sensitivity is indicated by a lower number of millivolts. The usual nominal settings of a ventricular IPG are 1.6 to 2.5 mV. This gives a margin of safety of 2 : 1 or 3 : 1, as the usual accepted R-wave amplitude is more than 5 mV. Lesser amplitude signals are usually not accepted and the lead is repositioned or a different configuration chosen.[17] Atrial sensitivity settings of 0.6 to 1 mV are usual, as the P-wave amplitude is 1.5 to 2.5 mV.

In patients with low-amplitude P- or R-wave signals, sensitivity settings may need to be increased (set to a lower millivolt value) (Fig. 15–8). They are decreased (set to a higher mV value) to prevent problems with myopotential tracking of the atrial channel (in DDD pacemakers) or inhibition of the ventricular channel (in DDD, DVI, or VVI pacemakers). In certain cases of myopotential inhibition, the ventricular channel may need to be made completely insensitive. This is accomplished by programming to the asynchronous mode (DOO, VOO, AOO) (Fig. 15–9). Use of bipolar pacing systems virtually eliminates this problem.[17,18]

REFRACTORY PERIOD

This is the time after a paced or sensed event during which the IPG sensing circuit is insensitive to incoming signals. It is lengthened to eliminate problems with T-wave sensing in VVI pacers. This will lead to prolonged inhibition and a very slow rate. Retrograde P-wave sensing in VDD or DDD pacemakers may initiate pacemaker-mediated tachycardias, unless the atrial refractory period is appropriately lengthened.

The usual settings are 250 to 325 msec for VVI pacemakers, and 400 msec for AAI pacemakers. For DDD systems, the atrial refractory period (postventricular atrial refractory period

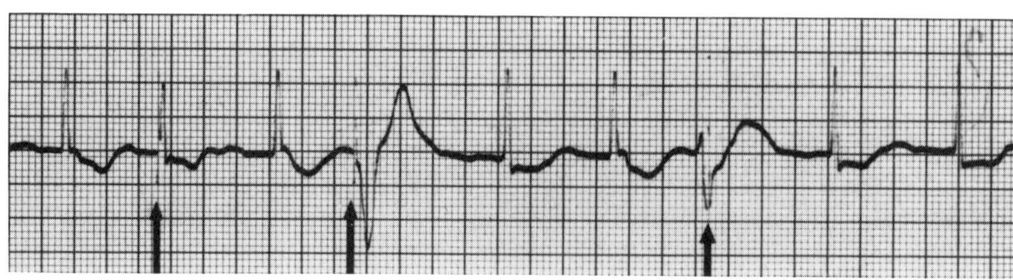

Fig. 15–8 Intermittent failure to sense. The pacing artifact occurs too soon after the previous intrinsic complex. The first two arrows show the pacing outputs after nonsensed complexes and denote the pacing interval. The next R waves is sensed properly, but the following one is not. The pacing interval is identical to the interval between the properly sensed R wave and the last pacing complex (last arrow).

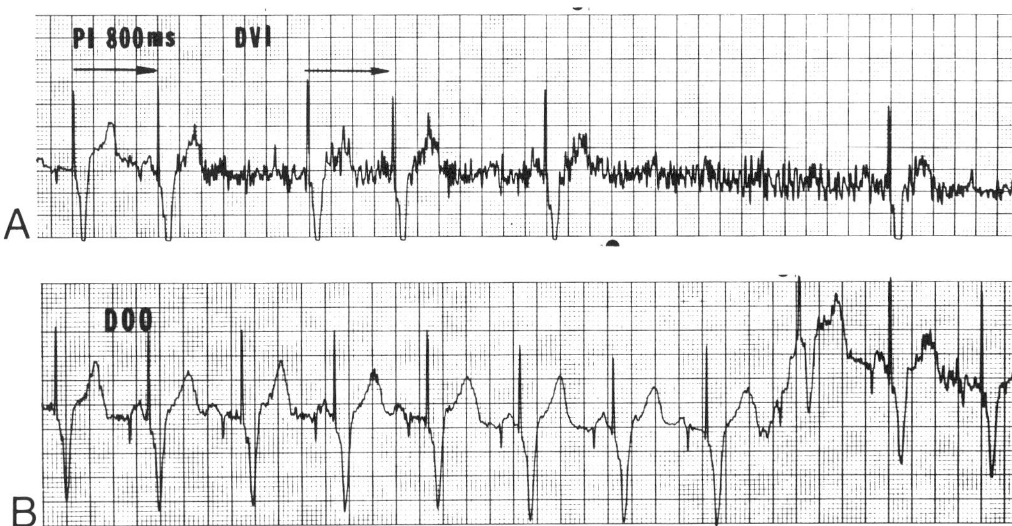

Fig. 15–9 (**A**) Myopotential inhibition in a DVI unipolar pacemaker set at the least sensitive setting. The pacing interval (PI) is 800 msec (arrow). With provocative maneuvers such as pressing both hands together in front of the chest, myopotentials are noted on the surface electrocardiogram and are of sufficient intensity to cause inhibition of the ventricular output. Note the longer pacing intervals without any intrinsic ventricular activity. This patient was symptomatic with syncopal episodes even after programming to the least sensitive setting. (**B**) The pacemaker has been programmed to the asynchronous mode (DOO). AV sequential pacing is noted throughout with uniform pacing intervals during provocative manneuvers. The patient's symptoms were abolished.

or PVARP) is set between 250 and 325 msec to eliminate tracking of retrograde P waves after a PVC or a ventricular paced event (Fig. 15–10). Retrograde VA conduction is measured during the implant procedure (Fig. 15–11), and the atrial refractory period is set at least 50 msec more than the measured value. It must be recognized that long atrial refractory periods will limit the maximum tracking rate of the pacemaker, since the pacing interval is equal to the sum of the AV interval and the atrial refractory period. Some pacemakers allow for faster tracking rates by a feature that extends the atrial refractory period after a PVC.

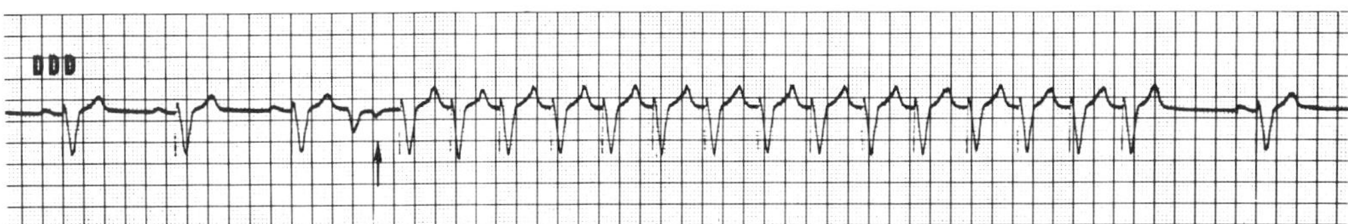

Fig. 15–10 Pacemaker-mediated tachycardia occurring in a patient with retrograde VA conduction. The fourth complex is a PVC, which produces a retrograde P wave (arrow). This P falls beyond the atrial refractory period and elicits ventricular pacing. With the loss of AV synchrony, retrograde P waves are produced with each ventricular paced complex. In this case, the tachycardia terminated spontaneously. Extension of the atrial refractory period would have obviated this problem.

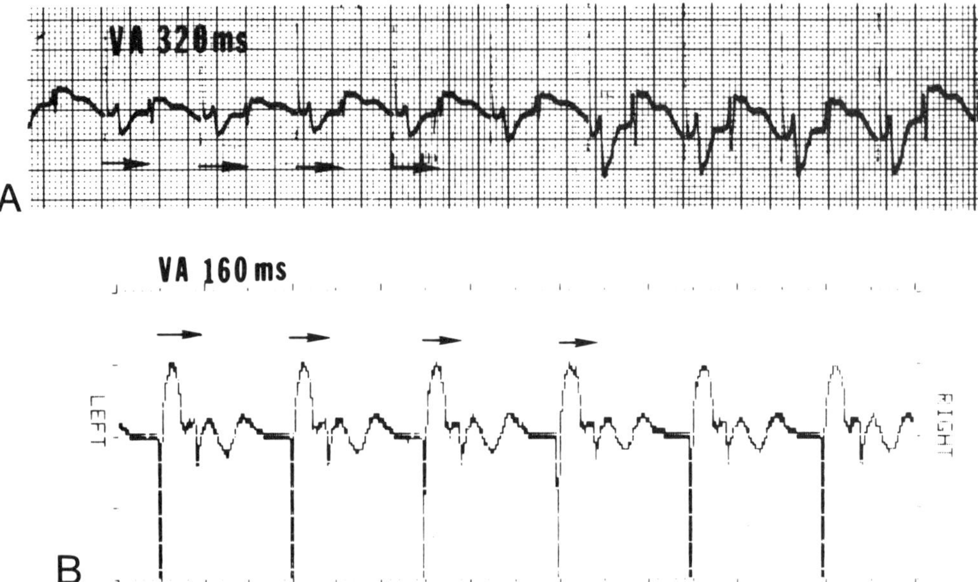

Fig. 15–11 (**A**) Intraoperative atrial endocardial electrogram during ventricular pacing. The arrows indicate the ventriculoatrial conduction interval between the ventricular pacing stimulus and the P wave intrinsic deflection. The amplitude of the tracing was increased on the right-hand side. (**B**) Telemetered atrial endocardial electrograms during ventricular pacing in a different patient. The large deflections are ventricular pacing stimuli. The arrows indicate the VA conduction interval, and the smaller sharp deflections are the telemetered intrinsic deflections of the P waves.

HYSTERESIS

This is a delay before the onset of ventricular pacing after sensing an intrinsic R wave. Actual pacing occurs at a faster rate. The pacing rate can be set at 50 ppm, for example, but hysteresis equivalent to a rate of 40 ppm may be programmed so that as long as the patient has an intrinsic rate above 40 ppm he will not be paced. If the intrinsic rate is less than 40 ppm the pacemaker starts to pace at 50 ppm until an intrinsic R wave is sensed (Fig. 15–12). In theory, this is a perfectly reasonable way of allowing the patient to have AV synchrony more often. However, some patients may be made uncomfortable with a slow hysteresis and a much

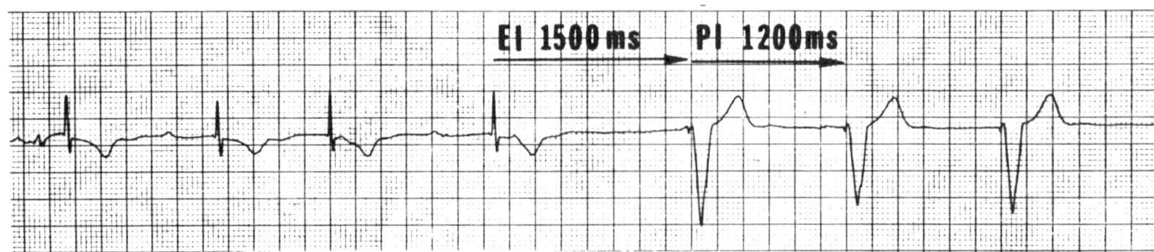

Fig. 15–12 Hysteresis. The pacing interval is 1,200 msec, or a rate of 50 ppm. The interval between the last sensed complex and the first paced one, the escape interval (EI) is 1,500 msec, longer than the pacing interval.

faster pacing rate and may stay in the pacing mode most of the time, so that the actual settings have to be tailored to the individual.

AV DELAY

This can be considered the equivalent of the PR interval on a nonpaced ECG. It is the time between the atrial pacing stimulus and the ventricular pacing stimulus or between the sensed P-wave intrinsic deflection and either a paced ventricular output or a sensed R wave intrinsic deflection. During this period, the atrial channel is refractory to any other atrial activity, while the ventricular channel is sensing. If there is normal conduction through the AV node or if a PVC occurs, the ventricular output is normally inhibited.

The usual setting is 150 to 175 msec. It may be temporarily shortened to test for ventricular capture in patients with normal AV conduction. In some situations it can be lengthened to test for AV conduction (Fig. 15–13), or to allow AV conduction to occur on a chronic basis. However, it has been found, using pulsed-doppler determination of cardiac output during DVI pacing, that it is usually preferable to pace the ventricle with an AV delay of around 150 to 175 msec rather than permit intrinsic AV conduction at AV delays of more than 225 msec.[19]

Patients who are paced primarily for sinus node dysfunction, however, may be more comfortable with longer AV delays to allow for intrinsic AV conduction. At the same time this saves the pacemaker battery since ventricular pacing occurs much less frequently than with a shorter AV delay.

Hemodynamic Effects of Cardiac Pacing

Initially, ventricular pacemakers provided a satisfactory hemodynamic alternative for patients with severe bradycardia and complete heart block. In the early days of cardiac pacing, most patients fell into this category.

As more reliable leads and pulse generators became available, pacemakers were used in prophylactic situations for patients with infrequent episodes of severe bradycardia or asystole who were otherwise in sinus rhythm most of the time. Ventricular pacing in these patients led to the elimination of syncopal episodes, but many would complain of fatigue, severe limitation in activity, and dizziness; and some were made worse than before the pacemaker implant, with signs of congestive heart failure and hypotension. These patients suffered from what has become known as the pacemaker syndrome. This syndrome is caused by several factors: (1) loss of AV synchrony, (2) retrograde ventriculoatrial conduction with atrial contractions

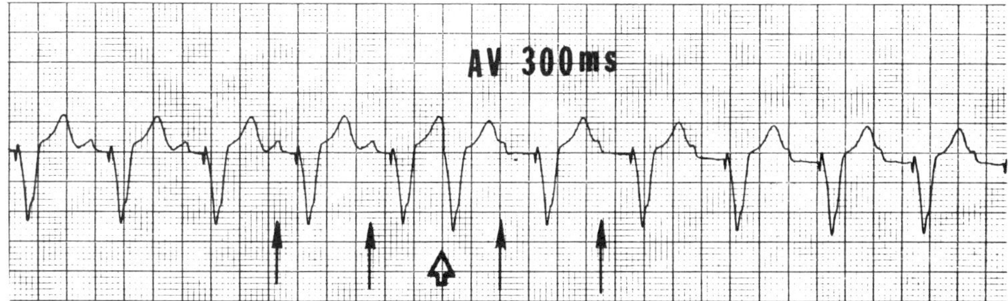

Fig. 15–13 The AV delay has been lengthened from 175 msec to 300 msec by programming (open arrow). The solid arrows point to the sensed P waves. Note that for the complexes following the programming to a longer AV delay the P waves are almost obscured by the preceding T waves. Intrinsic AV conduction did not occur in this trial.

against closed AV valves, resulting in cannon a waves or functional tricuspid and mitral regurgitation, and (3) the lack of ability to respond to changes in activity by a change in heart rate.[20]

Improved hemodynamic performance in these patients is usually achieved by one of the following maneuvers.

RATE AUGMENTATION

Increasing the ventricular pacing rate usually results in an increase in the cardiac output. However, there is a maximal heart rate beyond which the beneficial effects are lost and this limit varies from patient to patient. In a person at rest, once this limit is exceeded there is a progressive decrease in stroke volume as a result of a compromised diastolic filling period. During exercise, however, with improved contractility as a result of endogenous catecholamines, the limit is reached at a faster rate and a higher output.

Patients with ventricular pacemakers at a fixed rate can also increase cardiac output in periods of exercise or stress as a result of increased release of endogenous catecholamines and improved contractility. This method of response is slower than that obtained by increasing the heart rate. Increasing the rate with and without AV synchrony is clearly associated with a greater cardiac output within the limits mentioned above.[13,21] At rest, AV synchrony seems to play a greater role in improving the cardiac output; whereas with exercise, the faster rate is more important.

It may be useful in the perioperative situation to increase the pacing rate (provided the patient has a programmable generator) to meet the increased demands of the surgical stress. Because of the lack of AV synchrony, in ventricular-paced patients it will be necessary to use higher-than-usual filling pressures to achieve this goal as these patients depend exclusively on the passive ventricular filling phase of early to mid-diastole. The combination of these measures is likely to work best in patients with atrial fibrillation or junctional rhythms or in those with very slow atrial rates and complete heart block.

In patients with sick sinus syndrome who are usually in sinus rhythm and have an intact AV conduction, an increase in ventricular pacing rate can make the situation worse as AV synchrony and the atrial contribution to the cardiac output are eliminated. A vicious circle could be started in patients with a compromised ventricle if the cardiac output is reduced and the release of endogenous catecholamines results in increased afterload without improvement in contractility. Only atrial pacing is likely to significantly improve the cardiac output in these patients. However, if there is an AV block, AV sequential pacing (DVI) with an appropriate AV delay can accomplish the same goals.

AV SYNCHRONY

The atrial contribution to cardiac output has been measured at 10 to 30 percent of the total cardiac output. During atrial or AV-sequential pacing at any given rate, the cardiac output can be expected to be 10 to 30 percent greater than with ventricular pacing alone because the properly timed atrial contraction improves ventricular filling (Fig. 15–14).[13,22]

This is of particular importance in patients with decreased ventricular compliance, such as those with hypertension, aortic stenosis, or previous myocardial infarctions.[23] It has indeed been demonstrated that in these patients ventricular filling greatly depends on the late active phase of diastolic filling.

The proper timing is crucial. If a very short AV delay (less than 100 msec) is chosen, there may not be sufficient time for atrial contraction before the ventricular contraction occurs and the result may be worse than with ventricular pacing alone. With a long AV delay, the mitral and tricuspid valves will still be open during the initial isovolumic phase of ventricular contraction, and some regurgitation will occur, decreasing the cardiac output. There is a slight delay between the atrial pacing stimulus and

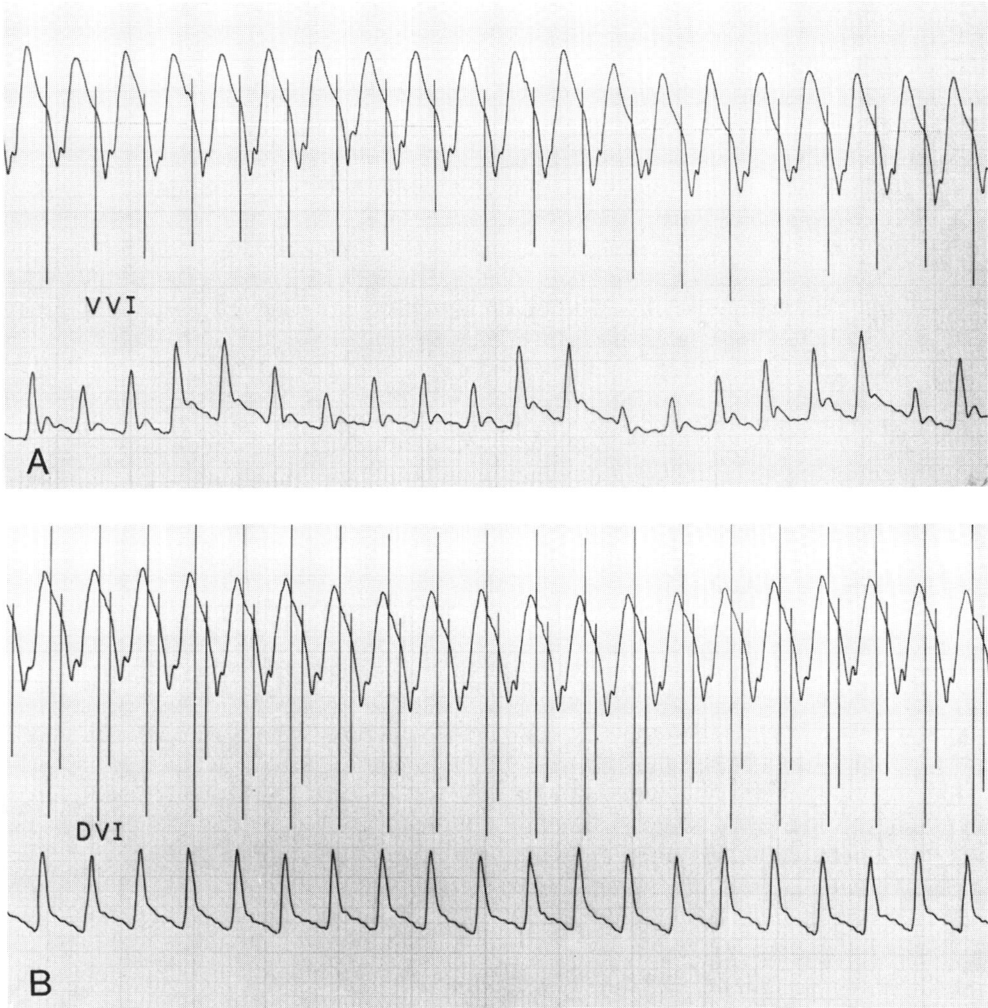

Fig. 15–14 (**A**) Arterial pressure tracing during VVI pacing shows beat-to-beat variation, which is dependent on the timing of the previous P wave. The P waves are not visible because of the wide QRS complex and the fast rate. (**B**) Arterial pressure tracing in the same patient during AV sequential pacing (DVI) at the same rate. The pulse tracing is very uniform, as AV synchrony as been restored.

the onset of the P wave (Fig. 15–15). In some patients the interval between the atrial impulse and the P wave can be considerably prolonged. As a result, the ventricular impulse must also be delayed to achieve an ideal physiologic interval between atrial and ventricular contractions. Some dual-chamber pacemakers achieve an optimal AV sequence by having variable AV delays which are longer after paced atrial impulses than after sensed P waves.

PREOPERATIVE ASSESSMENT OF PACEMAKER FUNCTION

In a patient with a pacemaker, a thorough preoperative evaluation includes preoperative assessment of pacemaker function. This assessment begins with the questions: Is the patient pacemaker dependent? What is the underlying intrinsic rhythm? What was the original indication for pacing? Is the pacemaker functioning

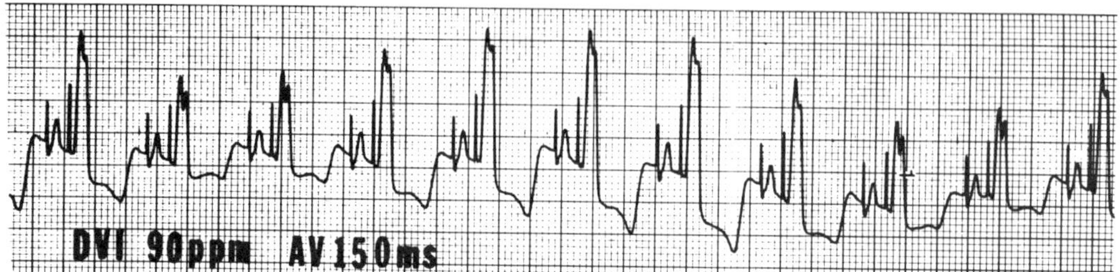

Fig. 15–15 AV sequential pacing with a AV delay of 150 msec. If the delay between the atrial stimulus and the P wave is longer than in this example, the interval between atrial and ventricular contractions could be too short for optimal hemodynamic benefit.

properly? Is the planned operation likely to interfere with pacemaker function? Is the generator a unipolar or a bipolar model? Is any adjustment advisable prior to the procedure?

Pacemaker Dependency

An estimate of pacemaker dependency can often be obtained from the history and knowledge of the initial indication for pacemaker insertion. Indeed, patients with complete heart block or those with severe bradycardia are more likely to be pacemaker dependent. They may become asystolic or extremely bradycardic, should the pacemaker suddenly be inhibited or malfunction as a result of intraoperative conditions. Those with sick sinus syndrome or bifascicular block are less likely to be dependent.

However, pacemaker dependency can be intermittent and is therefore best evaluated by programming. The pacemaker rate is set at 30 to 40 beats/min and the appearance of the patient's intrinsic rhythm is observed. If no intrinsic rhythm appears with this temporary reduction in pacing rate, it can be assumed that the patient is pacemaker-dependent, and that conditions which cause interruption of pacing are extremely hazardous and may lead to asystole.

Some pacemakers can also be temporarily

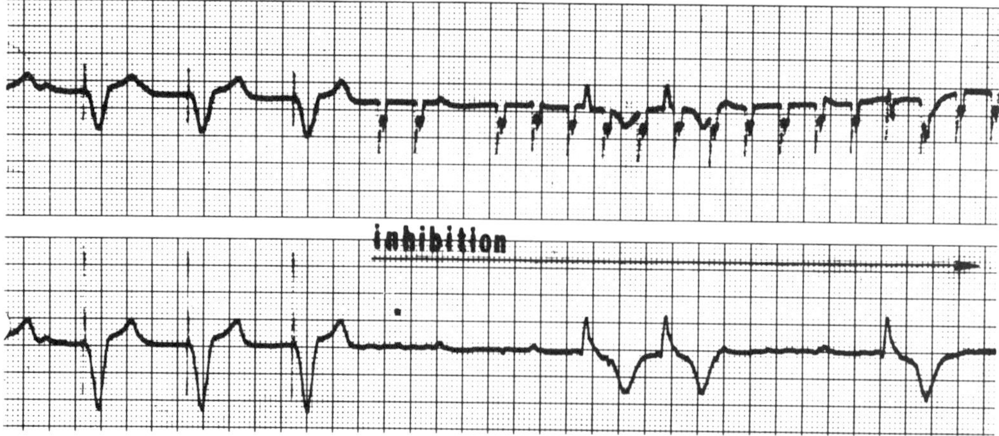

Fig. 15–16 Simultaneous two-lead ECG during pacemaker inhibition to assess the underlying rhythm. The top tracing shows the inhibiting impulses. These are not detectable in the bottom tracing, and the underlying rhythm can be easily seen.

inhibited by programming (Fig. 15–16). This may be of value in assessing the intrinsic complexes of the electrocardiogram for evidence of myocardial infarction.

Unipolar vs Bipolar Pacing Circuits

The unipolar pacing circuit has a lead with a single electrode in the chamber being paced. This is a stimulating electrode or cathode and is designated (−). The current path leads to the ground electrode or anode (+), which is located away from the heart, usually at the surface of the implanted generator. In a temporary pacemaker system, there may be an indifferent electrode within the subcutaneous tissue. The bipolar pacing circuit has both the cathode (−) or stimulating electrode and the anode (+) or ground electrode in the same lead within the paced chamber.

Each system has certain intrinsic advantages. In the unipolar circuit, the lead is of a smaller diameter, only a single set of thresholds needs to be obtained and the pacing artifact is easily identifiable on the surface electrocardiogram. A bipolar circuit requires a lead of a larger diameter that may be more difficult to insert. Its pacing artifact is much smaller and may be difficult to detect in some leads of the surface electrocardiogram (Fig. 15–2).

The most important difference between these two types of circuits is their susceptibility to electromagnetic interference. With the unipolar circuitry the lead forms a large antenna between the two electrodes and is much more susceptible to electromagnetic interference.[10,24] Electromagnetic interference (EMI) can be either exogenous,[25] from outside sources in the environment such as electrocautery, a powerful radio transmitter, spark-gap timers, diathermy, and nerve stimulators, or endogenous, from the patient, such as myopotentials.

This may not be clinically relevant if the patient has an adequate underlying rhythm most of the time, but is extremely important in the pacemaker-dependent individual.

Administration of depolarizing muscle relaxants can produce strong myopotentials during the period of fasciculation. These can inhibit the pacemaker and result in prolonged asystole.[9] If the patient has a programmable generator, the most reliable method of dealing with this potential problem is to program the pacemaker to an asynchronous mode (AOO, VOO, DOO) or to temporarily accomplish the same by applying a magnet over the generator. Using nondepolarizing agents is another alternative method. Still, during the course of an operation, the electrocautery can inhibit the pacemaker output or cause it to revert to asynchronous pacing, depending on the particular pacemaker model and the manner in which the cautery is applied. Use of nerve stimulators to monitor neuromuscular blockade can also have similar effects.[26] If they must be used, it is best to apply the stimulating electrodes to the side opposite the pacemaker. However, if the patient is grounded, the current path may

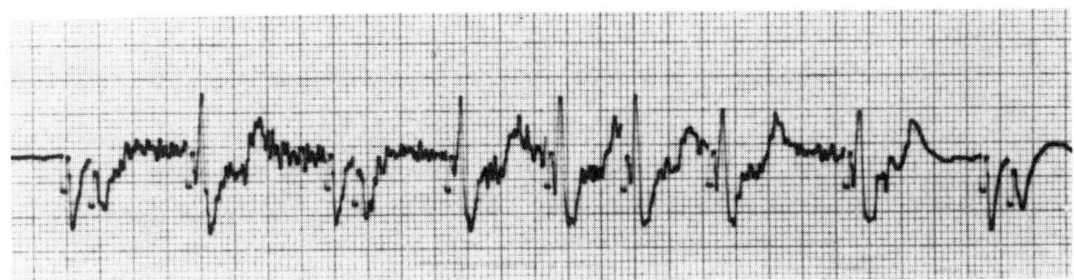

Fig. 15–17 Telephone-transmitted ECG of a patient with a dual-chamber (DDD) pacemaker who experienced palpitations while dressing. Ventricular pacing at or close to the maximum tracking rate was noted in the absence of P waves after the third complex. The problem was solved by decreasing the atrial sensitivity.

be such that its impulses are detected by the sensing amplifier and inhibit the pacemaker output.

In DDD pacemakers these same impulses can also be detected by the atrial channel and trigger ventricular pacing at fast rates to produce a type of pacemaker-mediated tachycardia due to EMI or myopotential tracking (Fig. 15–17).

Thus, for practical purposes, it is important to know the configuration (unipolar or bipolar) of the patient's pacemaker. If the operation will require one of the techniques that can result in inhibition of the ventricular output, appropriate programming should be done prior to surgery. If this is not possible, it is quite reasonable to monitor the patient with an arterial line or other pulse detector. Monitoring the ECG alone is not sufficient, since it is often sensitive to interference by electrocautery or may be difficult to interpret during fasciculations.

Capture and Thresholds

Once the patient's pacemaker model and the underlying rhythm have been defined, two other functions must be tested to document appropriate pacemaker function: capture and sensing.

Capture is readily confirmed by looking at the electrocardiogram. The ventricular pacing stimulus should always be followed by a ven-

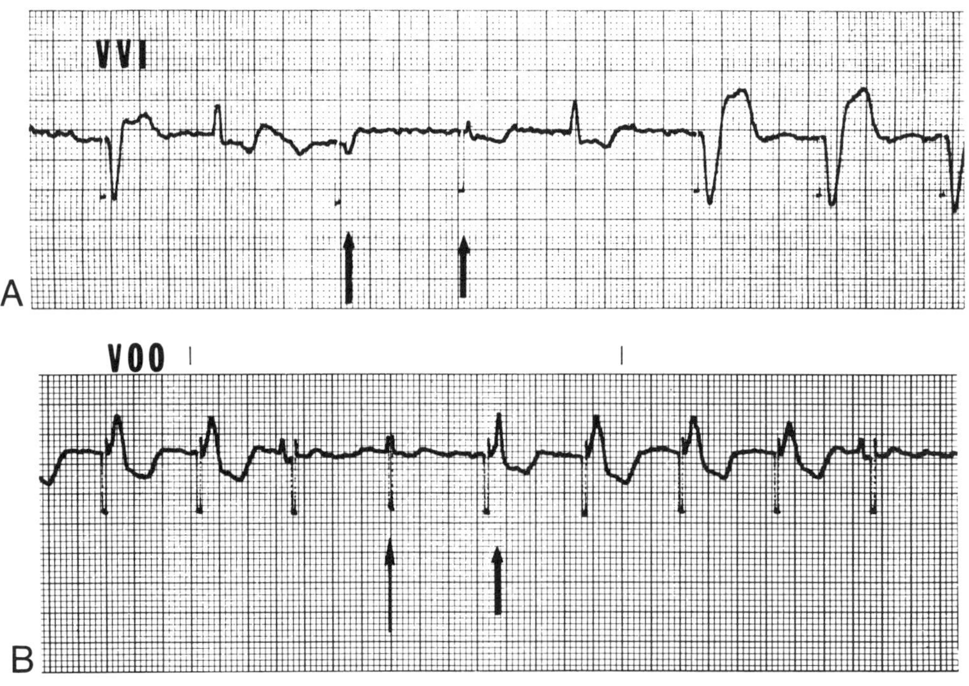

Fig. 15–18 (**A**) Fusion beats occurring during VVI pacing. The patient's intrinsic rhythm is close to the pacing rate. The first complex is paced, the second is an intrinsic beat. The third and fourth complexes (arrows) have a morphology that is almost isoelectric. This occurs when the paced and intrinsic complexes have opposite polarity on a given lead. (**B**) Fusion beat occurring during VOO pacing. In this case the appearance of the fusion beat (thick arrow) is intermediate between that of a paced and that of an intrinsic complex. The thin arrows show a pseudofusion beat with morphology similar to the intrinsic complex plus the ineffective pacing stimulus. The third and the last complexes are intrinsic complexes which are followed by pacing stimuli.

tricular depolarization with the typical LBBB pattern of right ventricular endocardial pacing. If the pacing rate is faster than the patient's intrinsic rhythm, complete capture is easily noted. If the two rates are close, some intrinsic impulses will inhibit the pacemaker and there will be no output. In this case another type of pattern is frequently seen. The fusion beat (Fig. 15–18) is a ventricular depolarization complex which occurs when the pacemaker stimulus falls just before the onset of the absolute refractory period and activates part of the ventricles. The resulting QRS morphology, due to activation from two different foci, is intermediate between that of a paced complex and the intrinsic rhythm. A pseudofusion beat occurs when the stimulus falls after the onset of the absolute refractory period. The QRS morphology is affected only slightly by the superimposed ineffective pacing stimulus.

Atrial capture is confirmed in two ways. One is by choosing a lead of the surface ECG in which the P waves are prominent, such as lead II, V_1, or a Lewis lead, and noting the P waves after each atrial pacing stimulus (Fig. 15–19). The other method is applicable only if the patient has intact AV conduction. Even if the P waves are not easily seen, the presence of an intrinsic ventricular depolarization after the PR interval is evidence of atrial capture. A dual-chamber pacemaker (DDD or DVI) may have to be programmed to a long AV delay in order to allow for AV conduction and use of this method of testing for atrial capture. With ventricular or atrial demand (VVI or AAI) or dual-chamber pacemakers (DDD, DVI), no pacemaker activity may be seen on the ECG (Fig. 15–6A) when the patient's intrinsic rhythm is faster than the lower rate limit of the pacemaker and sensing is adequate. To confirm capture, the pacemaker is transiently programmed to pace in the asynchronous mode (VOO, AOO, DOO) by application of a magnet (Figs. 15–6B and 15–18B). There may be some competition with the intrinsic rhythm, and pacing stimuli falling within the refractory period of the myocardium (phase 1 and 2 of the cardiac action potential) will be seen, but these cannot produce a second depolarization (third and last complexes, Fig. 15–18B). Stimuli that fall within the sensitive period will elicit depolarization and confirm capture. Sensing will be confirmed by transiently lowering the pacemaker rate or by programming to a triggered mode.

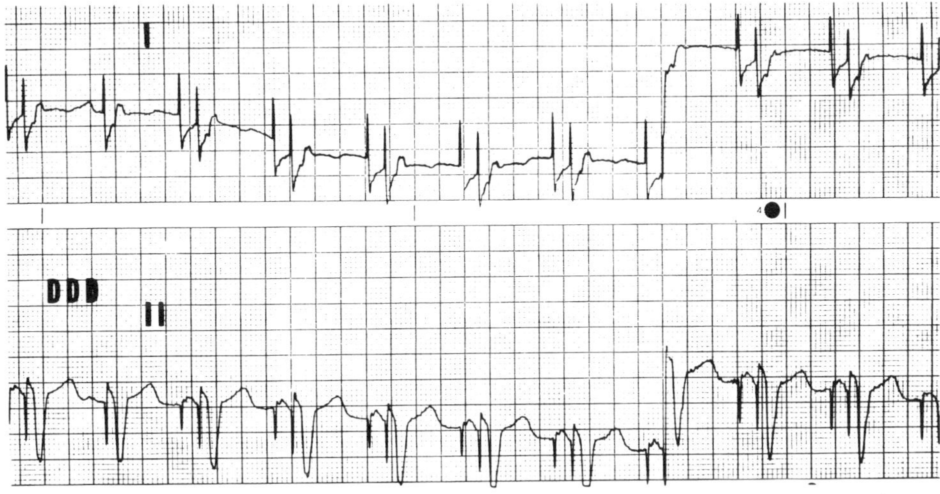

Fig. 15–19 The choice of lead is important in documenting atrial capture. Lead I shows an afterpotential that obscures the P wave. Lead II shows a P wave denoting capture on the atrial channel of this dual-chamber (DDD) pacemaker.

INTRAOPERATIVE ASSESSMENT OF PACEMAKER FUNCTION

Under most circumstances, the ECG and a blood pressure cuff will be adequate monitoring tools for the intraoperative monitoring of the patient with a pacemaker. However, in certain situations this type of monitoring alone will not be sufficient.

A pacemaker-dependent patient is vulnerable to interruption of pacing for even short periods, as the underlying rhythm is not sufficient to maintain an adequate cardiac output. For brief procedures during which the patient is awake and local anesthesia is used, a finger on the pulse may be adequate; but this will not be enough for major operations on such patients, particularly if nondepolarizing muscle relaxants, electrocautery, or a nerve stimulator are used. Patients with unipolar pacemakers that can be inhibited by myopotentials or electromagnetic interference are particularly vulnerable to these interferences. An arterial line is frequently indicated in these situations to gauge the beat-by-beat response to pacing throughout the procedure.

If the patient's intrinsic rhythm is slow, it is preferable to program the IPG to the asynchronous mode and at a faster rate to avoid competition and the possibility of inhibition of the IPG. This applies primarily to unipolar generators. If the patient's usual rate is adequate, it may not be possible to avoid competition entirely by increasing the rate, so it is preferable to leave the generator in the demand mode (VVI, DVI) and carefully monitor the arterial pressure during use of electrocautery to confirm that inhibition is not occurring, or to ensure that the underlying rhythm is adequate when inhibition occurs. During use of electrocautery, the ECG monitor is often impossible to interpret and the arterial pressure curve provides the most reliable indicator of safety. This problem might be avoided with the use of ECG monitors which adequately filter electrocautery artifacts.

The above recommendations apply to AAI, VVI, and DVI pacemakers, in which the mode of response is only inhibition. The situation is different for DDD or VDD pacemakers, in which the sensed activity in the atrial channel triggers ventricular pacing. Until recently, these IPGs have been of unipolar configuration and are thus susceptible to EMI and myopotential interference. To prevent the possibility of very rapid ventricular pacing, these IPGs are designed to track atrial activity or what is perceived as atrial activity up to a maximum tracking rate. They then block additional impulses by either a Wenckebach response or 2 : 1 block. The response to electrocautery may mimic this up to a point or may cause reversion to a safety or backup mode. In some instances this is ventricular demand or asynchronous pacing (VVI or VOO) at a specific recognizable rate. To prevent this, programming to an asynchronous mode (DOO) may be necessary. Some generators are particularly prone to this and are best explanted in situations such as a major thoracic or cardiac operation in which electrocautery will be used in the proximity of the IPG. On explanting the IPG, the lead terminals are connected to an external temporary dual chamber pacemaker (DVI) until the cautery is no longer used at the end of the procedure and then the IPG is reconnected.

REFERENCES

1. Zoll PM: Resuscitation of the heart in ventricular standstill by external electrical stimulation. N Engl J Med 247:768, 1952
2. Weirich WL, Gott VL, Lillehei CW: The treatment of complete heart block by the combined use of a myocardial electrode and an artificial pacemaker. Surg Forum 8:380, 1957
3. Furman S, Robinson G: The use of intracardiac pacemaker in the correction of total heart block. Surg Forum 9:245, 1958
4. Elmqvist R, Senning A: An implantable pacemaker for the heart. Proceedings of the Second International Conference on Medical Electronics. Lliffe & Sons, London, 1960
5. Chardack W, Cage A, Greatbatch W: A transistorized, self contained, implantable pacemaker for the long term correction of complete heart block. Surgery 48:543, 1960

6. Frye RL, Collins JJ, De Sanctis RW, et al: Guidelines for Permanent Cardiac Pacemaker Implantation. A report of the joint American College of Cardiology/American Heart Association Task Force on Assessment of Cardiovascular Procedures. J Am Coll Cardiol 4:434, 1984
7. Parsonnet V, Furman S, Smyth NPD: Revised code for pacemaker identification. PACE 4:400, 1981
8. Morse D, Steiner RM, Parsonnet V: A Guide to Cardiac Pacemakers. FA Davis, Philadelphia. 1983
9. Redd R, McAnulty J, Phillips S: Demand pacemaker inhibition by isometric skeletal muscle contraction. Circulation 49/50 (suppl III):957, 1974
10. Hauser, RG: Bipolar leads for cardiac pacing in the 1980's. A reappraisal provoked by skeletal muscle interference. PACE 5:34, 1982
11. Halperin JL, Camuñas JL, Stern EH, et al: Myopotential interference with DDD pacemakers: Endocardial electrographic telemetry in the diagnosis of pacemaker-related arrhythmias. Am J Cardiol 54:97, 1984
12. Levine PA: Why Programmability? Indications for and Clinical Utility of Multiparameter Programmable Pacemakers. Pacesetter Systems, Sylmar, California, February 1981
13. Samet P, Castillo C, Bernstein W: Hemodynamic sequelae of atrial, ventricular and sequential atrioventricular pacing in cardiac patients. Am Heart J 71:725, 1966
14. Waldo AL, Wells JL, Cooper TB, et al: Temporary cardiac pacing: Applications and techniques in the treatment of cardiac arrhythmias. Prog Cardiovasc Dis 23:451, 1981
15. Isicoff C: Understanding upper rate responses of DDD pacers. Heart Lung: J Crit Care 14:327, 1985
16. Furman S, Cooper JA: Atrial fibrillation during AV sequential pacing. PACE 5:133, 1982
17. DeCaprio V, Herzeler P, Furman S: A comparison of unipolar and bipolar electrograms for cardiac pacemaker sensing. Circulation 56:750, 1977
18. Fetter J, Hall DM, Hoff GL, Reeder JT: The effects of myopotential interference on unipolar and bipolar dual chamber pacemakers in the DDD mode. Clin Prog Electrophys Pacing 3:368, 1985
19. Estioko MR, Camuñas JL, Halperin JL, et al: Pulsed-doppler echocardiographic assessment of hemodynamic function during dual-chamber cardiac pacing. PACE 6:A87, 1983
20. Levine PA, Mace R: Pacing Therapy: A Guide to Cardiac Pacing for Optimum Hemodynamic Benefit. Futura, Mount Kisco, New York, 1983
21. Benchimol A, Ellis JG, Dimond EG: Hemodynamic consequences of atrial and ventricular pacing in normal and abnormal hearts. Am J Med 39:911, 1965
22. Hartzler GO, Maloney JD, Curtis JJ, Barnhorst DA: Hemodynamic benefits of atrioventricular sequential pacing after cardiac surgery. Am J Cardiol 40:232, 1977
23. Reiter MJ, Hindman MC: Hemodynamic effects of acute AV pacing in patients with left ventricular dysfunction. Am J Cardiol 49:687, 1982
24. Breivik K, Ohm OJ, Engedal K: Long-term comparison of unipolar and bipolar pacing and sensing using a new multiprogrammable pacemaker system. PACE 6:592, 1983
25. Warnowicz-Papp MA: The pacemaker patient and the electromagnetic environment. Clin Prog Pacing Electrophysiol 1:166, 1983
26. Barold S (ed): Modern Cardiac Pacing. Futura, Mount Kisco, New York, 1985

SUGGESTED READINGS

Council of Scientific Affairs, AMA: The use of cardiac pacemakers in medical practice. JAMA 254:1952, 1985

Furman S, Hayes DL: Implantation of atrioventricular synchronous and atrioventricular universal pacemakers. J Thorac Cardiovasc Surg 85:839, 1983

Ludmer PL, Goldschlager N: Cardiac pacing in the 1980's. N Engl J Med 311:1671, 1984

Moses HW, Taylor GJ, Schneider JA, Dove JT: A Practical Guide to Cardiac Pacing. Little, Brown, Boston, 1983

Parsonnet V, Furman S, Smyth NPD, Bilitch M: Optimal resources for implantable cardiac pacemakers. Circulation 68:227A, 1983

Zaidan JR: Pacemakers, p. 575. In Kaplan JA (ed): Thoracic Anesthesia. Churchill Livingstone, New York, 1983

16

Therapeutic ECG

Steven Konstadt, M.D.

Although primarily a diagnostic tool, there are situations in which the ECG also plays a therapeutic role. Two important therapeutic uses of the ECG are (1) to synchronize cardioversion, and (2) to provide the timing for aortic counterpulsation. In both settings, the R wave of the ECG provides the trigger for the therapeutic intervention. The R wave is used because of its location in the cardiac cycle and its relatively easy identification. The R wave is detected by a computer, recognizing its slope or slew rate, width, and amplitude in the following manner. The ECG electrodes detect potentials generated by the electrical activity of the heart. This voltage then passes through a bandpass filter, which is a combination of a lowpass filter that attenuates high-frequency signals and a high-pass filter that attenuates low-frequency information and amplifies the desired frequencies. The signal then passes through a threshold detector; if the signal exceeds the minimal set voltage, the criteria for an R wave are met and the intervention is triggered.[1] A more sophisticated method of R-wave detection depends on digital sampling and microprocessor interpretation. In this method, the signal is analyzed at a set frequency (usually at least twice as fast as the highest desired frequency to be sampled) and each point is assigned a discrete digital value according to its amplitude. The microprocessor analyzes the slope between the points, the total amplitude change in a set interval, and the width between significant changes in slope. These determinations precisely define the signal and the microprocessor then compares the signal to the strictly defined characteristics of an R wave. If the criteria for an R wave are satisfied, the system is triggered.[1]

SYNCHRONIZED CARDIOVERSION

Defining the role of electrical energy in therapeutic applications began more than 200 years ago. Abildgaard in 1775 recorded the earliest experiments demonstrating the use of electric shock in resuscitation.[2] After inducing fibrillation and apparent death of a bird with a single electric shock, he applied a second shock and revived the bird. Demonstrating its total recovery, the bird flew off and thereby eluded further experimentation. In 1947, during heart surgery, epicardial alternating current was first successfully used to defibrillate a human heart.[3] During the 1960s and 1970s it was shown that direct current was safer for the patient and that dysrhythmias other than ventricular fibrillation could be terminated by electric shock.[4] There are now two terms for this procedure. Electric shock applied to a heart in ventricular fibrillation is known as defibrillation, while cardioversion is the application of electric current to terminate other dysrhythmias. The major difference between the two is that cardioversion is synchronized to occur just after the R wave.

The physiologic basis of cardioversion can be explained as follows. Some dysrhythmias depend on self-sustaining reentrant pathways in which depolarization advances down the pathway and is separated from its tail by nonrefractory, fully recovered tissue known as the excitable gap. Externally applied electrical energy depolarizes the recovered tissue and closes the gap. The shock terminates the reentrant circuit, discharges automatic foci, and produces electrical homogeneity. However, it is still unclear why various dysrhythmias require different energy levels to accomplish this conversion.

The major risk of electrical shock for treatment of dysrhythmias is the induction of ventricular fibrillation; therefore, Lown et al.[5] introduced the technique of synchronized cardioversion in 1962 in an effort to avoid this complication. Previous physiologic studies and clinical observations had indicated the presence of a vulnerable period in animals and humans.[6] During this period, the application of external electrical energy has a high risk of producing ventricular fibrillation (Fig. 16–1). Studies in rabbits, cats, sheep, and lower primates using systematic shocks administered during all parts of the ECG cycle showed that the vulnerable period occurs at the terminal portion of the refractory state (i.e., at the apex of the T wave). In addition to the identical location in these various species, the vulnerable period had the identical duration of 30 msec (Fig. 16–2). Evidence for a vulnerable period in man stems from observations of pacer spikes which hit upon the T wave and produced ventricular fibrillation, and the correlation of sudden death (presumably ventricular fibrillation) with premature ventricular beats that occurred on the T wave.[6,7] The physiologic explanation for the vulnerable period is that during repolarization there is asynchronous recovery, hence an irregularly excitable electric field. Current applied to this irregular field follows tortuous slow pathways. This setting is conducive to fractionation of the impulse and electrical asynchrony. Reentrant phenomenon and further multiplication of the asynchrony can produce ventricular fibrillation.

Synchronized cardioversion delivers the current about 20 msec after the R wave (well before the T wave). Using synchronized cardioversion,

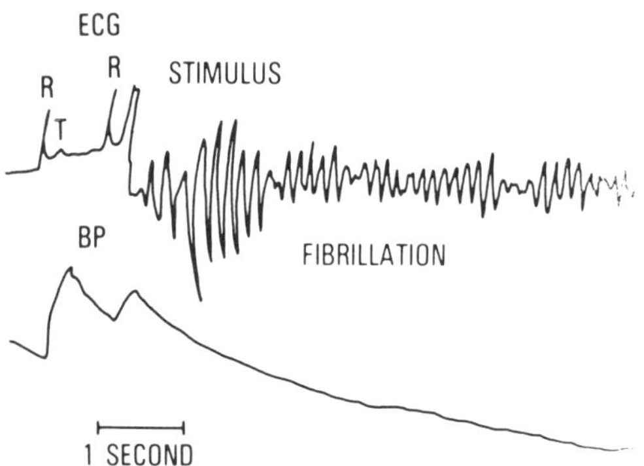

Fig. 16–1 An electrical stimulus delivered during the T wave produces ventricular fibrillation. (Karliner JS, Gregoratos G (eds): Coronary Care. Churchill Livingstone, New York, 1981.)

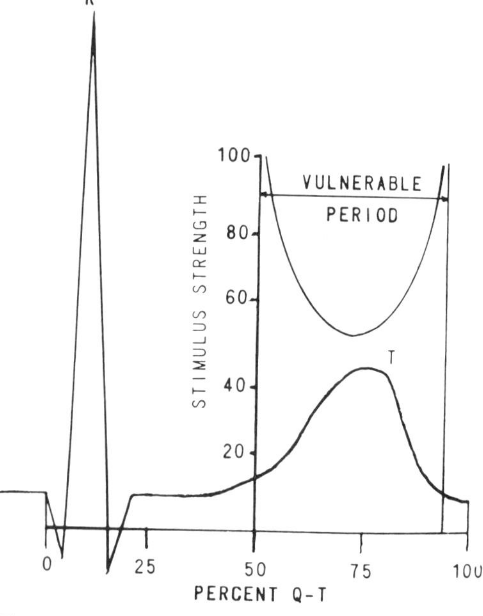

Fig. 16–2 The duration of the Vulnerable Period in Relation to the ECG. (Karliner JS, Gregoratos G (eds): Coronary Care. Churchill Livingstone, New York, 1981.)

the induction of ventricular fibrillation occurs with only 0.5 to 0.8 percent of the shocks delivered.[7,8] Despite the theoretical advantages of synchronized cardioversion, other investigators have obtained similar rates of successful rhythm conversion and ventricular fibrillation induction using nonsynchronized current.[9–11] One possible explanation for the similar safety of nonsynchronized current is that the vulnerable period is extremely short and therefore easily missed. For example, if the patient's heart rate is 150 beats/min there are 2½ cycles/sec. Each cycle has a 30-msec vulnerable period. Multiplying the cycles per second by the milliseconds vulnerable per cycle yields 75 msec vulnerable per second. This, random chance of hitting the vulnerable period is about 0.8 percent or the observed rate for both synchronized and nonsynchronized current. It is not clear why synchronization does not further reduce the rate of induction of ventricular fibrillation, but it may have to do with the intensity of the shock.

Although this controversy exists, it has become standard practice to synchronize cardioversion for the treatment of all dysrhythmias except ventricular fibrillation. A cardioverter is diagrammatically shown in Figure 16–3. The ECG signal passes through an analog switch to an amplifier, which augments the signal and displays it on an oscilloscope. It then passes through a filter to a threshold detector, and when the detector notes an R wave, a 30-msec delay circuit is activated. This in turn activates the trigger circuit, and the current is discharged to the patient while a switch prevents discharge into the cardioverter.

Practically, the technique is performed in the following manner:[12]

1. ECG electrodes are placed on the patient in the usual fashion.
2. The lead with the tallest R wave is chosen. If no tall R wave is obtained, it is necessary to reposition the electrodes and improve skin contact by an alcohol rinse and mild abrasion. The ECG should also be examined for tall positive deflections other than the R wave that may trigger the cardioverter. Several examples of interfering deflections are pacer spikes, RR′ waves seen with bundle branch blocks, wire

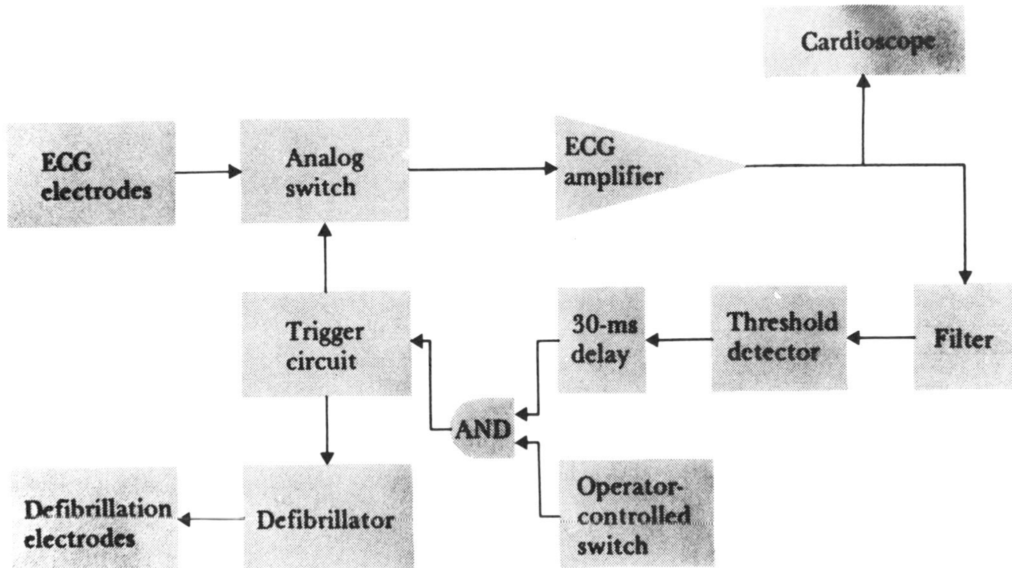

Fig. 16–3 Diagram of a defibrillator. (Webster JG (ed): Medical Instrumentation. P. 640. Houghton-Mifflin, Boston, © 1978. Used by permission.)

movement, and line isolation monitor switching. Alternative leads may not have these deflections, or if possible, the pacer may be turned off prior to cardioversion.

3. The patient is anesthetized with a barbiturate or benzodiazepine.[13,14]

4. The paddles are coated with conductive gel, particularly along the edges and placed on the patient. The anteroposterior position seems to require lower energy than the anterolateral position, but is more difficult to place. The anterior paddle is placed along the right sternal border at the level of the second and third interspaces. The posterior paddle is placed at the angle of the left scapula. If a lateral position is used, the paddle is placed in the anterior axillary line at the level of the xiphoid process.

5. For elective cardioversion, a low energy

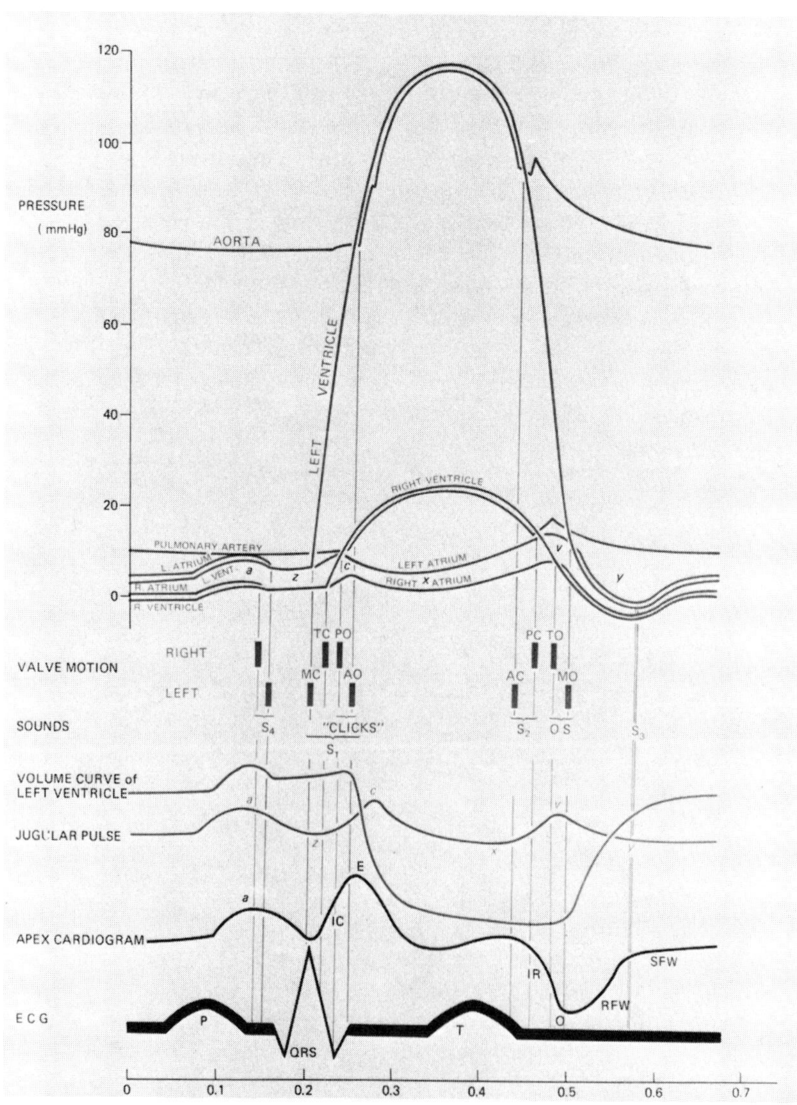

Fig. 16–4 Diagram and timing of the cardiac cycle. (Hurst JW (ed): The Heart. © 1982 McGraw-Hill, New York. Reproduced with permission.)

(i.e., 5 watt-sec) is chosen and the paddles are activated. Discharge will occur after the cardioverter senses the R wave.

6. Monitoring lead II or V_1 will most often show if the cardioversion was successful. If the patient's rhythm has not responded, the energy is increased to 10, 25, 50, 100, 200, or 400 watt-sec, successively. If the patient develops ventricular fibrillation, the synchronizing mode must be deactivated and the patient defibrillated immediately with 100 to 400 watt-sec.

AORTIC COUNTERPULSATION

The intraaortic balloon pump (IABP) is a synchronized left ventricular (LV) assist device placed in the descending thoracic aorta. The balloon inflates during diastole after closure of the aortic valve and deflates just before the start of the next ventricular systole. Inflation during diastole increases coronary blood flow, while deflation immediately prior to systole creates a sink that decreases aortic impedance and left ventricular work. The IABP is indicated for the treatment of the low-output syndrome, unstable angina, and ischemic ventricular dysrhythmias.[15,16]

In order for the IABP to function effectively, the inflation and deflation must be properly coordinated with the cardiac cycle. Experimentally, variables such as aortic blood flow and coronary blood flow have been used to adjust the IABP, but for clinical purposes the easily obtained ECG or arterial pressure tracing are used. The R wave of the ECG is most often used to trigger the IABP. A brief description of the cardiac cycle in both electrical and hemodynamic terms will clarify the rationale of this technique.

The cardiac cycle starts with atrial depolarization represented by the P wave (Fig. 16–4). The atrium then contracts filling the ventricle. During this time, the wave of depolarization is passing through the conduction system producing the PR interval and then the ventricle depolarizes during the QRS complex. At the peak of the R wave, ventricular isovolumic contraction begins. When the LV pressure exceeds

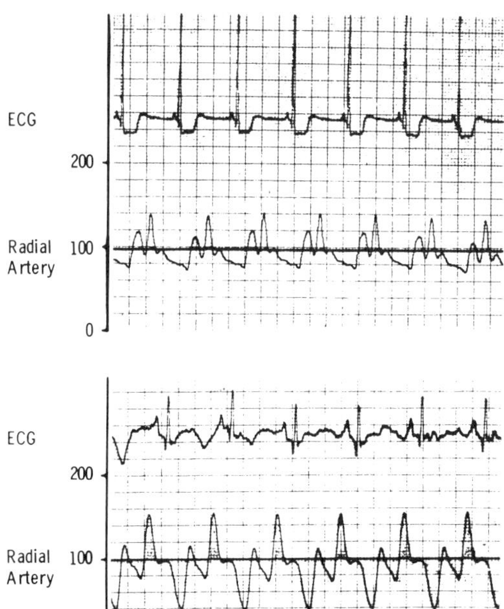

Fig. 16–5 Incorrect intraaortic balloon pump (IABP) inflation is shown in the upper two panels and correct timing in the lower two panels.

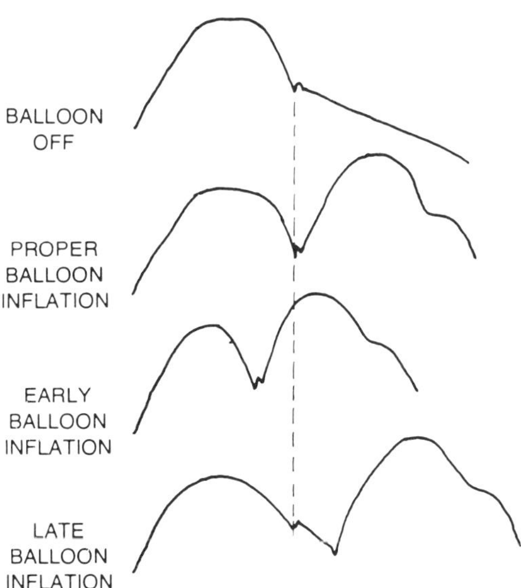

Fig. 16–6 Setting balloon inflation. (Reproduced from the Roche Operators Manual with permission.)

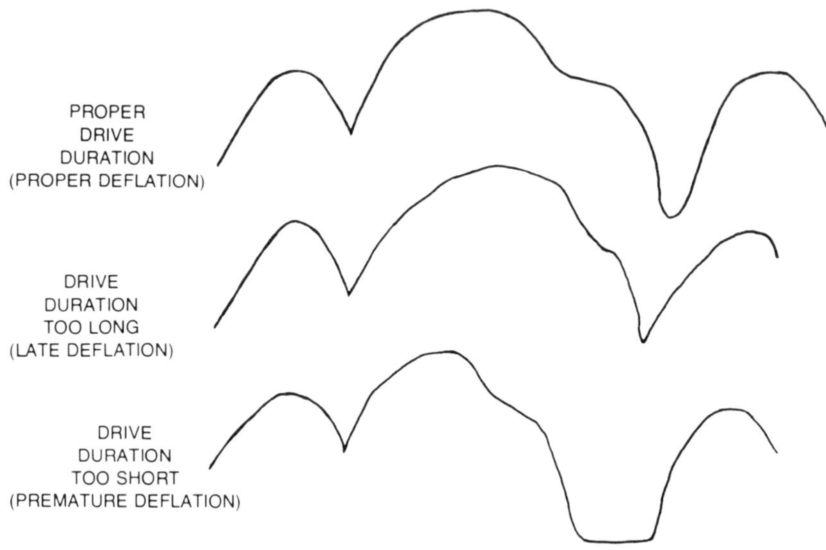

Fig. 16–7 Setting balloon deflation. (Reproduced from the Roche Operators Manual with permission.)

Table 16–1. Common Operating Problems with the IABP

Problem	Probable Cause	Remedy
ECG MONITORING		
ECG waveform not displayed	1. Defective patient connections.	Check electrodes and cable connections.
	2. Remote monitor not connected to console property.	Check connections from remote monitor to ECG MON IN connector.
	3. Defective ECG skin amplifier.	Monitor ECG externally and bring signals to display via ECG MON IN connector.
	4. Defective display.	Monitor ECG via strip chart (if console has this option) or external monitor (via ECG OUT connector).
Ac interference in waveform	1. Detached reference electrode	Reattach electrode wire.
	2. Poor electrode contact	Apply new electrodes.
	3. Lead wires too close to radiating AC source	Bundle wires together and reroute them close to patient's body.
Noisy display	1. Excessive muscular artifact	Administer therapy.
	2. Inadequate skin preparation	Repeat skin preparation; use new electrodes.
	3. Electrodes improperly positioned	Reposition new electrodes.
ECG baseline wander	1. Poor electrode contact.	Apply new electrodes.
	2. Patient cable yoke is on patient's abdomen and is picking up respiratory movement.	Reposition the patient cable yoke.
	3. Electrodes improperly positioned.	Reposition new electrodes.

IABP, intraaortic balloon pump.
(Reproduced from the Roche Operators Manual with permission.)

aortic pressure, the aortic valve opens and ejection occurs. Ejection will continue until the pressure in the ventricle falls below that of the aorta (at the end of the T wave on the ECG). The ventricle then relaxes until the next R wave. From this discussion and Figure 16–4, it can be seen that the R wave heralds ventricular systole and is the appropriate signal for deflation of the IABP. The T wave is often used as the signal for balloon inflation. Incorrect and correct balloon timing are shown in Figure 16–5.[17]

Alternatively, the arterial pressure tracing may be used for balloon deflation timing. However, the R wave is the preferred signal,[16] since it is easily identifiable by the computer. The arterial pressure changes that occur with systole are later in the cardiac cycle and have a lesser slope, both of which make identification more difficult. This is particularly true in patients with aortic stenosis or poor myocardial contractility.

There are situations in which even an easily identifiable R wave is inadequate to time the IABP. In some patients, the interval between the R wave and systole is too short to allow total deflation. This results in loss of the presystolic drop (Fig. 16–5, upper panel). It most commonly occurs in patients with rapid heart rates, but may also occur at normal rates. Since balloon deflation is also dependent on diastolic arterial pressure, patients with a low diastolic pressure will not adequately deflate the balloon, and they also lose the presystolic drop. In these situations, the intervals of inflation and deflation are empirically set and adjusted to obtain optimal

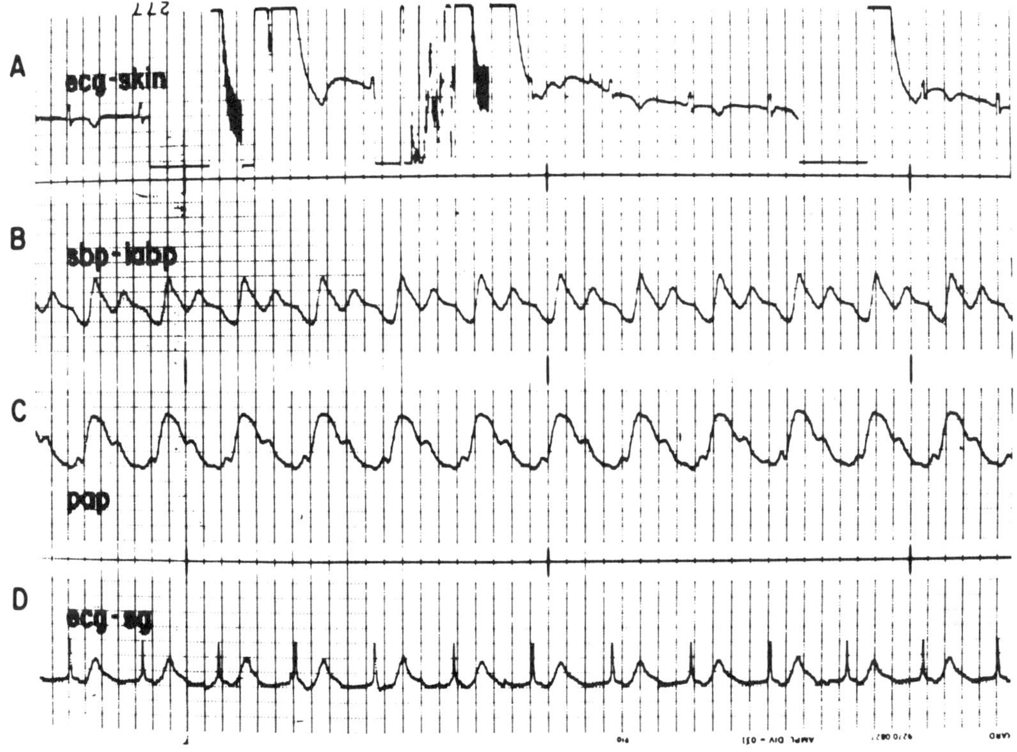

Fig. 16–8 Use of the multipurpose pulmonary arterial catheter to record an intracardiac ECG and trigger the intraaortic balloon pump (IABP). Note the lack of interference. A, skin ECG with interference from the electrocautery; B, radial artery pressure; C, pulmonary artery pressure; D, intraventricular electrogram recorded from the ventricular leads of the multipurpose catheter. (Lichtenthal PR: Multipurpose pulmonary artery catheter. Ann Thorac Surg 36:493, 1983.)

pressure tracings (Figs. 16–6 and 16–7). To improve IABP function in these settings, closed-loop central algorithims have been developed using central aortic root pressure tracings and a microprocessor to evaluate and control IABP function.[18] If this technique proves both efficacious and affordable in clinical trials, it may provide a significant advance in IABP technology.

Although the above problems exist, the more common difficulty in clinical practice is obtaining an adequate ECG signal. Frequent causes and remedies for this difficulty are shown in Table 16–1. During surgery there are additional sources of ECG interference, including (1) electrocautery, (2) line isolation monitor switching, and (3) cardiac pacing. To combat this interference, several of the IABP consoles are equipped with filters capable of suppressing some of these signals. A second method of eliminating interference is to use a multipurpose pulmonary arterial catheter with pacing electrodes in the right atrium and ventricle. An intraventricular ECG can be obtained by attaching the right arm lead to the proximal ventricular wire and the left arm lead to the distal ventricular wire. When lead I is selected, a reliable ECG signal that is relatively insensitive to electrocautery is obtained (Fig. 16–8).[19] It should be mentioned that this procedure carries the risk of microshock. If the ECG monitor is not totally isolated, the catheter electrodes will serve as a ground for the electrocautery. Current passing through the small electrodes of the catheter will have a high density and will create the risks of an electrical burn or ventricular fibrillation.

Pacing can also interfere with IABP timing. Payne and Cleveland[20] showed that bipolar atrial pacing requires a lower current than unipolar pacing, and, therefore, creates a smaller pacing spike. This smaller spike does not pass the threshold detector and will not trigger the IABP (Fig. 16–9). Another technique to avoid pacer or electrocautery interference is to simultaneously pace the patient and the IABP. This requires a special pacing box with multiple electrically isolated outputs. One set of outputs is connected either to epicardial or to transvenous pacing wires, and the other ventricular output is connected to the ECG input of the IABP console. Atrial, ventricular, or atrioventricular pacing may be selected. The IABP console will read the ventricular spike as an R wave and properly trigger balloon deflation. Once again, if the electrical isolation is faulty, the risk of microshock is present.

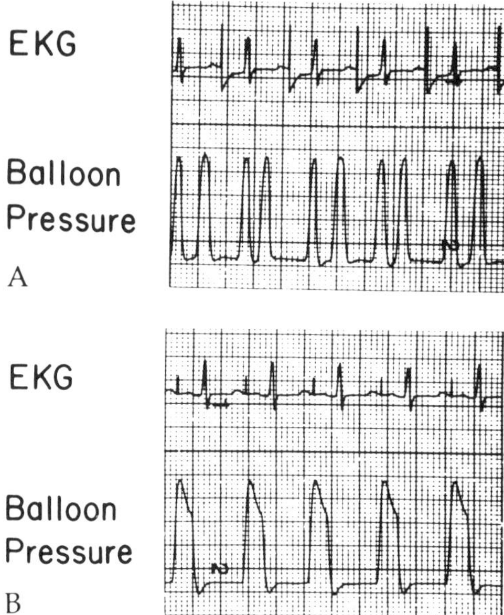

Fig. 16–9 Bipolar atrial pacing (**B**) produces a smaller pacing spike than unipolar atrial pacing (**A**) and does not trigger the IABP. (Payne DD: Atrial pacing during IABP. Ann Thorac Surg 30:191, 1980.)

REFERENCES

1. Webster JG: Medical Instrumentation. Houghton-Mifflin, Boston, 1978
2. Abildgaard PC: Tentamina electrica in animalibus instituta. Soc Hauniemsis Collect 2:1157, 1775
3. Beck CS, Pritchard WH, Feil SA: Ventricular fibrillation of long duration abolished by electric shock. JAMA 135:985, 1947
4. Glassman E: Direct current cardioversion. Am Heart J 82:128, 1971
5. Lown B, Amarasingham R, Neuman J: New method for terminating cardiac arrhythmias—

Use of synchronized capacitor discharge. JAMA 182:548, 1962
6. Bellet S: Defibrillation and countershock. p. 426. In Bellet S (ed): Essentials of Cardiac Arhythmias. WB Saunders, Philadelphia, 1972
7. DeSilva RA, Graboys TB, Podrid PJ, Lown B: Cardioversion and defibrillation. Am Heart J 100:881, 1980
8. Lown B: Electrical reversion of cardiac arrhythmias. Br Heart J 29:469, 1967
9. Kreus KE, Salokannel SJ, Waris EK: Non-synchronized and synchronized direct-current countershock in cardiac arrythmias. Lancet 2:405, 1966
10. Waris EK, Scheinin TM, Kreus KE, et al: Non-synchronized direct current countershock. Acta Med Scand 178:309, 1965
11. Kavanagh-Gray D: Non-synchronized direct current countershock in cardiac arrythmias. Can Med Assoc J 96:1460, 1967
12. Lown B, Kleiger R, Wolff G: The technique of cardioversion. Am Heart J 67:282, 1964
13. Orko R: Anesthesia for cardioversion. Br J Anaesth 46:947, 1974
14. Orko R: Anesthesia for cardioversion. Br J Anaesth 48:257, 1976
15. Ionescu MI: Techniques in Extracorporeal circulation. Butterworths, London, 1981
16. Bolooki H: Clinical Application of Intra-aortic Balloon Pump. Futura, Mt. Kisco, New York, 1984
17. Kaplan JA, Craver JM: Assisted circulation. p. 441. In Kaplan JA (ed): Cardiac Anesthesia. Grune & Stratton, Orlando, Florida, 1979
18. Philippe E, Clark JW, Lande A, Ellis JR: Microprocessor control of intra-aortic balloon pumping. Ann Biomed Eng 8:209, 1980
19. Lichtenthal PR, Collins JT: Multipurpose pulmonary artery catheter. Ann Thorac Surg 36:493, 1983
20. Payne DD, Cleveland RJ: Atrial pacing during intra-aortic balloon pumping. Ann Thorac Surg 30:191, 1980

Index

Page numbers followed by *f* denote figures; those followed by *t* denote tables.